D1398471

MARKETING HEALTH SERVICES

Richard K. Thomas

MARKETING HEALTH SERVICES

THIRD EDITION

AUPHA

Health Administration Press, Chicago, Illinois

Association of University Programs in Health Administration, Arlington, Virginia

Your board, staff, or clients may also benefit from this book's insight. For more information on quantity discounts, contact the Health Administration Press Marketing Manager at (312) 424–9470.

Library of Congress Cataloging-in-Publication Data

Thomas, Richard K., 1944–
  Marketing health services / Richard K. Thomas. — Third edition.
    p. cm.
  Includes bibliographical references and index.
  ISBN 978-1-56793-678-0 (alk. paper)
  1. Medical care—Marketing. I. Title.
  RA410.56.T48 2015
  362.1068'8—dc23
                          2014017261

The paper used in this publication meets the minimum requirements of American National Standard for Information Sciences—Permanence of Paper for Printed Library Materials, ANSI Z39.48-1984. ∞ ™

Acquisitions editor: Tulie O'Connor; Project editor: Jane Calayag; Cover designer: Marisa Jackson; Layout: BookComp, Inc.

Found an error or a typo? We want to know! Please e-mail it to hapbooks@ache.org and put "Book Error" in the subject line.

For photocopying and copyright information, please contact Copyright Clearance Center at www.copyright.com or at (978) 750–8400.

Health Administration Press
A division of the Foundation of the American
   College of Healthcare Executives
One North Franklin Street, Suite 1700
Chicago, IL 60606–3529
(312) 424–2800

Association of University Programs
   in Health Administration
2000 North 14th Street
Suite 780
Arlington, VA 22201
(703) 894–0940

BRIEF CONTENTS

DETAILED CONTENTS

PREFACE TO THE THIRD EDITION

Since the publication of the second edition of *Marketing Health Services* a little more than five years ago, the world of healthcare has changed significantly—and with it the practice of healthcare marketing. Healthcare is now in the era of the Affordable Care Act (ACA), the healthcare reform law passed in 2010 whose most publicized and controversial provision—the health insurance exchange—has just taken effect in 2014. The ACA provisions emphasize value over volume and population health over episodic healthcare delivery. These are difficult mandates for healthcare organizations, many of which lack the financial, staffing, and other resources needed just to stay open.

Beyond the ACA and amid many threats in the environment lie opportunities—such as social media channels, healthcare globalization, and consumer engagement, to name a few—that an organization can explore and benefit from with guidance from the marketing function. As always, marketing is an indispensable partner in healthcare, especially in the uncertain period between the blanket implementation of new rules and the rush to adopt compliant strategies and adjust existing approaches.

In other words, each time the paradigm has shifted in healthcare, marketing has been there to move the organization in the ideal direction. That was true when reimbursement infrastructures changed in the 1970s, when competition between providers skyrocketed in the 1980s, when mergers and consolidations surged in the 1990s, and when technology and customer relationship became a force in the 2000s. This list drives home the point that the trends and challenges that emerged in the past decades have remained fixtures in the healthcare environment of the 2010s.

This book, like the first two editions, enumerates the forces that are changing and challenging healthcare. It also chronicles the evolution of healthcare marketing—from one purely associated with advertising or promotion to one that counts research, education, and strategy formulation as major responsibilities. Such comprehensive coverage of healthcare marketing illustrates its value and deep contributions to the goals of the healthcare system.

A Little History

Most marketing insiders consider 1977 to be the year in which healthcare marketing was officially launched. In that year, the American Hospital Association sponsored the first conference on healthcare marketing, and the first book on healthcare marketing was published. However, hospitals and other healthcare organizations had been engaging in public relations, physician relationship development, community service, and promotional activities long before that time—just that few people equated these efforts with marketing.

Since then, healthcare marketing has gone through a series of highs and lows. In the 1980s, marketing was formally recognized as an appropriate activity for healthcare providers, an important milestone given that it was initially perceived as an inappropriate—even an unethical—discipline for the helping profession. In addition, some healthcare organizations began to establish marketing departments; set marketing budgets; create new positions, such as vice president for marketing; outsource marketing activities to agencies; adopt marketing concepts and methods from other industries; launch aggressive marketing campaigns; and, most important, learn that marketing healthcare goods and services was not the same as marketing hamburgers and widgets—thus, the approaches that are required and effective in the healthcare arena are expressly different from those in other industries.

The reception that healthcare marketing received in those early years wasn't always warm, however. It was the first to get cut when budgets were tight. It caused tension between those who eagerly accepted it and those who doggedly resisted it. It suffered through periods of marketing frenzy followed by periods of neglect and retrenchment.

Through the 1990s and 2000s, healthcare marketing continued to prove itself as a legitimate organizational function. More full-service marketing departments were being established in house. More healthcare marketers were being appointed as heads of marketing departments and thus as part of management or administration. More sophisticated and healthcare-specific marketing techniques (such as Internet marketing) were being developed and implemented. More trained and experienced healthcare marketers were emerging.

This proliferation of marketers dedicated to the business of healthcare imparted several lessons that still resonate today. First, marketing is so much broader than mass media advertising, a realization that prompts organizations to reassess their marketing efforts. Second, understanding the market in which the business operates; the customers who live in that market; and those customers' needs, wants, behaviors, and motivations is critical.

Conclusion

Although healthcare is a service industry, it is still a business that needs marketing interventions. However, these interventions must be unique and appropriate for healthcare products and their consumers—not a copy of the prevailing techniques used in other industries. This book walks readers through both traditional and contemporary processes and approaches that healthcare marketers rely on and that enable healthcare organizations and providers to rise above current trends and turmoil and to position themselves for the future healthcare environment.

INTRODUCTION TO THE THIRD EDITION

This book explores the history, perspectives, concepts, processes, and role of marketing in the healthcare industry—particularly the health services delivery setting. This third edition retains the features that readers found useful in previous editions, such as the examples, case studies, discussion questions, key points, and additional resources. In this edition, however, new examples, exhibits, recommendations, and statistics have been added; the cases have been revised; and the most current resources have been included. Plus, definitions of important terms and concepts now appear in the margins, supplementing the full-length discussions.

The content itself—although it remains true to its original intent of being a comprehensive guide—has been updated at every possible turn to reflect the present and distant-future realities of the Affordable Care Act (ACA) and social media. In fact, in Chapter 8 the potential effects on healthcare marketing of ACA provisions and the voluntary accountable care organization infrastructure are examined, while Chapter 11 (new to this edition) surveys social media and their enormous contributions to disseminating healthcare information and narrowing the gap between consumers, providers, and marketers.

The Target Audience

Students in healthcare administration and healthcare marketing programs as well as students in business administration programs with a healthcare marketing component compose the primary audience for this book. It could also serve as a reference text for professors or instructors of healthcare administration or marketing courses and for academicians who conduct research in these topics but are not marketing practitioners themselves.

Health professionals (including physicians, nurses, and other clinicians) are the secondary audience for this book. The same can be said of healthcare executives and administrators, health planners, and other facility staff and contractors involved in marketing activities. In this ultra-competitive environment, most health professionals—regardless of official titles or span of responsibilities—are expected to be at least familiar with marketing concepts, not only to support the organization's marketing efforts but also to promote their own departments to those who set the budget.

The third category of audience is composed of marketing professionals —whether they work for a marketing or related consulting firm or as independent agents—who want to do business in the healthcare arena. Whether they are new to the marketing field or are seasoned marketing veterans, they will find something in the book that would prove useful for their healthcare clients.

The Content

At times, the topics covered in the chapters overlap or appear in more than one chapter. That is intentional—to emphasize and review the basic points or to put them in context. Following are summaries of the content of each chapter:

Part I: History and Concepts

- Chapter 1 presents an overview of the history of marketing—from its introduction to healthcare to its contemporary incarnation. The ways in which healthcare differs from other industries and the ways in which healthcare marketing is different from other types of marketing are examined. In addition, the chapter sheds light on the factors that have helped marketing become accepted in healthcare and the contribution that marketing can make to the industry. Finally, it reviews current developments in healthcare and their implications for marketing.
- Chapter 2 defines the key terms and concepts that form the foundation of marketing and reviews their application to healthcare. The four Ps of marketing and their expansion to the seven Ps (for the healthcare industry) are discussed. Marketing functions, techniques, and approaches are enumerated, and the challenge of adapting marketing processes from other industries to healthcare is addressed.
- Chapter 3 focuses on marketing as a function in healthcare organizations. It identifies the types of marketing techniques typically used by different types of organizations. The factors that influenced healthcare's adoption of marketing are reviewed along with the factors that are affecting the contemporary nature of healthcare marketing.

Part II: Healthcare Markets

- Chapter 4 discusses how a healthcare market is described and delineated. Among the concepts addressed are geographic and nongeographic boundaries, consumer demand, market profiling, mass marketing and micromarketing, and effective markets.

- Chapter 5 answers the questions "who are healthcare customers?" and "how are they similar and dissimilar from other customers?" It explains consumer behavior and attitudes, the different types of market segmentation (e.g., geographic, demographic, psychographic), and the consumer decision-making process.

- Chapter 6 is all about the healthcare product—the goods sold and services provided by various healthcare organizations. The product mix is explained, as well as the different types of goods and services available in the market. The common classifications and coding systems used in healthcare are highlighted.

- Chapter 7 addresses the factors that contribute to the demand for health services. It touches on healthcare wants and needs, recommended standards for healthcare, and utilization patterns. It also proposes methods marketers can use to measure demand and introduces various indicators of health services utilization. The numerous factors that determine the demand for and ultimate consumption of health services are identified.

Part III: Healthcare Marketing Techniques

- Chapter 8 focuses on marketing strategies. The need to align marketing strategies with the organization's overall strategic plan is emphasized. It summarizes the steps in strategic planning, the processes for developing and selecting a strategy, and the strategic approaches that may be taken. Branding as a strategy is discussed as well. The possible implications for healthcare marketing of the ACA and emerging accountable care organizations are highlighted.

- Chapter 9 details the traditional marketing techniques commonly used by healthcare marketers, such as public relations, advertising, personal sales, sales promotion, and direct marketing. It provides an overview of media options, social marketing, and integrated marketing. It also explains the modifications marketers must make to adapt traditional promotional approaches to the healthcare arena.

- Chapter 10 presents contemporary marketing techniques. One set is based on traditional marketing programs and includes direct-to-consumer marketing, business-to-business marketing, internal marketing, and concierge services. The other set is based on technology and includes database marketing, customer relationship management, and Internet marketing. Consumer engagement as an emerging theme in marketing is addressed.

- Chapter 11 focuses on social media and their application to healthcare marketing. It identifies the common types of social media, their value to consumers and marketers, and their healthcare-specific uses.

- Chapter 12 examines healthcare marketing from a global perspective. As the pace of healthcare globalization increases, international healthcare marketing is expected to grow in importance. Among the topics explored in this chapter are the trends in medical tourism, the four categories of medical tourists, and strategies and techniques useful to international healthcare marketers.

Part IV: The Marketing Effort

- Chapter 13 explores the ins and outs of managing a marketing campaign. It breaks down the steps involved—from concept to plan to implementation to evaluation. It pinpoints the players (including both internal and external marketing agents, suppliers, and consultants) and departments (including creative, production, and media planning and buying departments) of the marketing function. The financial aspects—the marketing budget and return on investment—are also described.

- Chapter 14 presents an overview of the healthcare marketing research process. It describes the types, steps, and methods researchers undertake to collect data and information on markets, products, prices, promotions, and distributions. Geographic information systems, quantitative and qualitative research, and surveys and interviews are among the tools discussed.

- Chapter 15 offers a comprehensive look at marketing planning. It presents the common steps in the planning process and examples of how the steps are applied in real-world marketing scenarios.

- Chapter 16 examines marketing data, particularly the sources of such data. It discusses the complications of mining and using patient/customer information under HIPAA rules as well as the dimensions/traits that make data useful to healthcare marketers. Methods for generating population data and estimating demand in the absence of actual data are included, along with data compendia collected and released by the federal government.

Part V: The Future of Healthcare Marketing

- Chapter 17 summarizes where healthcare marketing is at present and where it is headed in the near future. The discussion revolves around the current trends and factors that are likely to influence the future characteristics of both healthcare and marketing.

The Instructor Ancillaries

Instructor resources are located in a secure area on the Health Administration Press website and are available to adopters of this book. These resources include an instructor's manual, PowerPoint slides, answers to selected case study questions, and a test bank. For access information, e-mail hapbooks@ache.org.

HISTORY AND CONCEPTS

Part I places the field of marketing and its applications to healthcare in a historical context. Chapters 1 through 3 introduce basic marketing concepts.

THE ORIGIN AND EVOLUTION OF MARKETING IN HEALTHCARE

S ince the notion of marketing was introduced to healthcare providers during the 1970s, the field has experienced periods of growth, decline, retrenchment, and renewed growth. This chapter reviews the history of marketing in the US economy in general and traces its evolution in healthcare over the last quarter of the twentieth century. The chapter then turns to the challenges marketers have faced in their efforts to gain a foothold in healthcare.

The History of Marketing

Marketing, as the term is used today, is a modern concept. The term was first used around 1910 to refer to what is called *sales* in the contemporary sense. Marketing is a uniquely American concept, but the word itself has been adopted into the vocabulary of other languages that lack a word for this activity. Although the 1950s mark the beginning of the marketing era in the United States, the marketing function within the US economy took several decades (in stages) to become established, and marketers had to overcome a number of factors that slowed the field's development.

Many of these factors reflected economic characteristics carried over from the World War II period. In the 1950s, America was still in the Industrial Age, and the economy was production oriented until well after the war. Because essentially all aspects of the economy were geared to **production**, the prevailing mind-set emphasized the producer's interests over the consumer's. This production orientation assumed that producers already knew what consumers needed. Products were made to the manufacturer's specification, and then customers were sought. A "here is our product—take it or leave it" approach characterized most industries during this period.

Production
A focus on generating (rather than distributing) goods that deemphasizes the role of marketing

Stage 1: The Rise of Product Differentiation and Consumerism
A wide variety of new products and services emerged during the postwar period, particularly in consumer goods industries. Newly empowered consumers demanded a growing array of goods and services. This development contributed to the emergence of marketing for three primary reasons. First,

consumers had to be introduced to and educated about these new goods and services. Second, the entry of new producers into the market gave rise to a level of competition unknown in the prewar period. Mechanisms had to be developed to make the public aware of a new product and to distinguish that product (in the eyes of potential customers) from that offered by competitors. Consumers had to be made aware of purchase opportunities and then persuaded to buy a certain brand. Third, the standardization of existing products during this period further contributed to the need to convince newly empowered consumers to choose one good or service over another. Where few differences existed between the products in a market, the role of marketing became crucial. Marketers were enlisted to highlight and, if necessary, create differences between similar products.

As a result of these developments, the seller's market was transformed into a buyer's market. Once the consumer market began to be tapped, the highly elastic demand for many types of goods became evident. The prewar mentality had emphasized meeting consumer needs and assumed that a population could purchase only a finite amount of goods and services. With the increase in discretionary income and the introduction of consumer credit after World War II, consumers began to satisfy wants. Fledgling marketers discovered that not only could they influence consumers' decision-making processes but they also could create demand for certain goods and services.

Culture
A society's tangible and intangible aspects reflecting its beliefs, values, and norms

The growing acceptance of marketing was aided and abetted by changes in American **culture**. The postwar period was marked by a growing emphasis on consumption and acquisition. The frugality of the Depression era gave way to a degree of materialism that shocked older generations. The availability of consumer credit and a mind-set that emphasized "keeping up with the Joneses" generated demand for a growing range of goods and services. This period witnessed the birth of the first generation of Americans with a consumer mentality.

By the 1970s, there was a growing emphasis on self-actualization in American culture. This development called for additional goods and services and even created a fledgling market for consumer health services (e.g., psychotherapy, cosmetic surgery). A growing consumer market with expanding needs, coupled with a proliferation of products, created a fertile field for marketing activity.

Underlying these developments was the growing emphasis on change itself. As society continued to undergo major transformations, change had not only become accepted as inevitable but also began to take on a positive connotation. Newly empowered consumers demanded an ever-growing array of goods and services. The future orientation emerging within society further underscored the importance of change in forging a path to a better future. People began changing jobs, residences, and even spouses at a rate unheard of to their forebears. The social and economic advancement of each generation improving over the previous one became a maxim—a part of the American dream.

Stage 2: The Shifting Role of Sales

The second stage of marketing evolution focused on **sales**. Many US producers had enjoyed regional monopolies (or at least oligopolies) since the dawn of the Industrial Age. Under these conditions, sales representatives took orders from what were essentially captive **audiences**. Marketing would have been considered an unnecessary expense under this scenario. However, as competition increased in most industries after World War II, these regional monopolies began to weaken.

The emphasis on sales that characterized the economy during the last third of the twentieth century continued to reflect the production orientation of society. Sales representatives eventually served as a bridge between the production economy and the service economy as they developed and maintained relationships. Their roles progressed from being "order takers" to being "consultants" to their clients, sending information from customers back to producers and facilitating the emergence of a market orientation in American business. Even so, the emphasis on sales continued to overshadow the nascent emphasis on services.

Stage 3: The Emergence of the Consumer's Point of View and the Service Economy

By the last quarter of the twentieth century, the industrial economy had given way to a service economy, and the remaining production industries became increasingly standardized. This shift from a product orientation to a service orientation represented a sea change for marketing. Service industries tend to be market driven, and American corporations began abandoning their "father knows best" mind-set in favor of a market orientation. For the first time, progressive managers in a wide range of industries sought to determine what consumers wanted and then strived to fulfill those needs. This shift opened the door to market research and to the exploitation of consumer desires by professional marketers. The new market-driven firms adopted an outside-in way of thinking that viewed service delivery from the customer's point of view.

The emergence of a service economy had important implications for both marketing and healthcare. Services are distinguished from goods in that they are generally consumed as they are produced and cannot be stored or taken away. The marketing of services is different from the marketing of goods, representing a different set of challenges for marketers in any field, including healthcare. A new mind-set accompanied by new promotional

Sales
An approach to business that emphasizes transactions rather than promotions

Audience
People or organizations that read, view, hear, or are otherwise exposed to a promotional message

approaches to the marketing of services had to be developed as the United States became a service-oriented economy.

Stage 4: The Rise of the Electronic Age

As the twenty-first century dawned, healthcare marketing like marketing in other sectors of the economy experienced an electronic revolution. Electronically empowered consumers could now research, compare, and buy health-related products on the World Wide Web and, with the advent of social media, instantaneously share their healthcare experiences and opinions on the services they received. In addition, consumers could consult websites for information on medical conditions, healthcare providers, and healthcare facilities. Healthcare organizations, too, began to increasingly incorporate electronic health records and other secure data systems into their operations. Healthcare organizations also started to offer a growing number of options for interacting with their patients online—through websites, blogs, and social networks, among others.

Social networking sites like Facebook—through profiles "owned" by an organization, a provider, or an individual consumer—have become forums for consumers to discuss the quality of care at a facility, a doctor's characteristics or expertise, general information about a provider or a group, disease symptoms and diagnoses, treatment options, pricing or cost of services, and healthcare industry news. For example, when the **Patient Protection and Affordable Care Act (ACA)** was enacted in 2010, social networks were abuzz with information (and misinformation) on the healthcare reform's provisions and implementation. (This edition devotes Chapter 11 to social media, reflecting this topic's ascendancy in American society.)

Patient Protection and Affordable Care Act (ACA)
2010 legislation that aims to expand health insurance coverage and improve healthcare delivery and quality

The Introduction of Marketing in Healthcare

Healthcare did not adopt marketing approaches to any significant extent until the 1980s, although some healthcare organizations in the retail and supplier sectors had long employed marketing techniques to promote their products. Well after other industries had adopted marketing, these activities were still uncommon among organizations involved in patient care.

Nevertheless, some precursors to marketing were well established in the industry. Every hospital and many other healthcare organizations had long-standing public relations functions that disseminated information about the organization and announced new developments (e.g., new staff, equipment purchases). The public relations staff worked mainly with the media—disseminating press releases, responding to requests for information, and dealing with the press when a negative event occurred.

Most large provider organizations also had communications functions (often under the auspices of the public relations department). Communications staff would develop materials to disseminate to the public and to the employees of the organization, such as internal—and, later, patient-oriented—newsletters and patient-education materials.

Some of the larger healthcare organizations also established government relations offices. Government relations staff was responsible for tracking regulatory and legislative activities that might affect the organization, served as an interface with government officials, and acted as lobbyists when necessary. Government relations offices frequently became involved in addressing the requirements of regulatory agencies.

Healthcare organizations of all types were involved in informal promotional activities to an extent. Hospitals sponsored health education seminars, held open houses at new facilities, or supported community events. Hospitals marketed themselves by making their facilities available to the community for public meetings and otherwise attempting to be good corporate citizens. Physicians marketed themselves through such activities as networking with colleagues at the country club, sending letters of appreciation to referring physicians, and providing services to high school athletic teams. See Exhibit 1.1 for a discussion of some of the key developments in the history of healthcare marketing.

EXHIBIT 1.1
A Brief History of Healthcare Marketing

Although the 1970s marked the formal emergence of marketing in the health services industry, few healthcare organizations—as organizations—had yet bought into marketing. For-profit hospital chains like Columbia and HCA may have had more of a marketing orientation, while Evanston (Indiana) Hospital had a vice president of marketing in 1976. However, many observers of the field would cite the publication of Philip Kotler's (1975) *Marketing for Non-Profit Organizations* as the event that legitimized marketing within the **not-for-profit** healthcare sector.

The emergence of marketing in healthcare was driven by a handful of assertive and creative people who took the initiative and, often against great odds, established marketing programs. True, a few healthcare organizations developed permanent marketing programs early on, but the inroads marketing made in the 1970s and 1980s were a result of the tenacity of a handful of true believers.

The field was given impetus by the pioneering activities of Scott MacStravic and popularized through his 1977 book *Marketing Health Care*. MacStravic served as an officer in various professional organizations for healthcare marketers and strategists and helped establish

(continued)

Not-for-profit
An organization granted tax-exempt status by the Internal Revenue Service

healthcare marketing as a separate profession. In the academic arena, Eric Berkowitz, a marketing professor at the University of Massachusetts, built on Kotler's early work and helped establish healthcare marketing as a legitimate component of academic marketing through numerous books and articles on the topic. Other academics who contributed to the establishment of healthcare marketing were Steven W. Brown, who contributed numerous publications in the 1980s, and Roberta Clark, who collaborated with Kotler in applying marketing principles to healthcare.

By the end of the 1980s, marketing was being incorporated into the structure of healthcare organizations. Marketing departments were being established, and marketing expenses were being factored into organizational budgets. Marketers were being promoted to managers, directors, and, ultimately, vice presidents. Marketing was moving from the periphery of the organization to the boardroom. Once technical resources who were consulted as needed, marketers were becoming full partners in the corporate decision-making process. The most progressive healthcare organizations developed a marketing mind-set to ensure that marketing was a consideration in every initiative and that marketers provided input on the direction of the enterprise.

By the 2000s, the marketing activities of hospitals were beginning to look more like those of their counterparts in the for-profit sector (e.g., pharmaceutical companies, medical device companies). The typical hospital marketing department included a staff of five or more with budgets in the millions of dollars. Marketing executives were increasingly at the vice president level, earning salaries comparable with those of other healthcare executives.

The importance of marketing in healthcare is also reflected in the emergence of publications devoted to the topic, including *Marketing Health Services* (the healthcare journal of the American Marketing Association) and *Health Marketing Quarterly*. Articles on healthcare marketing regularly appear in other marketing publications as well (such as in *Advertising Age*). Numerous newsletters are devoted to healthcare marketing or some component of it, such as health communications or public relations.

Associations for healthcare marketers have been established, such as the **Society for Healthcare Strategy & Market Development** of the American Hospital Association. The **American Marketing Association** has an active healthcare marketing division, and one of its eight special interest groups is devoted to healthcare.

Society for Healthcare Strategy & Market Development
A division of the American Hospital Association that serves marketing and planning professionals in healthcare

American Marketing Association
The primary organization devoted to the marketing field

Textbooks on healthcare marketing began appearing in the 1980s, and healthcare marketing courses are part of the marketing curriculum in many US universities. Courses on the topic are now standard in healthcare administration programs. Numerous universities and educational programs offer specialized training courses on various aspects of healthcare marketing.

All of these developments reflect the growing importance of marketing in the healthcare arena and its changing role. The ways in which marketing is being transformed as it matures in the healthcare industry are discussed throughout this book.

Periods of Growth for Healthcare Marketing

The periods through which marketing has evolved in the healthcare setting are outlined in this section. Exhibit 1.2 summarizes the implications of this evolution for the hospital industry.

The 1950s

Although the 1950s are often viewed as the "age of marketing," marketing did not appear on healthcare's radar screen until much later. The emerging pharmaceutical industry, however, was beginning to market to physicians, and the fledgling insurance industry was beginning to market health plans to consumers. In the healthcare trenches, providers were light-years away from formal marketing activities. Hospitals and physicians, for the most part, considered marketing (read: advertising) to be inappropriate and even unethical. This stance, however, did not preclude hospitals from offering free educational programs or implementing public relations campaigns, nor did it prevent physicians from cozying up to potential referring physicians and networking with colleagues at the country club. At the time, these activities were not thought of as marketing.

EXHIBIT 1.2
The Evolution of Marketing in Healthcare

Business Orientation	Manufacturer	Hospital
Production	Produce quality product	Deliver quality care
Sales	Generate volume	Fill hospital beds
Marketing	Satisfy consumer needs/wants	Satisfy consumer needs/wants

As the hospital industry came of age and many new facilities were established, the industry continued to reflect a production orientation, which was by then waning throughout the rest of the economy. The demand for physician and hospital services was considered inelastic, and little attention was paid to the characteristics of either current patients or prospective customers. The emphasis was on providing quality care, and most providers held **monopolies** or **oligopolies** that shielded them from competition within their markets.

Monopoly
One organization controls the total market for a good or service

Oligopoly
A few organizations dominate a market or an industry

The 1960s

As the health services sector expanded during the 1960s, the role of public relations was enhanced. Although the developments that would force hospitals and other healthcare organizations to embrace marketing were at least a decade away, the public relations field was flourishing. This relatively basic marketing function was the healthcare organization's primary means of keeping in touch with its various stakeholders.

The stakeholders of this period were primarily the physicians who admitted or referred patients to healthcare facilities and the donors who made charitable contributions to the organization. Consumers were not considered an important constituency because they did not directly choose hospitals but were referred by their physicians. The use of media to advance strategic marketing objectives had not evolved, and media relations in this era often consisted of answering reporters' questions about patients' conditions.

Electronic media
Media that transmit content electronically, such as radio, TV, and the Internet

Print was the medium of choice for communications throughout the 1960s, despite the increasingly influential role that **electronic media** (TV and radio, at that time) were playing for marketers in other industries. This era was marked by polished annual reports, informational brochures, and publications targeted to the community. Healthcare communications became a well-developed function, and hospitals continued to expand the role of public relations.

Some segments of the healthcare industry not involved in patient care entered the sales stage (stage 2 in the evolution of the marketing function) during this decade. For example, pharmaceutical companies and insurance plans established sales forces to promote their drugs to physicians and market insurance plans to employers and individuals, respectively.

The 1970s

During the 1970s, urgency began to grow among hospitals with regard to promoting their services within the community. The desire for greater market presence was reinforced by the growing conviction that, in the future, healthcare organizations were going to have to be able to attract customers. Many organizations expanded their public relations functions to include a broader marketing mandate. These types of activities appeared to be particularly common in parts of the country where health maintenance organizations were emerging.

The for-profit hospital sector also grew in importance during the 1970s. With few limits on reimbursement, both not-for-profit and for-profit hospitals expanded their services. Continued high demand for health services and the stable payment system created by Medicare made the industry attractive to investor-owned companies. Numerous national for-profit hospital and nursing home chains emerged during this period.

Some early attempts at **advertising** health services were made, and interest in marketing research was beginning to emerge. These activities by the healthcare establishment were "officially" recognized—and given legitimacy—at a conference on marketing sponsored by the American Hospital Association during the mid-1970s. The marketing movement in healthcare was given further impetus by rulings that relaxed the restrictions on advertising, imposed early on by various regulatory agencies, for healthcare providers.

Advertising
Any paid form of presentation or promotion of ideas, goods, or services

For hospitals, the sales era began in the mid-1970s with the changes that occurred in reimbursement. Under cost-based reimbursement (e.g., Medicare), competition with other hospitals had not been a major concern. Hospitals had ample patients, and occupancy rates were high. The top priority was to attract as many customers as possible by enticing physicians to admit their patients. To this end, hospitals developed physician relations programs and offered other enticements to encourage physician loyalty (Berkowitz 2010).

When hospitals recognized that patients might play a role in the hospital selection decision, a second strategy for selling to the public emerged. In the mid-1970s, some hospitals adopted mass advertising strategies to promote their programs, including billboard displays and television and radio commercials that touted a particular service. The goal of the marketer was to convince prospective patients to use his hospital when presented with a choice between competing hospitals (Berkowitz 2010). Communication efforts were beginning to be targeted toward patients, and patient satisfaction research grew in importance. Even so, marketing in the sense of managing the flow of services between an organization and its customers was still not a recognized function of most healthcare organizations. See Exhibit 1.3 for a chronology of the development of healthcare marketing.

The 1980s

If healthcare marketing was born in the 1970s, it came of age in the 1980s. The healthcare industry had evolved from a seller's market to a buyer's market, a change that was to have a profound effect on the marketing of health services. Employers and consumers had become purchasers of healthcare, and

EXHIBIT 1.3
Healthcare Marketing Timeline

	1950	1960	1970	1980	1990	2000	2010
Stage	Premarketing ――――――――→			Introduction ―→	Growth ―→	Maturity ―→	
Primary techniques	Public relations Communication		Government relations	Advertising Marketing research Direct marketing Personal sales	Direct-to-consumer Relationship marketing Social marketing Internet marketing	Social media	
Main theme	Publicity Information management		Regulatory influence Consumer research	Sales Technology applications	Relationship management	Consumer engagement	
Marketing target*	General public		Government agencies Health plans	Physicians Employers	Referral agents Businesses	Consumers Market segments	

*Patient care organizations

the physician's role in referring patients for hospital services was beginning to diminish. The hospital industry continued to grow during the 1980s, as centrally managed health systems (both for-profit and not-for-profit) expanded and national chains of hospitals, nursing homes, and home health agencies were established.

Marketers had to begin looking at target audiences in an entirely different way, and the importance of consumers was heightened by changes in insurance reimbursement patterns. Hospitals began to think of medical care in terms of product or service lines, a development that had major consequences for the marketing of health services. Hospitals realized that marketing directly to consumers for such services as obstetrics, cosmetic surgery, and outpatient care could generate revenue and enhance **market share**.

Although marketing was beginning to be accepted in healthcare, the industry suffered from a lack of professional marketing personnel. Few marketers had experience with healthcare, and attempts at importing marketing techniques from other industries were generally unsuccessful. Many healthcare administrators still saw marketing as an expensive gimmick and considered marketers to be outsiders with no place in healthcare.

The rise of service-line marketing launched the great hospital advertising wars of the 1980s. Barely a blip on the healthcare marketing radar screen a decade earlier, advertising grew dramatically during this decade. In 1983, hospitals spent $50 million on advertising; by 1986, that figure had risen to $500 million, a tenfold increase in three years. Once an enterprise of dubious respectability, advertising was now hailed as a marketing panacea for hospitals (Berkowitz 2010).

A growing number of **health professionals** who suddenly found themselves in competition for patients came to see marketing as a key to competitive success. This perception brought about a surge in advertising activity by large healthcare organizations. Unfortunately, much of the advertising of the mid- to late 1980s was ineffectual at best and disastrous at worst. Many campaigns were poorly conceived and wasted an enormous amount of money. Ad copy tended to be institutionally focused, and healthcare marketing initiatives lacked the impact of the advertising produced in other industries—in large part because of the conservative, risk-averse culture of hospitals.

Advertising came to be the activity that epitomized marketing for many in healthcare during this period. Marketers themselves perpetuated this notion, and even today, many healthcare executives equate marketing with advertising. Ultimately, the surge in advertising was both a blessing and a curse. On the one hand, advertising campaigns were something relatively concrete; an organization could invest in them and reasonably expect to incur some benefit as a result. On the other hand, the ineffectiveness of much of this advertising and the negative fallout it often generated were setbacks for

Market share
The percentage of the total market captured by a company

Health professional
A trained individual who performs a clinical, an allied health, an administrative or a managerial, or a technical duty

the proponents of healthcare marketing. After experiencing the initial rush of seeing their billboards and television commercials, hospital administrators began to question the expense and, more important, the effectiveness of the marketing initiatives they were funding.

During the 1980s, healthcare organizations faced serious financial retrenchment. Hospitals were looking for cuts wherever they could find them, and marketing expenditures were easy targets. Budgets were cut and marketing staff were laid off. Although the marketing function was not entirely eliminated, it was often incorporated under the umbrella of business development or strategic planning. In many organizations, marketing was squeezed out of the budget and kept alive by just a few dedicated marketing professionals. In some healthcare organizations, marketing disappeared as a corporate function and was never reinstated. On the positive side, this retrenchment allowed healthcare marketers to reassess the field and concentrate on developing baseline data that could be used when a marketing revival occurred.

Despite these setbacks, consumer research in healthcare came into its own during this decade. Most hospitals had conducted patient satisfaction research for some time, but consumer research was virtually unknown until the 1970s. By the mid-1980s, a majority of hospitals were conducting physician and consumer research. The latter was crucial in developing advertising messages and monitoring the success of marketing programs.

The 1990s

Healthcare became more market driven in the 1990s, and the marketing function grew in importance in healthcare organizations. The institutional perspective that had long driven decision making gave way to market-driven decision making. Every hospital was trying to win the hearts and minds of healthcare consumers.

Health/healthcare system
A multifacility healthcare organization; also may refer to the overall healthcare system

Advertising by healthcare organizations resurged during the mid-1990s, spurred by the massive wave of hospital mergers. The consolidation of healthcare organizations into ever-larger **healthcare systems** resulted in the creation of larger organizations with expanded resources and more sophisticated management. Many executives entered the field from outside of healthcare, bringing a more businesslike mind-set with them.

Direct to consumer
A marketing approach that targets the end user rather than referral agents or intermediaries

The consumer was rediscovered during this process, and the **direct-to-consumer** movement was initiated. The popularity of guest relations programs during the 1990s solidified the transformation of patients into customers. As consumers gained influence, marketing became increasingly integrated into the operations of healthcare organizations. The consumers of the 1990s were better educated and more assertive about their healthcare needs than were consumers of the previous generation. The emergence of the Internet as a source of health information further contributed to the rise of **consumerism**. Newly empowered consumers were taking on an increasingly influential (if informal) role in reshaping the US healthcare system.

During the 1990s, health professionals developed a new perspective on the role of marketing, aided by a new generation of healthcare administrators who were more business oriented. A more qualified corps of marketing professionals emerged that brought ambitious but realistic expectations to the industry. Pharmaceutical companies began advertising directly to consumers, which made everyone in the industry more aware of marketing's potential. In addition, everyone in healthcare was becoming more consumer sensitive, and new data gave health professionals a better understanding of the healthcare customer.

Marketing research grew in importance during this decade. The need for information on consumers, customers, competitors, and the market demanded an expanded research function. Patient and consumer research was augmented, and newly developed technologies brought the research capabilities of other industries to healthcare.

Business practices in general came to be more accepted in healthcare during this period, and marketing was an inevitable beneficiary. Marketing was repackaged in a more professional guise, and the shift away from advertising was noticeable. Marketing ended the decade as a more mature discipline, emphasizing market research and sensitivity to the needs of the consumer. Healthcare had finally reached stage 3 in the evolution of the marketing function.

By the end of the twentieth century, healthcare marketing had changed substantially. In the 1990s, the emphasis shifted from sick people to well people in response to the emergence of **managed care** and capitated payments. There was a new focus on patient satisfaction and increased efforts at generating consumer data. The baby boomers who were coming to dominate the healthcare landscape viewed marketing as a source of valuable information rather than hucksterism and were disinclined to use an organization that did not cater to their interests.

Image advertising was deemphasized in favor of targeted promotions for specific services, making for more content and less fluff. Techniques from other industries, like customer relationship marketing, began to be explored. The new generation of healthcare administrators seemed to be more comfortable with marketing and considered this function an inherent aspect of healthcare operations.

With the repackaging and maturation of marketing in the 1990s, the field became more sophisticated overall. The market was in many ways more

Consumerism
A movement in which consumers participate in defining their healthcare needs and how those needs are met

Managed care
Health insurance plans that contract with providers and healthcare organizations to provide care for members at negotiated rates

Image advertising
A promotional focus on the overall attributes (rather than specific services) of an organization

competitive, and even the managed care environment held opportunities for promotional activities. In addition, mergers not only created more potential marketing clout but also often involved for-profit healthcare organizations that were inherently more marketing oriented.

The 2000s to the Present

By the end of the 1990s, a new cohort of healthcare administrators was in place and began exhibiting a greater acceptance of business practices, including marketing. The industry had witnessed a massive turnover in hospital administrators through retirement, mergers, and downsizing. Many of the new wave of administrators came from other, often more profit-oriented industries where marketing was considered a normal corporate function. These administrators instilled a marketing mind-set in keeping with the more strategic orientation they brought to the industry.

Although some still focus on advertising and sales, twenty-first century marketing executives have expanded their toolboxes to address the full range of activities to support the marketing function. Market segmentation and target marketing techniques have been adapted from other industries. Reliable and effective public, media, and community relations; customer service; and reputation and relationship management are making a comeback, demonstrating the effectiveness of carefully designed low-cost methods for reaching audiences and swaying public opinion.

The consumer is increasingly considered the key to success, and various data-management and customer-relations techniques have been put into place. *Consumer engagement* is a current buzzword in healthcare, and efforts aimed at getting healthcare consumers to buy in are growing. The new healthcare environment—influenced in part by the ACA—demands a new approach that includes a population component that generates measurable community benefit. As healthcare providers are increasingly paid for performance rather than volume, a more thoughtful approach to marketing will be required.

Considered by some as the major development of the twenty-first century, social media are playing a growing role in the marketing of health services. By the end of the twentieth century, virtually all healthcare providers had established an Internet presence; for many, this was not only a core component of their marketing initiative but also a means of interacting with customers and prospective customers. This electronic communication capacity has been expanded with the explosion of social media. Patients are able to instantaneously communicate with each other and, increasingly, with health professionals. Prospective customers can interact with existing customers before using health services. The flooding of cyberspace with healthcare "chatter" requires close monitoring by marketers.

Why Healthcare Is Different from Other Industries

Healthcare as an industry is set apart from the other sectors of the economy because of its specific characteristics. In particular, healthcare providers behave in a manner often inconsistent with that of organizations in other industries. Health professionals, especially clinicians, fall into a special category, and the fact that clinicians—not administrators or businesspeople—make most of the decisions regarding patient care creates a dynamic unique to healthcare. The nature of healthcare goods and services sets them apart from the goods and services offered in other industries. Further, significant differences exist between healthcare consumers and the consumers of virtually any other goods or service. These differences are particularly apparent with regard to the consumer's decision making (see Chapter 5 for more discussion on the decision-making process).

Characteristics of the Healthcare Industry

The development of a marketing culture in any industry is predicated on certain assumptions about that industry and the marketing enterprise, including the existence of a rational market for the goods and services proffered by the organizations in that industry. The market is presumed to involve organized groups of sellers, informed buyers, an orderly mechanism for carrying out transactions between sellers and buyers, and a straightforward process for transferring payment for products between buyers and sellers.

The existence of a market is also predicated on the assumption that buyers are driven primarily by economic motives and seek to maximize their benefits from the exchange. In healthcare, however, a number of factors operate to prevent the buyers and sellers of health services from interacting in the same manner as buyers and sellers in other industries.

The existence of a market also presumes that there are sellers competing for the consumer's resources and that this competition determines the price of goods and services. In healthcare, however, healthcare providers often maintain monopolies over particular services in particular markets—or, more commonly, oligopolies of healthcare organizations may dominate particular markets. Thus, buyers of health services are often limited in their options. In view of these prerequisites for the existence of a market, one could argue that, to the extent that any type of market for health services exists, it is not "rational" in the way that the markets for other goods and services are.

As an industry, healthcare also differs from other sectors of the economy in that its key organizations have diverse goals. In other industries, the intent is to sell as many units as possible while extracting the maximum profit from the transactions. Anything other than making a profit is secondary to the single-minded goal of selling consumer products. Most healthcare organizations, on the other hand, are obligated to accept clients whether or not they can pay for the services. Emergency departments cannot turn away anyone needing emergency care until that person has at least been stabilized. Physician offices may require some payment up front from those who do not have insurance, but there are ethical considerations associated with turning a clearly symptomatic individual away. Thus, the economic considerations that apply to other industries may be compromised as a result of factors unique to healthcare.

Unlike other industries, healthcare lacks a straightforward means of financing the purchase of goods and services, particularly patient care services. Customers in other industries typically pay directly—either out of pocket or through some form of credit—for the goods and services they consume. While healthcare consumers may pay some small portion of the cost out of pocket, most fees are paid by a third party, whether a private insurance plan or a government-sponsored plan such as **Medicare** or **Medicaid**. The seller may have to deal with thousands of different insurance plans, and the cost of health services is reimbursed using a combination of different payment mechanisms. Thus, it would not be unusual for an elderly patient to have the costs of one hospital visit paid for with Medicare reimbursement, supplementary private insurance reimbursement, and out-of-pocket payments. This arrangement is not found in any other industry and creates a much more complicated financial picture for healthcare.

Finally, healthcare is different from other industries in that the normal rules of supply and demand seldom apply. An increase in the supply of health services, for example, does not necessarily result in a decrease in price, nor does increased demand invariably drive up prices. For one thing, the availability (supply) of services dictates, to a certain extent, the demand for these services. Pent-up demand for health services often surfaces when more facilities become available. As a result, neither the increased supply of beds nor the increase in demand has a significant impact on prices.

The factors that govern supply, demand, and price in healthcare are complex and unique to this industry. The supply of health services is affected by the vagaries of health professional training programs, restrictions enforced by regulatory agencies, and even fads. The level of demand—arguably the most problematic of the three—is typically not controlled by the end user. Except for elective procedures for which the consumer pays out of pocket, most decisions that affect the demand for health services are made by **gatekeepers**, such as physicians and **health plans**. Thus, the level of demand is more often a function of such factors as insurance plan provisions, the availability of resources, and physician practice patterns than a function of the level of sickness in the population. Exhibit 1.4 describes the emergence of healthcare as a major institution within US society.

Medicare
The federal health insurance program for Americans aged 65 or older

Medicaid
The joint federal–state health insurance program for low-income individuals

Gatekeeper
An individual or organization that makes decisions on behalf of an end user or otherwise controls the purchase of goods and services

Health plan
Public or private medical insurance

Characteristics of Healthcare Organizations

Healthcare organizations tend to be multipurpose organizations. Although some purveyors of healthcare goods or services are single-minded in their intent, large healthcare organizations like hospitals are likely to pursue a number of goals simultaneously. Indeed, the main goal of an academic medical center may not be to provide patient care at all. It may be education, research, or community service, with direct patient care as a secondary concern. Even large specialty practices are likely to be involved in teaching and research, and although they are not likely to neglect their core activity, they often have a more diffuse orientation than do organizations in other industries.

Further, a large proportion of healthcare organizations—most notably hospitals—are chartered as not-for-profit organizations. Although physician groups are usually incorporated as for-profit professional corporations, many community-based clinics, faith-based clinics, and government-supported programs operate on a not-for-profit basis. This "charitable" orientation creates an environment that is much different from that of other industries. The governmental financial support provided to some health facilities and programs also creates a different dynamic. For some organizations, the unpredictability of government subsidy is an unsettling factor. For others, the assurance of government support means they may not be as vulnerable to the vagaries of the market.

Characteristics of Healthcare Products

The goods and services that constitute healthcare products are also unique. Although many health-related goods (e.g., adhesive bandages, fitness equipment, over-the-counter drugs) may be marketed like any other products, most **consumer health products** do not fall into this category. Even the most common consumer health product—pharmaceuticals—must often be prescribed by an intermediary before it can be acquired and consumed.

Consumer health products
Healthcare goods distributed through retail outlets and directly purchased by the customer

---

Several developments in US society and in healthcare over the last quarter of the twentieth century laid the foundation for the emergence of healthcare marketing. Current trends in healthcare have now brought marketing to center stage. Changes in demographic characteristics, lifestyles, and other population attributes have all contributed to the growing importance of healthcare marketing. Trends in the healthcare arena that are anticipated to continue for the foreseeable future indicate that the role of marketing in healthcare is growing.

(continued)

EXHIBIT 1.4
The Emergence of Healthcare as an Institution in the United States

A healthcare system can be understood only within the sociocultural context of the society in which it exists, and no two healthcare delivery systems are exactly alike. Differences between healthcare systems are primarily a function of differences in context. The social structure of a society, along with its cultural values, establishes the parameters for the healthcare system. In this sense, the form and function of the healthcare system reflect the form and function of the society in which it resides. Ultimately, the development of marketing in healthcare (or any industry) reflects the characteristics of both that industry and that society.

The ascendancy of the healthcare institution in the twentieth century was given impetus by the growing dependence on formal organizations of all types. The industrialization and urbanization of the United States reflected a transformation from a traditional, agrarian society to a complex, modern society in which change, not tradition, was the central theme. In such a society, formal solutions to societal needs take precedence over informal responses.

Healthcare provides possibly the best example of this emergent dependence on formal solutions because it is an institution whose very development was a result of this transformation. Our great-grandparents would have considered formal healthcare to be the last resort when faced with sickness and disability. Few of them ever entered a hospital or regularly saw a physician. Today, in contrast, the health-care system is often seen as the first resort when health problems arise. Traditional, informal responses to health problems have given way to complex, institutionalized responses. Healthcare has become entrenched in the fabric of American life to the point that Americans turn to it not only for clear-cut health problems but also for a broad range of psychological, social, interpersonal, and spiritual problems.

The restructuring of institutions during the twentieth century was accompanied by a cultural revolution that resulted in an extensive **value** reorientation in American society. The values associated with traditional societies (such as kinship, community, authority, and primary relationships) were overshadowed by the values of modern industrialized societies (such as secularism, urbanism, and self-actualization). Ultimately, the restructuring of American values was instrumental in the emergence of healthcare as an important institution.

The modern values that emerged after World War II supported the emergence of an institutional structure, which would subsequently spawn the development of modern Western medicine. These values shifted the emphasis in American society to economic success,

Value
Anything—usually intangible—a society considers important, such as freedom and economic prosperity

educational achievement, and scientific and technological advancement and supported the ascendancy of healthcare as a dominant institution. The conceptualization of health as a distinct value in society represented a major development in the emergence of the healthcare institution. Before World War II, health was generally not recognized as a value by Americans but was vaguely tied to other notions of well-being. Public opinion polls before the war did not identify personal health as an issue for the populace, nor was healthcare delivery considered a societal concern. By the 1960s, however, personal health had climbed to the top of public opinion polls as an issue, and the adequate provision of health services became an important issue in the mind of the American public (Thomas 2003a). By the last quarter of the twentieth century, Americans had become obsessed with health as a value and with the importance of institutional solutions to health problems.

By any measure, healthcare could be considered a dominant institution in contemporary American society. Other institutions—such as politics, the military, and the arts—receive comparatively fewer resources. Further, Americans have become increasingly obsessed with their health. In public opinion polls, respondents frequently cite health as one of their most pressing personal concerns and healthcare as a leading national concern. The following graph (the most recent issued at the time of this writing) prepared by the Centers for Medicare & Medicaid Services displays trends in healthcare costs as a proportion of the gross domestic product (GDP):

US Healthcare Costs as a Percentage of GDP

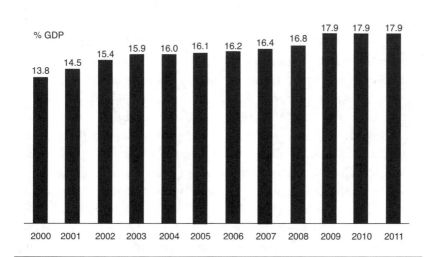

Healthcare providers are generally concerned with promoting a service, yet the nature of their services is difficult to describe. A physician might break down services by procedure code (e.g., CPT [current procedural terminology] codes), but few services stand alone. Services come in bundles, such as the group of services that surrounds a surgical procedure. Although clinicians (and their billing clerks) may see them as discrete services, the patient perceives them as a complex mix of services related to a heart attack, diabetes management, or cancer treatment.

As discussed in Chapter 6, the products generated by a healthcare organization are difficult to conceptualize. The things healthcare organizations and health professionals think they provide (e.g., quality care, prolonged life, elimination of pathology) are often hard to define or measure. The difficulty in specifying the services provided becomes obvious when a marketer asks a hospital department head what services the department provides.

Healthcare services are also characterized by their inability to be substituted or replaced by other goods or services. For example, although one form of transportation might be substituted for another, a surgical procedure can seldom be substituted for another. Unlike other industries, healthcare often provides only one solution to a particular challenge.

Characteristics of Health Professionals

Historically, the healthcare industry has been dominated by professionals rather than by administrators. Clinical personnel (usually physicians, but other clinicians as well) define much of the demand for health services and are directly or indirectly responsible for most healthcare expenditures. This setup is comparable to the systems in other industries in which technicians rather than administrators run the organization. The situation in healthcare is complicated by the fact that clinicians and administrators may not share the same goals.

Ethics
A code of behavior that specifies a moral stance, particularly in professional dealings

The medical **ethics** that drive the behavior of health professionals exist independently of system operations. Clinicians are bound by oath to do what is medically appropriate, whether or not it is cost-effective or contributes to the organization's efficiency. Decisions made in the best interests of the patient may not reflect the best interests of the organization. Although health professionals have had to become more realistic regarding indiscriminate use of resources, clinical interests continue to outweigh financial considerations in most cases. Conflict between the goals of clinicians and administrators is inherent in healthcare organizations, and no comparable situation can be found in any other industry.

The conflict between the clinical and business sides of the healthcare operation is exacerbated by the antibusiness orientation of many health professionals. Most healthcare workers entered the field because they wanted to be in a profession not a business, and physicians and other clinicians often have a distorted perception of the business world. If health professionals cannot appreciate the business side of the operation, they are not likely to appreciate the importance of marketing. Even among nonclinicians, many common business practices may be considered inappropriate for the not-for-profit healthcare world.

Characteristics of Healthcare Consumers

What probably most sets the healthcare field apart from other industries is the nature of its consumers. In healthcare, the term *consumer* refers to any person with the potential to consume a good or service. Everyone is likely to use healthcare goods or services and, thus, be involved in the healthcare system at some time or another. Despite this unique attribute, healthcare organizations historically failed to perceive their consumers in this manner. Until recently, the assumption was that a person was not a prospect for health services until he or she became sick. Thus, healthcare providers made no attempt to develop relationships with nonpatients. Today, however, numerous parties cater to nonpatients. Major industries have developed around prevention, fitness, and lifestyle management. Much of the social marketing that takes place in US society is geared toward nonpatients.

Healthcare consumers are perhaps most distinguished from consumers of other goods and services by their insulation from the price of the products they buy. Because of healthcare's unusual financing arrangements and lack of access to pricing information, healthcare consumers seldom know the price of the services until after they have received those services. In typical cases, the physician or clinician providing the service is also not likely to know the price of that service. Because **third-party payers**—and not the end users—usually pay for the service performed, healthcare consumers may not even notice how much their care costs. As a result, clinicians are likely to provide or recommend the services they believe to be medically necessary, regardless of price. However, this situation presents at least two problematic consequences.

Third-party payer An entity—other than the provider and patient—that pays for the cost of goods or services

First, consumers are not likely to willingly limit their resource utilization. If they do not know the amount of the fees being charged—and, further, do not have to pay them anyway—they have no incentive to consider the cost. Similarly, physicians or clinicians have no incentive to provide services efficiently if cost is not a consideration. In fact, under traditional fee-for-service arrangements, the incentives available to physicians have encouraged greater use of resources because physicians receive an additional fee for each additional service they perform. Second, few healthcare providers are able to use price as a means of competition or as a basis for marketing. With the exception of organizations that provide elective services or that serve a retail market, providers cannot compete on the basis of price. Few healthcare organizations make their fee schedules public, and even when they do, they are likely to employ varying mechanisms for determining the price of a service. For example, the per diem rates for a hospital room may be determined on the basis of different factors by two competing hospitals, thereby making comparisons meaningless.

Another factor setting healthcare consumers apart from other consumers is the personal nature of the services involved. Most healthcare encounters involve an emotional component that is absent in other consumer transactions. Every diagnostic test is fraught with the possibility of a "positive" finding, and every surgery—no matter how minor—carries the potential for complications. Today's well-informed consumers are aware of not only the severity of medical errors that occur during a hospital stay or procedure but also the rate of system-induced morbidity. Even if consumers can remain stoic about their own care, they are likely to exhibit emotions when the care concerns a parent, a child, or some other loved one.

Initial Barriers to Healthcare Marketing

Given the pervasiveness of marketing in the United States, how can one explain the relative lack of marketing in an industry that accounts for as much as 18 percent of the gross national product? This section discusses some of the barriers that have slowed the acceptance of marketing in the healthcare arena.

No (Real or Perceived) Need

Until the 1980s, most healthcare organizations thought they had no competitors. They had plenty of patients, and revenues were essentially guaranteed by third-party payers. Competition had often been minimized through unwritten agreements among various healthcare providers. If providers did not overtly collude among themselves to carve up the patient market, they respected informal boundaries that were set to reduce competition. They often maintained monopolies or oligopolies in their market areas.

These factors contributed to the perception (and, in many cases, the reality) that marketing was an unnecessary activity for healthcare organizations. From the perspective of mainstream providers, physicians referred their patients to the hospital and insurance plans steered their enrollees to the facility. Why market to end users who were not going to make the decision anyway? This mind-set perpetuated the impression that marketing was not needed and overlooked such important marketing tasks as physician relationship development and health plan contract negotiation.

Resistance to Business Aspects of Healthcare

Much of health professionals' resistance to marketing reflected their misconceptions about the nature of business and marketing. For health professionals, business practices carried an unfavorable connotation—that is, clinical concerns were subjugated by business priorities. A similar misperception existed regarding the nature of marketing. "Marketing equals advertising" was the dominant perception early in the history of healthcare marketing, and even today (as mentioned earlier) many health professionals retain that narrow (and negative) perception of marketing. The concern over contaminating a helping profession with business principles led to healthcare organizations enacting various provisions against advertising.

Concerns Over Marketing Costs

Concerns related to the cost of marketing also played a role in healthcare organizations' slow acceptance of marketing practices. Marketing (again, primarily advertising) was seen as an expensive proposition. While more commercial operations, like pharmaceutical companies, saw marketing expenses as a normal cost of doing business, hospitals and physicians with no previous experience in this regard suffered sticker shock at the marketing price tag. This lack of experience with marketing also caused them to overlook numerous aspects of marketing that involved little or no expense.

Even today, healthcare organizations are seldom able to measure the cost of providing a service, making **cost–benefit analyses** difficult to perform. Further, so many factors come into play (e.g., referral patterns, consumer attitudes) in determining the use of services that isolating the impact of marketing activities (or doing an **impact evaluation**) is hard. Even if marketing is grudgingly accepted, there is widespread concern that marketing can do little to alter practice patterns, market shares, or any other indicator of importance to the provider. Thus, given a chronic shortage of resources, many health professionals question the appropriateness of expending scarce resources on an activity perceived to have limited benefit. These concerns have been reinforced by disgruntled patients who have linked their high hospital bills to excessive spending on expensive advertising. Even if the spending does not affect the patient's bill, the negative fallout from highly visible marketing efforts could affect the public image of many healthcare organizations.

Cost–benefit analysis
An evaluation technique that compares the cost of a project with its anticipated benefits

Impact evaluation
An assessment of the changes brought about by the marketing effort

Ethical and Legal Constraints

Ethical and legal constraints have also posed a major barrier to the incorporation of marketing into healthcare. The nature of health-related goods and services has made them the target of restrictions not found in other industries. As stated earlier, until recent years, it was considered unethical for physicians and many other clinicians to advertise. Although other types of marketing were generally accepted, overt advertising initiatives were discouraged if not prohibited. Physicians were restrained by professional considerations, and hospitals often imposed internal constraints on their marketing activities.

In some cases, legal restraints have been put in place to prohibit advertising and other overt forms of marketing. The Federal Trade Commission, for example, limits the types of advertising and the advertising content pharmaceutical companies and other healthcare consumer products companies can provide. Congressional legislation also has been enacted to limit the marketing activities of providers reimbursed under the Medicare and Medicaid programs. Exhibit 1.5 presents additional ethical issues in healthcare marketing.

EXHIBIT 1.5
Ethical Issues
in Healthcare
Marketing

Concerns over the marketing practices for various medical remedies can be traced to 200 years ago—the days when patent medicines were sold on street corners, at carnivals, and by traveling salesmen. The claims made for such potions were often exaggerated or clearly false. Eventually, government regulations were put into place to control the claims of purveyors of such products; with the support of the American Medical Association (AMA), the first medicine labeling laws were passed in 1938. Today, in the United States, the federal Food and Drug Administration and the Federal Trade Commission serve as watchdogs over health-related products and medical devices.

Since the advent of the marketing era in the United States after World War II, ethical issues have nagged the healthcare industry. In the post–World War II period, physicians commonly endorsed various products in exchange for payment from the manufacturer. Physicians were paid to endorse various pharmaceutical products, for example, by indicating that one drug was superior to its competitors. During this period, physicians sometimes strayed from their areas of expertise and endorsed other products as well. The most controversial of these actions involved physicians who endorsed various cigarette brands. Doctors were paid to attest that Brand X was healthier for consumers to smoke than Brand Y. The influence of the AMA and other forces was eventually brought to bear, and such practices were discontinued.

These experiences led the AMA to enforce a virtual prohibition of marketing by physicians. In 1947, the AMA forbade physicians from advertising for self-promotion. This prohibition continued through 1957, when it was modified to only restrict physicians from soliciting patients. These restrictions did not affect such traditional marketing activities as networking and entertaining would-be referrers, and it was even customary at that time for doctors to provide kickbacks (called "fee splitting") to referring physicians.

By the 1960s, the strict injunction against advertising had been eased somewhat and physicians were allowed to cite their name, address, and specialty in telephone directories and similar publications as a means of demonstrating their professionalism and distinguishing themselves from other health professionals. The AMA eventually back-pedaled from its strong stance against physician advertising, and in the 1990s many physicians initiated aggressive marketing campaigns. Even so, such physicians are often perceived in a bad light by their colleagues.

Although hospitals were not constrained to the same extent, many hospital administrators also had ethical qualms concerning marketing (or at least advertising). These qualms did not restrict marketing activities such as public relations, educational activities, and communication strategies, but they did discourage many hospitals from overt media advertising. Ultimately, the combined effect of increasing competition, reduced revenues, and more demanding consumers overcame any lingering reluctance of hospitals and health systems to engage in marketing.

Much of the controversy surrounding marketing in healthcare has involved the pharmaceutical industry. The marketing of over-the-counter drugs, of course, is covered by federal regulations that control the claims that can be made regarding the drugs' efficacy. The marketing of prescription drugs directly to consumers is tightly controlled by federal regulation, and until the end of the twentieth century, pharmaceutical companies were prohibited from marketing directly to consumers. Even with relaxed rules concerning pharmaceutical marketing, there are still strict limits on the claims that can be made in drug advertisements.

Drug manufacturers have stirred up the most controversy by focusing their marketing activities almost exclusively on the physicians who prescribe drugs to their patients. Pharmaceutical companies spend up to 25 percent of their budgets on marketing and sales activities, and the bulk of this sum has historically been allocated to advertising in medical journals, supporting educational programs for potential subscribers, and making sales calls to physicians.

The pharmaceutical companies' long-standing practice of providing free samples of drugs to physicians eventually came under fire and is facing restrictions. More controversial, however, have been the blatant attempts to "buy" physician support by providing gifts, free trips, and other incentives designed to encourage physicians to endorse a particular drug through their prescribing practices. Congress eventually reacted to the perceived excesses by pharmaceutical companies in an

(continued)

attempt to influence the decision making of physicians, and legislation was enacted that severely limited the ability of drug companies to provide incentives to physicians.

Although the marketing activities of health professionals will continue to be guided by self-imposed ethical standards, regulations governing the marketing of health-related products are not likely to disappear. Because of the nature of healthcare products and services, continued oversight by various regulatory agencies can be expected. As marketing activities expand in healthcare, they will continue to be affected by a combination of ethical restraints and legal regulations.

Why Healthcare Marketing Requires a Unique Approach

Because marketing philosophies and techniques cannot be readily transferred from other industries to healthcare, healthcare marketing requires its own unique approach and takes on characteristics unlike those of marketing in other industries. While some of these issues are addressed in later chapters, the following summarize the main reasons:

- *Health services are more of a challenge to market than goods.* Most of the products marketed in healthcare are services rather than goods. Health services are extremely difficult to segregate, and most episodes of care involve the consumption of both goods and services.
- *The demand for many health services is relatively rare and highly unpredictable.* Except for patients who suffer from chronic conditions and require ongoing care, significant health episodes are infrequent occurrences. The current hospital admission rates suggest that only 10 percent of the US population are hospitalized in a year's time, and even that number overstates hospital use because some patients are admitted more than once during a year. Further, the onset of significant health episodes is hard to predict, with the conditions that require the most intensive resources typically arising unexpectedly.
- *The healthcare end user may not be the target for the marketing campaign.* The situation in healthcare is unique in that the end user may not be the decision maker regarding the consumption of services and goods. Further, the consumer may not be the party responsible for paying for the services and goods consumed. For these reasons, the marketing challenge is more difficult than for typical consumer products, and price—a critical differentiating factor for most products—may not be relevant to healthcare marketing.

- *The healthcare product being marketed may be highly complex and may not lend itself to easy categorization.* With a few exceptions, healthcare products cannot be easily separated from other goods and services involved in an episode of care. For reimbursement purposes, costs are divided between professional fees and facilities fees, and a procedure for which marketing is desired (e.g., a hip replacement) is a complex procedure involving many parties and cost centers. Pricing is particularly a challenge when so many overlapping aspects of care exist.

- *Not all prospective customers for a health service are considered desirable.* While most healthcare providers have a moral, if not a legal, responsibility to care for all patients, the fact is that not all patients are considered desirable from a business perspective. Given the complexity of reimbursement for services, the availability of insurance coverage and the type of coverage may determine the desirability of a patient from a financial perspective. The marketer's challenge is made even greater in that the organization cannot appear to be "skimming" the most profitable patients and neglecting the less profitable.

- *The outcome of health services is difficult to measure.* Promoting a service on the basis of superior outcomes represents a challenge for healthcare marketers. Although there is a growing movement toward "standardizing" the medical episode, the fact is a number of factors could contribute to a favorable or unfavorable **outcome** of a clinical episode. While the provider may be perceived as providing high-quality care, one or two adverse episodes could distort this perception and increase the challenge for the marketer.

- *The impact or outcome of healthcare marketing efforts is difficult to measure.* Perhaps the greatest difference in healthcare marketing is its inability to definitively demonstrate that it is responsible for any observed change in organizational outcome (e.g., increased patient volume, higher revenues). Many different factors contribute to the flow of new patients to health services providers, so it is difficult to parse out the role of marketing. Referral patterns of clinicians and steering by insurance plans are just two examples of these factors that could mitigate any perceived marketing benefit.

- *The differences between healthcare organizations and their services are difficult to quantify.* Over time, various providers have become increasingly similar in the services they offer and the resources they bring to bear. Even differences in pricing may not be distinguishing factors in that cost data are hard to acquire and, even if acquired, may be calculated in a variety of ways, thereby making comparison impossible. When all hospitals, for example, offer the same services, have the same equipment, and possibly have overlapping medical staffs,

Outcome
In healthcare, the consequences of a clinical episode; in marketing, the results of a promotional campaign

the marketer is challenged in making the case for a superior or even a different organization.

Developments That Encouraged Healthcare Marketing

Despite the barriers to incorporating marketing into healthcare, during the 1980s and 1990s significant progress was made toward establishing marketing as an integral function of healthcare organizations. Marketing was finally accepted by various healthcare organizations as a legitimate corporate function—because of a number of developments that reflected changes in society overall, trends in the healthcare industry, and changes in the nature of consumers. These key developments, many of which are discussed in later chapters, included the following:

- Introduction of competition
- Overcapacity in the hospital industry
- Rise of the consumer
- Introduction of new services
- Growth of elective procedures
- Introduction of a retail component
- Entry of entrepreneurs
- Mergers and acquisitions
- Need for social marketing
- Consumer engagement movement
- Affordable Care Act

All of these developments occurred within the framework of a changing healthcare paradigm. Exhibit 1.6 describes the ongoing evolution from medical care to healthcare.

EXHIBIT 1.6
From Medical
Care to
Healthcare

Medical model
The traditional paradigm of Western medicine that is based on germ theory and emphasizes a biomedical approach

Since the 1970s, there has been a movement away from medical care toward healthcare. The growing awareness of the connection between health status and lifestyle and the realization that medical care is limited in its ability to control the disorders of modern society have prompted a move away from a strictly **medical model** of health and illness to one that incorporates more of a social and psychological perspective. Originally noted by Engel (1977), this paradigm shift, in which medical care was redefined as healthcare, gained momentum during the 1980s and 1990s.

Medical care is narrowly defined as the formal services provided by the healthcare system that are under the control of a physician. This concept focuses on the clinical or treatment aspects of care and excludes the nonmedical dimension. **Healthcare,** on the other hand, consists of any function that might be directly or indirectly related to preserving, maintaining, and/or enhancing **health.** This concept includes not only formal activities (such as visiting a health professional) but also informal activities such as preventive care (e.g., brushing teeth), exercise, proper diet, and other health maintenance activities.

Since the beginning of the twentieth century, the dominant paradigm in Western medical science has been the medical model of disease. Built on the germ theory formulated late in the nineteenth century, the medical model provided an appropriate framework within which to address and respond to the acute health conditions prevalent well into the twentieth century. By the 1970s, however, enough anomalies had been identified to bring the prevailing paradigm into question. Despite the ever-increasing sophistication of medical technology, the importance of the nonmedical aspects of care was increasingly recognized.

Clearly, the **epidemiologic transition**—by which acute conditions were displaced by chronic disorders—has played a major role. As acute conditions waned in importance and chronic and degenerative conditions came to the forefront, the medical model began to lose some of its salience. Once the cause of most health conditions ceased to be environmental microorganisms and became aspects of lifestyle, a new model of health and illness was required. The chronic conditions that had come to account for most health problems did not respond well to the treatment-and-cure approach of the medical model. Chronic conditions could not be cured but had to be managed over a lifetime, and this called for a different approach.

Independent of this trend, patients had been expressing growing dissatisfaction with the operation of the healthcare system. The traditional approach to care was not a comfortable fit with the attitudes baby boomers were bringing to the doctor's office. This population—more than any other group in US society—has led the movement toward the changing emphasis in healthcare. This cohort emphasizes convenience, value, responsiveness, patient participation, and other attributes not traditionally incorporated into the medical model. Further, the runaway costs of the system have led all observers to question the wisdom of pursuing the one-size-fits-all approach to solving health problems that is traditional in medical care.

The transition from the medical care model to the **healthcare model** has affected every aspect of care—from the standard definitions of

(continued)

Healthcare
Any informal or formal activity intended to restore, maintain, or enhance the health status of individuals or populations

Health
Traditionally, a state reflecting the absence of biological pathology; today, a state of overall physical, social, and psychological well-being

Epidemiologic transition
A change in a population's epidemiologic profile—from acute to chronic health problems—as a result of aging and changing demographic characteristics

Healthcare model
A holistic view of health and illness that includes biological, social, and psychological dimensions

Health status
The degree
to which an
individual or a
population is
characterized by
health problems;
the level of ill
health within a
population

health and illness to the manner in which healthcare is delivered. **Health status** is now defined as a continuous process rather than as a specific episode of care. Causes of ill health are now sought in the environment, and the patient's social context is now often under the microscope. The importance of the nonmedical component of therapy has come to be recognized to the point that fathers are now allowed to participate in childbirth and families are encouraged to participate in the treatment of cancer patients. This paradigm shift calls for a significant change in the manner in which healthcare organizations structure their marketing activities.

Why Healthcare Should Be Marketed

Today—with marketing firmly established as a legitimate function within healthcare—it may seem unnecessary to justify healthcare marketing efforts. However, there are still reluctant healthcare administrators and financial managers who question the need for and importance of marketing. The following arguments have been offered in defense of marketing throughout the years:

- *Building awareness.* With the introduction of new products and the emergence of an informed consumer, healthcare organizations needed to build an awareness of their services and expose target audiences to their capabilities.
- *Enhancing visibility or image.* With the increasing standardization of healthcare services and a growing appreciation of reputation, healthcare organizations needed to initiate marketing campaigns that will improve top-of-mind awareness and distinguish their organizations from their competitors.
- *Improving market penetration.* Healthcare organizations were faced with growing competition, and marketing was a means for increasing patient volumes, growing revenues, and gaining market share. With few new patients in many markets, marketing was critical for retaining existing customers and attracting customers from competitors.
- *Increasing prestige.* Many healthcare organizations, especially hospitals, believed success hinged on being able to surpass competitors' prestige. If prestige could be gained through having the best doctors, the latest equipment, and the nicest facilities, these factors needed to be conveyed to the general public.

- *Attracting medical staff and employees.* As the healthcare industry expanded, competition for skilled workers increased. Hospitals and other healthcare providers needed to promote themselves to potential employees by marketing the superior benefits they offered to recruits.
- *Serving as an information resource.* As healthcare became more complex and the array of services offered by healthcare organizations grew, these organizations needed to constantly inform the general public and the medical community about the products they offered. Whether through press releases or recorded telephone announcements, the pressure to get the word out was growing.
- *Influencing consumer decision making.* Once healthcare organizations realized that consumers had a role to play in healthcare decision making, the role of marketing in influencing this process was recognized. Whether it involved convincing consumers to decide on a particular organization's services or to speed up the decision-making process, marketing was becoming increasingly important.
- *Offsetting competitive marketing.* Once healthcare organizations realized their competitors were adopting aggressive marketing approaches, they began to adopt a stance of defensive marketing. They felt compelled to respond to the gambits of competitors by out-marketing them.
- *Demonstrating community involvement.* Not-for-profit healthcare organizations should demonstrate their contribution to improving the health of their communities, especially in light of the ACA's focus on population health management. Increasing scrutiny of tax-exempt institutions should encourage them to use marketing techniques that would showcase how they address unmet health needs in their respective service areas.

Summary

Since the concept of marketing was introduced to healthcare providers in the 1970s, the field has undergone periods of growth, decline, retrenchment, and renewed growth. Initial resistance to healthcare marketing had to be overcome by an industry that was primarily not-for-profit and averse to self-promotion. The healthcare industry is unique in a number of ways, and numerous barriers prevented the immediate acceptance of marketing as an essential function.

Healthcare organizations slowly adopted marketing concepts and techniques from other industries and eventually developed approaches more suited to the unique nature of healthcare. Early on, marketing was often equated with advertising, so many healthcare organizations mounted major advertising campaigns during the 1980s. Realizing the limitations of advertising in a service industry, healthcare organizations added direct-sales capabilities and technology-based marketing approaches to supplement their more traditional public relations and communication marketing techniques.

Today, a new generation of health professionals more oriented to business principles is in place, positions for marketing directors and vice presidents are well established, and marketing is an accepted part of healthcare administration. Marketers are increasingly part of the corporate inner circle, converting marketing from an external activity to a core function of the progressive healthcare organization.

Healthcare, like any other infrastructure for meeting US society's needs, has evolved to address the needs and wants of a population that is increasingly turning to it as the solution for a wide range of problems. The fact that healthcare now accounts for as much as 18 percent of the gross national product reflects, among other trends, the population's growing concern for their health.

Key Points

- Although US industry accepted marketing in the 1950s, a number of factors prevented the healthcare industry from adopting marketing initially.
- The pioneers in healthcare marketing can be traced back to the 1970s, but marketing was not widely accepted as a legitimate function for healthcare organizations until much later.
- Early on, there were no experienced healthcare marketers, and marketing experts had to be imported from other industries.
- Changes in the healthcare arena over time (particularly the increase in competition) resulted in a surge of interest in marketing; this interest has been fostered with each new development in the field.
- Once health professionals accepted marketing, the field underwent various periods of growth and contraction in response to market developments.
- Initially, healthcare marketing was often equated with advertising, and healthcare organizations underwent considerable trial and error before accepting other promotional techniques.
- By the 1990s, healthcare marketing was maturing as a field, and a new generation of healthcare administrators and healthcare marketers was on board.

- By the turn of the twenty-first century, healthcare organizations had come to consider marketing as an essential function, and marketing resources were increasingly wed to strategic planning and development efforts.
- Since 2000, social media has heavily affected marketing in healthcare and all other industries.

Discussion Questions

1. Why didn't healthcare professionals consider marketing to be important until the 1980s?
2. What factors mitigated the introduction of marketing into healthcare?
3. Why do health professionals view marketing in a different way than do their counterparts in other industries?
4. How do ethical and legal constraints affect marketing in healthcare more than in other industries?
5. What factors ultimately forced the incorporation of marketing into healthcare?
6. Why is today's healthcare environment more hospitable to marketing and marketers than past environments were?
7. What indicators attest that marketing has matured as a legitimate function in the healthcare field?

Additional Resources

American Marketing Association: www.ama.org

Health Marketing Quarterly: www.tandfonline.com/toc/whmq20/current#.Uzh LE1so7IU

Marketing Health Services: www.ama.org/publications/MarketingHealthServices

Omran, A. R. 1971. "The Epidemiologic Transition: A Theory of the Epidemiology of Population Change." *Milbank Memorial Fund Quarterly* 49: 509–38.

Society for Healthcare Strategy & Market Development: www.shsmd.org

Thomas, R. K. 2003. *Society and Health: Sociology for Health Professionals.* New York: Springer.

BASIC MARKETING CONCEPTS

This chapter introduces the basic marketing concepts used in healthcare and other industries. Standard marketing terminology is presented, and relationships between the various concepts are outlined. Many of these concepts are foreign to healthcare, and some are problematic in the healthcare setting. However, these definitions lay the groundwork for an understanding of the marketing endeavor and help health professionals understand the language marketers use. Most of the concepts considered in this chapter are addressed in more detail in later chapters.

Defining Fundamental Concepts and Terms

Far too often, authors of textbooks dive straight into the intricacies of their subject matter without clearly defining the concepts with which they are working. They assume that the reader already has an appreciation of the basics. This assumption is often not valid and certainly not likely to be the case for those approaching healthcare marketing for the first time. For this reason, the fundamentals are presented here, along with a discussion of their applications in the healthcare arena.

Marketing

Marketing can be defined in a variety of ways. According to the American Marketing Association, marketing is "the process of planning and executing the conception, pricing, promotion, and distribution of ideas, goods, and services to create exchanges that satisfy individual and organizational objectives" (Bennett 1995). Another definition depicts marketing as a management process that identifies, anticipates, and supplies customer requirements efficiently and profitably. Philip Kotler (1999), one of the early proponents of marketing in healthcare, defines marketing as a social and managerial process by which individuals and groups obtain what they need and want by creating and exchanging products and value with others.

   A parsing of the first definition provides some important information about marketing. First, marketing is a process, which implies that the marketing operation involves several systematic steps. The definition specifies planning as part of the process. In other words, marketing should not be done

Marketing
A multifaceted process that involves research, planning, strategy formulation, promotion, and other activities

Marketing campaign
A formal, organized effort to promote a product to a target audience

impulsively; the execution of a **marketing campaign** should be well thought out. This definition notes four components of the marketing process (elsewhere referred to as the four Ps): product conception, pricing, promotion, and the distribution channels (or "place") through which the products are distributed.

Products
Ideas, goods, and services

Goods
Tangible products typically purchased in an impersonal setting on a one-at-a-time basis

Services
Activities or processes (or sets thereof) that meet the needs of a consumer

    Products include the ideas, goods, and/or services the organization is promoting. Ideas may involve such concepts as a hospital's image or the notion that pregnant women should receive prenatal care. **Goods** and **services** combined are thought of as products. In healthcare, products include tangible goods (e.g., crutches, hospital beds, adhesive bandages) and intangible services (e.g., physical examinations, immunizations, cardiac catheterizations).

    The economic aspect of the marketing transaction is demonstrated by the fact that an exchange is seen as the end result of the marketing process. Thus, a physician offers medical services in exchange for money (directly from the patient or from a third party), a hospital offers physicians staff privileges in exchange for their admissions, and an insurance plan offers healthcare coverage in exchange for the insured's premiums. All of these exchanges are facilitated through marketing at some level. Ultimately, the intent of marketing is to meet the goals of the organization (as the seller) while, at the same time, meeting the needs of the customer (as the buyer). Unless the goals of both parties are met, the marketing process is considered unsuccessful.

Healthcare Marketing

When marketing is extended to the healthcare field, not all components of the original definition fit comfortably, and the process must often be modified for application to the healthcare environment. For example, providers may have limited ability to use pricing as a marketing tool because third-party payers are willing to pay only a specified amount, regardless of the provider's fee. Or, hospitals may be limited in their ability to change their locations in response to consumer demand. Thus, one challenge for healthcare marketers is to adapt marketing principles to the unique characteristics of the healthcare industry. Exhibit 2.1 moves beyond the standard definitions and talks about what marketing really is.

Market

Market
A setting in which (actual and potential) buyers and sellers come together to exchange goods and services

The concept of marketing implies the existence of a market. In its original premarketing form, a **market** referred to a real or virtual setting in which potential buyers and potential sellers of goods or services came together for the purpose of exchange. In this sense, it refers to both function (as in the system for exchange) and form (as in a marketplace). The notion of a marketplace has been modified to refer to the individuals or organizations in a

EXHIBIT 2.1
What Marketing
Really Is

Most health professionals tend to think of marketing in terms of advertising, public relations, direct mail, or any number of other promotional techniques. All too often in healthcare, the term *marketing* is used to reference one of these specific functions, masking the range of activities carried out under the banner of marketing and the extent to which marketing should pervade an organization.

Marketing has been defined as any activity related to the development, packaging, pricing, and distribution of healthcare products along with any mechanisms used for promoting these products. This definition, however, does not capture the essence of marketing. Marketing is a multifaceted process that involves a wide range of activities of which the promotional piece (e.g., advertising) is a small—albeit highly visible—part. Marketing involves research, planning, strategy formulation, and a number of activities that have little to do with promotion. (Indeed, promotion is only one of the four Ps that constitute the marketing mix.)

Looked at in a less pecuniary light, marketing serves the healthcare consumer as a force for health education, an information resource, a guide to decision making, and an opportunity to make the customer's perspective known. From the organization's perspective, the marketing program can provide input into strategic direction, coordinate a wide range of corporate activities, and support the development of a customer service organization. Marketing can make or break the organization's reputation and can serve as the driving force in relationship development efforts.

Marketing—and marketers—are often looked at in a less-than-favorable light, not only in healthcare but in other industries as well. However, if one understands the true functions of marketing, marketing clearly can make a more significant contribution to the success of the organization than is generally acknowledged.

market that are potential customers. Thus, to marketers, a market is a set of people (or organizations) who have an actual or a potential interest in a good or service or, according to Kotler (1999), a set of actual and potential buyers of a product. Alternatively, a market is defined as a group of consumers who share some characteristic that affects their needs or wants and makes them potential customers for a good or service.

Markets are often thought of in terms of a **market area**—that is, a geographic area containing the potential customers for a particular organization's goods or services. Markets may also be defined in nongeographic terms and may refer to segments of the population independent of geography. The

Market area
The actual or desired area from which organizations draw or intend to draw customers; also known as *service area*

market, however defined, is thought to generate a measurable level of *market demand*, which represents the total volume of a product or service likely to be consumed by specific groups of customers in a specified market area during a specified period. (Demand is a problematic concept in healthcare. Chapter 7 is devoted to this topic.)

Marketing Functions

Now that the basic definitions are out of the way, it may be worthwhile to consider what the functions of marketing in healthcare (or any other industry) actually are. The functions of marketing form a hierarchy—with the broad, big-picture functions at the top and the narrow-focused functions at the bottom. This section describes the types of marketing functions at the various levels of the hierarchy.

Enterprisewide Functions

The most expansive marketing operations carried out by a healthcare organization affect the entire enterprise (i.e., hospital, health system, health plan). At this level, marketers have the following functions:

- *Conceptualizing the market.* From the perspective of the organization, a marketer's primary function may be to conceptualize the market in which the organization operates. Conceptualization involves profiling the organization in terms of its attributes, determining the market it serves (and the characteristics of the market area population), assessing the environment in which healthcare functions, and otherwise determining where the organization fits into the overall scheme of things.
- *Determining strategic direction.* The marketer's functions include identifying the organization's strategic thrust (if one has been stated), examining the organization's position in the market, and identifying opportunities that might exist in the marketplace. The marketer considers various strategic options and chooses the approach that best fits the organization and the market it seeks to cultivate.
- *Supporting business goals.* The marketer supports the organization's business development by identifying segments of the market on which to focus, clarifying opportunities that exist in the marketplace, revealing the organization's position in relation to its competitors, and otherwise determining the nature of the services the market desires. A range of promotional techniques can be used to support this function.

- *Establishing a reputation.* Some marketers would argue that the essence of marketing is building and enhancing an organization's reputation. All organizations are assigned a reputation by the consuming public, whether they want one or not. Marketers are responsible for proactively creating a positive reputation, enhancing it through an integrated marketing approach, and protecting it against the efforts of competitors.

Operational Functions

Enterprisewide marketing addresses the needs of the organization through strategy development and reputation management. Marketing also supports the narrower concerns related to the operations of the organization, as indicated by the following functions:

- *Performing marketing research.* Marketing research provides the foundation for all other marketing functions. On an ongoing basis, the marketer should delineate the service area for the organization, specify the service area's characteristics and population, and analyze the competition. Marketing research should identify opportunities in the market in terms of growing demand, underserved populations, and new product potential.
- *Developing a marketing plan.* Health professionals often neglect to develop systematic plans for accomplishing their goals, and in marketing, there is a tendency to rush into a marketing campaign without an overarching plan. The marketing plan should reflect the goals and objectives established by the organization, not just for marketing but also for overall organizational advancement. The marketer's primary responsibility is to ensure that a well-conceived marketing plan is in place before any promotional activities are implemented.
- *Coordinating enterprisewide promotional efforts.* One of the first things any marketer should do is to identify all existing promotional efforts that are under way on the part of the organization. Existing marketing efforts should be evaluated and standards should be developed to ensure a consistent message across all promotional activities. The marketer should coordinate the marketing efforts of the various entities in the organization and serve as a liaison between internal marketing efforts and external marketing resources.
- *Developing relationships.* Many would argue that the primary goal of marketing is to develop relationships, which is also an area of emphasis in contemporary healthcare. Relationships may involve patients and

other customers, referring physicians, health plans, business partners, government representatives, and a host of other entities with whom the healthcare organization needs to maintain relationships. The marketer has a key role in most aspects of developing and maintaining relationships.

- *Creating a marketing organization.* Organizations' marketing efforts often overlook their own employees. Healthcare organizations can establish a marketing mind-set among their employees via internal marketing, thereby turning every associate into a salesperson and creating a marketing organization. Ideally, every employee should have some marketing skills, and every decision should be made with marketing implications in mind. The marketer is responsible for ensuring that marketing is incorporated into the organization's DNA.

Educational Functions

An important but sometimes overlooked function of marketing is educating the public. As indicated by the following list, providing information to existing and prospective customers, referring physicians, potential donors, and other constituent groups is a major responsibility of marketing professionals.

- *Educating patients and the general public.* With the introduction of new products and the emergence of informed consumers, healthcare organizations must build awareness of their services and expose target audiences to their capabilities. Healthcare consumers have short attention spans, and the public must be continually reminded of the organization's availability. For some, the educational function of marketing takes precedence over all other functions.
- *Providing information and referral resources.* Healthcare organizations are considered an important resource for the community. Not only does marketing make consumers aware of the organization's services, but it also fulfills the organization's responsibility to educate the community regarding positive health behavior. In community after community, the most trusted healthcare organizations are those that are perceived as reliable sources of health information.
- *Enhancing visibility and corporate image.* With the increasing standardization of healthcare services and a growing appreciation of reputation, healthcare organizations find it necessary to initiate marketing campaigns that improve top-of-mind awareness and distinguish them from their competitors. Consumers are bombarded by ever-increasing message "clutter," and marketers must be able to communicate the organization's message effectively to maintain a high level of visibility and promote a positive corporate image.

- *Differentiating the organization and its services.* At a time when it is increasingly difficult for healthcare consumers to distinguish one healthcare organization from another, a marketer needs to impress upon the target audience how the organization is different from its competitors and why consumers should care about the difference. In the unlikely case that little or no differences exist, the marketer must make a creative case that establishes a competitive advantage.

Promotional Functions

Promotional activities are generally the first things that come to mind when the topic of marketing comes up. The following functions relate to the day-to-day activities of marketers in a healthcare setting:

- *Influencing consumer decision making.* With consumers now taking a more active role in healthcare decision making, marketers have an unprecedented opportunity to make a case for their organization. After building awareness among consumers, the marketer's next responsibility is to influence consumer behavior. Marketers should be sensitive to the stage of readiness of various customer groups and implement marketing techniques accordingly.
- *Improving market penetration.* Healthcare organizations faced with growing competition can use marketing as a means of increasing patient volumes and growing market share. With few new patients in many markets, marketing becomes critical for retaining existing customers and attracting competitors' customers. Marketers are well positioned to identify opportunities in the marketplace and implement programs that will attract customers and increase market penetration. If the organization cannot establish a favorable position in the market, its competitors will dictate its position.
- *Increasing profit.* On the surface, we might assume that the raison d'être for healthcare marketing should be to increase profits and, hence, should be first among marketing functions. The obvious conclusion may not be the most appropriate conclusion in healthcare, given the high proportion of not-for-profit organizations in the industry and the need to satisfy other goals in addition to bottom-line profits. More important perhaps is the need to perform a wide range of other functions before the profit motive can even be considered.
- *Winning awards versus being effective.* Note that the previous statements say nothing about winning awards for marketing campaigns. For many marketing professionals who entered healthcare from other industries, the goal was to sponsor award-winning media campaigns that involved flashy promotional materials or television

spots. Unfortunately, there appears to be little correlation between receiving accolades for marketing campaigns and the success of the organization being promoted. For whatever reason, decision makers and those paying for services in healthcare are less influenced by slick advertising campaigns than they are by the actual substance offered by the healthcare organization.

Marketing Techniques

The action dimension of marketing is embodied in the techniques marketers use to support the various marketing functions. On a day-to-day basis, marketers are likely to pay less attention to the lofty goals of the marketing endeavor and more attention to concrete marketing activities. The techniques marketers use to achieve their objectives are summarized in this section and described in detail in chapters 9 and 10.

Public Relations

Public relations (PR)
The management of communication that uses publicity and other persuasive techniques to influence feelings, opinions, or beliefs

Public relations (PR) is a form of communication management that uses publicity and other forms of promotion and information to influence feelings, opinions, or beliefs about an organization and its products. The PR function is carried out through press releases, press conferences, distribution of feature stories to the media, public service announcements, and other publicity-oriented activities. In the past, healthcare organizations have used PR to manage crises and control damage, justify questionable actions, explain negative events, and so forth. Over time, however, PR has been cast in a more proactive light as healthcare organizations have come to appreciate the benefits of a strong PR program.

Communication

Communication
The process of conveying information to internal and external audiences

Large healthcare organizations typically establish mechanisms for communicating with their stakeholders (internal and external). Communications staff develops materials to disseminate to the public and to the employees of the organization, generates internal newsletters and publications geared to relevant customer groups (e.g., patients, enrollees), and develops patient-education materials. Separate communications departments may be established, or this function may overlap with the public relations or community outreach functions. Marketers expend a great deal of effort in determining the best approaches to communication. Exhibit 2.2 discusses **communication** concepts applied to healthcare marketing.

EXHIBIT 2.2
Communication
Theories in
Marketing

Communication refers to the transmission or exchange of information and implies the sharing of meaning among those who are communicating. Students of marketing have expended considerable effort on specifying models of communication that relate to the marketing process. Communication in marketing may be directed at (1) initiating actions; (2) making needs and requirements known; (3) exchanging information, ideas, attitudes, and beliefs; (4) advancing understanding; and/or (5) establishing and maintaining relations.

Communication in marketing can occur in a variety of ways:

- *Face-to-face communication* includes formal meetings, interviews, and informal contact.
- *Oral communication* includes telephone contact, public address systems, and video conferencing systems.
- *Written communication* includes letters (external), memoranda (internal), e-mails, reports, forms, notice boards, journals, bulletins, newsletters, and manuals.
- *Visual communication* includes charts, films, slides, videos, and video conferencing.
- *Electronic communication* includes Internet chat, voice mail, and electronic data interchange.

A number of communication models have been developed for application to marketing, and Berkowitz (2010) has adapted one of these models for healthcare. According to Berkowitz, this marketing communication model has the following nine components in healthcare. An understanding of each of these components is important for effective marketing communication.

1. *Sender*. The sender is the party sending the message to the other party. Also referred to as the communicator or the source, the sender is the "who" of the process and takes the form of a person, company, or spokesperson for someone else.
2. *Message*. The message is the combination of symbols and words the sender wishes to transmit to the receiver. The message is the "what" of the process and indicates the content the sender wants to convey.
3. *Encoding*. Encoding is the process of translating the meaning of the message into symbolic form (e.g., words, signs, sounds). At this point, a concept is converted into something transmittable.

(continued)

4. *Channel*. The channel is the means used to deliver a marketing message from sender to receiver. The channel is the "how" of the process and connects the sender to the receiver.

5. *Receiver*. The receiver is the party receiving the message, also known as the audience or the destination. Marketing efforts are directed toward a receiver.

6. *Decoding*. Decoding refers to the process carried out when the receiver converts the "symbols" transmitted by the sender into a form that makes sense to him or her. This process works under the assumption that the receiver is using the same basis for decoding that the sender used for encoding.

7. *Response*. Response refers to the receiver's reaction to the message. At this point, the effect of the message is gauged in terms of the meaning the receiver attaches to it.

8. *Feedback*. Feedback refers to the aspect of the receiver's response that the receiver communicates back to the sender. The type of feedback depends on the channel, and the effectiveness of the effort is gauged in terms of the feedback.

9. *Noise*. Noise refers to any factor that prevents the receiver from decoding a message in the way the sender intended. Noise can be generated by the sender, the receiver, the message, the channel, the environment, and so forth.

The marketing communication process could be unsuccessful for any number of reasons. Factors that might influence this process include selective attention of the receiver, selective distortion by the receiver (e.g., changing the message to fit preconceptions), selective recall (i.e., the receiver absorbs only part of the message), and message rehearsal (i.e., the message reminds the receiver of related issues that tend to distract from the point of the message).

Communication experts indicate that effective communication requires certain attributes: It must contain value for the receiver; be meaningful, relevant, and understandable; and be transmittable in a few seconds. Further, the communication must lend itself to visual presentation, if possible; be relevant to the lives of everyday people; and stimulate the receiver emotionally. Marketing communication must also be interesting, entertaining, and stimulating.

Source: Adapted from Berkowitz (2010).

Community Outreach

Community outreach is a form of marketing that seeks to present the organization's programs to the community and establish relationships with community organizations. Community outreach may involve episodic activities, such as health fairs or educational programs for community residents, or it may involve ongoing initiatives carried out by outreach workers who are visible in the community. This aspect of marketing emphasizes the organization's commitment to the community and its support of local organizations. Community outreach initiatives seek to generate word-of-mouth communication concerning the organization and/or its services.

Community outreach
A presentation of an organization's programs and services to the community to establish a relationship

Government Relations

Long before most healthcare organizations considered incorporating a formal marketing function, they were involved in **government relations** activities. Healthcare organizations are typically regulated by state and federal government agencies. Decisions related to adding, eliminating, or changing a service may be constrained by government regulations, and the reimbursement available to healthcare providers may be controlled by government agencies. Not-for-profit organizations must continually demonstrate that they deserve their tax-exempt status. For these reasons, healthcare organizations must maintain discourse with a variety of government agencies, cultivate relationships with politicians and other policymakers, and often initiate lobbying activities directed toward various levels of government.

Government relations
Organizational liaison with government agencies that enact regulations, determine reimbursement levels, provide funding, and monitor activities

Networking

Networking involves developing and nurturing relationships with individuals and organizations with which mutually beneficial transactions can be carried out. Physicians and other clinicians—who, until recently, would never deign to advertise—actively network with their colleagues. Networking may take the form of a specialist casually running into potential referring physicians at the country club or a hospital administrator attending meetings that might involve potential clients, partners, or referral agents. Networking is particularly effective when dealing with parties who are reluctant to provide "face time" or when one prefers an informal setting involving personal interaction for getting to know prospective business associates.

Networking
The process of establishing and nurturing relationships that may result in a mutual benefit

Sales Promotion

Sales promotion involves any activities or materials that act as a direct inducement to customers by offering added value to a product. Sales promotions are more likely to be associated with the sale of consumer health products (e.g., rebates) or business-to-business healthcare sales (e.g., low-interest financing) than with the provision of health services. The sales promotion

Sales promotion
The process of highlighting the value of a product to induce a purchase

mix might involve health fairs and trade shows, exhibits, demonstrations, contests and games, premiums and gifts, rebates, low-interest financing, and trade-in allowances. Sales promotion is separate from, but often an adjunct to, personal sales.

Advertising

Advertising refers to any paid form of nonpersonal presentation or promotion of ideas, goods, or services by an identifiable sponsor transmitted via mass media for purposes of achieving marketing objectives. The advertising mix might include print advertisements, electronic advertisements, mailings, catalogs, brochures, posters, directories, outdoor advertisements, and displays. These activities are organized in the form of an advertising campaign that involves designing a series of advertisements and placing them in various advertising media to reach a target market.

Personal Sales

Personal sales
An oral or conversational presentation of promotional material to a prospective purchaser for the purpose of sales

Personal sales involve the presentation of promotional material in a conversation with one or more prospective purchasers for the purpose of making sales. The salesperson attempts to foster a mutually profitable economic exchange between buyer and seller through interpersonal contact. The success of personal sales depends on the seller's ability to communicate the product's qualities and its benefits for the buyer. The personal selling mix might include sales presentations, sales meetings, incentive programs, distribution of samples, and participation in health fairs and trade shows.

Database Marketing

Database marketing
The use of a data set of past, current, and prospective customers to promote an organization's products

Database marketing involves establishing and exploiting data on past and current customers and future prospects in a way that allows effective marketing strategies to be implemented. Database marketing can be used for any purpose that can benefit from access to customer information. These functions may include evaluating new prospects, cross-selling related products, launching new products to potential prospects, identifying new distribution channels, building customer loyalty, converting occasional users to regular users, generating inquiries and follow-up sales, and establishing niche marketing initiatives. The database established for this purpose often provides the basis for customer relationship management and may be an integral part of an organization's call center.

Direct Marketing

Direct marketing
The process of targeting groups or individuals with specific characteristics and transmitting promotions directly to them

Direct marketing targets groups or individuals with specific characteristics and transmits promotional messages straight to them. These promotional activities may take the form of direct mail or telemarketing as well as other approaches aimed at specific individuals. Increasingly, the Internet is being used for direct marketing. An advantage of direct marketing is that the message can be customized to meet the needs of target populations.

Customer Relationship Management

Customer relationship management (CRM) is a business strategy designed to optimize profitability, revenue, and **customer satisfaction** by focusing on relationships rather than transactions. Although long used in other industries, CRM is relatively new to healthcare. The industry's lack of focus on customer characteristics and its limited data management capabilities have slowed the acceptance of CRM in healthcare. However, the new market-driven environment is encouraging healthcare organizations to develop and use customer databases.

Social Marketing

In healthcare, **social marketing** involves applying commercial marketing techniques to influence the attitudes, knowledge, and behavior of target audiences related to the improvement of individual and community health status. Social marketing differs from other types of marketing only with respect to the objectives of marketers and their organizations. Social marketers seek to influence social behaviors for the benefit of their target audience and general society, not for the benefit of the marketing organization. In contrast to the top-down approach of traditional marketing, social marketers listen to the needs and desires of the target audience and build the marketing campaign from the bottom up.

Case Study 2.1 describes a marketing campaign that uses a variety of marketing techniques.

Marketing Approaches

Marketers employ marketing strategies that reflect the audience they are soliciting. A campaign aimed at the general population will involve a different approach than one targeting a population subgroup. Depending on the circumstances, the approach may include mass marketing, target marketing, or micromarketing.

Mass Marketing

Mass marketing involves the development of generic messages that are widely broadcast to the entire service area. There is no attempt to target specific audiences, identify likely best customers, or tailor the message to a particular subgroup. This approach involves the use of mass media (e.g.,

Customer relationship management
A business strategy designed to optimize profitability, revenue, and customer satisfaction by focusing on customer relationships rather than transactions

Customer satisfaction
The degree to which customers' wants and needs are fulfilled

Social marketing
An approach to effecting behavioral change in the general population through public relations, advertising, and other techniques

Mass marketing
An approach that targets the total population — typically through network TV or newspapers — as if it were one undifferentiated conglomeration of consumers

CASE STUDY 2.1
Capturing the "Older Adult" Market

Many healthcare organizations came to see the aging of the baby boom generation as an opportunity to expand their services. Regional Medical Center (RMC, a fictional organization on which this case study is based) responded to this opportunity by establishing a service line devoted to older adults. The intent was to capture the business—and the loyalty— of this large, relatively affluent, and increasingly needy segment of the population. The service line was designed to meet the emerging needs of this population for specialty services such as cardiology, orthopedics, ophthalmology, and urology in a manner that was appealing to this relatively demanding consumer segment.

Because this service was considered innovative in the community served by RMC, an aggressive promotional campaign was undertaken. RMC's marketing department considered a wide range of marketing options and decided on a multipronged campaign to approach the target population from a variety of directions. The first phase of the promotional campaign focused on internal marketing. It was important that RMC's employees be familiar with this new program and be able to articulate its merits to potential customers. Many of the customers for the new program were likely to be existing patients of RMC.

Well before the new program was scheduled to open for enrollment, an aggressive PR campaign was initiated. Press releases were distributed, articles were prepared for local publications and professional journals, and celebrity spokespersons were lined up. Simple yet attractive **collateral materials** (e.g., business cards, letterhead, envelopes, brochures) were developed for distribution to prospective customers and to referral agents who might channel customers to RMC. Information was distributed to providers and organizations that might serve other needs of the target population, and the community's major insurance plans were made aware of the new program and its benefits. Tours of the facility housing the new program were provided to key constituents (such as referring physicians and health plan representatives), and open houses were scheduled for both medical professionals and the general public.

The marketing initiative also involved direct solicitation of members of the target population. RMC extracted data from its internal database on existing customers and purchased mailing lists of households that included members aged 50 to 65. Using the findings from previous research on the "buttons to push" in this age cohort, marketing staff

Collateral material
Material used to reinforce an organization's image or support a media advertising campaign

prepared materials that would appeal to the particular needs of older adults. The address lists were then used to mail materials directly to targeted individuals.

While RMC did not want to rely on expensive media advertising for attracting customers, its marketers felt that some media presence was necessary—not only to attract customers who might be missed through the direct-mail campaign but also to make the general public aware of this new program. In some cases, other family members might be making decisions for the older adult population, and awareness of this program on the part of the general public was considered important. After careful research on the communication attributes of family caregivers, a series of newspaper, radio, and television advertisements were produced. These advertisements were placed in the sections of the local newspaper that members of this age group read, aired on the radio stations they preferred, and presented on the television channels they viewed most often. For the electronic media, particular attention was paid to the time of day and day of the week members of the target population were expected to be engaged.

The success of RMC's new older-adult service line during the first year exceeded the expectations of the organization's administrators. While it was difficult to determine which of the various promotional techniques used had the most impact on the program's early success, the marketing staff concluded, on the basis of its evaluation of the campaign, that it was the integrated approach—a variety of coordinated activities—that led to the successful program launch.

Case Study Discussion Questions

1. Why did RMC think that older adults presented enough of an opportunity to establish an entirely new program?
2. What information did RMC need to gather about this target population before the program could be established?
3. What information did RMC need to gather about this target population before the marketing campaign could be planned?
4. What were the different paths through which RMC attempted to reach the target audience?
5. Which marketing techniques did RMC use to reach the target population?
6. Why was internal marketing an important first step in marketing this new program?

newspaper, radio, television) to blanket the market area. The message has to be general and typically touts the merits of the organization rather than any specific services.

Hospitals' use of mass marketing in the past reflected their desire to promote the organization overall (rather than specific services) and their belief that they could be all things to all people. No attempt was made to distinguish between different segments of the population, and only the crudest distinction based on geography was made between markets. This type of approach is effective at disseminating a small amount of information to a large number of people and can be useful when marketing a basic product that appeals to a homogenous audience.

Target Marketing

Target marketing
An approach that focuses on a market segment to which an organization desires to offer goods or services

Target marketing refers to marketing initiatives that focus on a market segment to which an organization desires to offer goods and/or services. Target marketing stands in contrast to mass marketing, which aims promotional efforts at the total market. Target markets in healthcare may be defined on the basis of geography, demographics, lifestyle, insurance coverage, usage rate, and other customer attributes. Thus, target marketing is likely to involve the use of customer segmentation systems.

Micromarketing

Micromarketing
An approach that breaks the market down to the household or even the individual level to target those most likely to consume a product

Micromarketing is a form of target marketing. Companies that use micromarketing tailor their marketing programs to the needs and wants of consumers narrowly defined in terms of geography, demographics, psychographics, or the benefits they desire. Customers and potential customers are identified at the household or individual level and directly marketed to using customized communication techniques. Micromarketing is most effective when marketers want to reach consumers with a narrow range of attributes.

Healthcare Products and Customers

The definition of marketing offered early in this chapter refers to the promotion of ideas, goods, or services. (The term *product*, used throughout the text, is often used interchangeably with *service*.) As mentioned, the product to be marketed in healthcare is often difficult to specify, unlike the products of other industries. Most of what healthcare organizations offer takes the form of services, and, unlike goods, they tend to be harder to precisely describe.

In addition, the nature of the product in healthcare has changed dramatically over the past couple of decades. Twenty years ago, one could define the product simply as a medical procedure, an orthotic device to correct a physical disability, or a consumer health product. In today's climate, healthcare products include not only these traditional products but also prepaid health insurance plans offered by health maintenance organizations or a group purchasing contract offered by a provider network. (The nature of healthcare products is discussed further in Chapter 6.)

Many healthcare organizations offer a variety of products to their customers. Certainly, the hospital is an example of an organization that offers a wide range of services and goods. A major hospital offers hundreds, if not thousands, of different procedures. In addition, hospitals offer a variety of goods (in the form of drugs, supplies, and equipment) that are charged to the customer. One can describe an organization's product mix in terms of the combination of ideas, goods, and services it offers.

Ideas

Much of what healthcare organizations promote takes the form of *ideas*—intangible concepts that are intended to convey a perception to the consumer. The organization's image is an idea that is likely to be conveyed through marketing activities. The organization may want to promote the perception of quality care, professionalism, value, or some other subjective attribute. The development of a brand, for example, involves the marketing of an idea. The intent is to establish a mind-set that places the organization at the top of the consumer's mind on the assumption that familiarity will encourage consumer action.

When healthcare organizations first incorporated advertising, most of the attention was focused on promoting ideas. In particular, early marketers attempted to promote the organization's image and establish it as the preferred provider in its market. Although the trend has shifted away from image advertising and toward service advertising, many healthcare organizations continue to market ideas to their target audiences.

Goods

For the purposes of this text, products can refer to goods or services. *Goods* are tangible products typically purchased in an impersonal setting on a one-at-a-time basis. The purchase of goods tends to be a one-shot episode, while the purchase of services may be fulfilled through an ongoing process. Although healthcare is generally perceived in terms of a service, the sale of goods is ubiquitous in the industry. Consumer health products (e.g., soap, condoms, toothpaste) are household products. Pharmaceuticals—whether prescription or over the counter—are purchased by nearly everyone at some point. Consumers are even gaining access to home-testing kits (e.g., pregnancy and ovulation tests) and therapeutic equipment (e.g., hearing aids), and the sale/rental of durable medical equipment (e.g., wheelchairs) is a major industry. Even in a hospital setting, the bill for care is likely to include a number of goods among the itemized charges.

Services

Relative to goods, *services* are difficult to conceptualize. Services (e.g., physical examinations) are intangible in that they do not take the concrete form of goods (e.g., drugs). Services are more difficult to quantify, and consumers evaluate them differently from tangible products. Because services are often more personal (especially in the case of healthcare), they are likely to be assessed in subjective rather than objective terms. They are variable in that they cannot be subjected to the quality controls placed on goods but reflect the variations that characterize the human beings who provide the services. They are inseparable from the producer in that they are dispensed on the spot without separation from the provider. They are perishable in that they cannot be stored and, once provided, have no residual value. Finally, they defy ownership rules in that, unlike goods, they do not involve transfer of tangible property from the seller to the buyer.

Consumers

Consumer, as the term is usually used in healthcare, refers to any individual or organization that is a potential purchaser of a healthcare product. (This definition differs from the more economics-based notion of a consumer as the entity who actually uses the product.) Theoretically, everyone is a potential consumer of health services; consumer research, for example, is generally aimed at the public at large. The consumer is often the end user of a good or service but may not necessarily be the purchaser. The term **consumer behavior** refers to the utilization patterns and purchasing practices of the population of a market area.

Customers

In healthcare, the **customer** is typically thought of as the actual purchaser of goods or services. Although a patient may be a customer for certain goods and services, the **end user** (e.g., the patient) is often not the customer. Someone else may make the purchase on behalf of the patient. Further, treatment decisions may be made by someone other than the patient. For this reason, hospitals and other complex healthcare organizations are likely to serve a range of customers, including patients, referral agents, admitting physicians,

Consumer
In healthcare, any individual or organization that is a potential purchaser of goods and services

Consumer behavior
The consumer's pattern of consumption of goods and services

Customer
In healthcare, the actual purchaser (but not necessarily the end user) of goods or services

End user
The person or organization that ultimately consumes a good or service, regardless of who makes the purchase decision or pays for the product

employers, and a variety of other parties who may purchase goods or services from the organization. For this reason, the customer identification process in healthcare is more complicated than it is in other industries.

Clients

A **client** is a type of customer that consumes services rather than goods. A client relationship implies personal (rather than impersonal) interaction and an ongoing relationship (rather than a single encounter). Professionals typically have clients, whereas retailers have customers or purchasers. The relationships between service providers and clients are likely to be more symmetrical than the relationships between service providers and patients, who are typically dependent on and powerless relative to the service provider. Many also believe the term *client* implies more respect than the term *patient*.

Client
In healthcare, a customer that consumes services rather than goods; in advertising, the entity being served by the advertising agency

Patients

Although the word **patient** is used loosely in informal discussion, a patient is someone who has been defined as sick by a physician. This definition almost always implies formal contact with a clinical facility (e.g., physician's office, hospital). Technically, a symptomatic individual does not become a patient until a physician officially designates the individual as such, even if the prospective patient has consumed over-the-counter drugs and taken other measures for self-care. Under this scenario, an individual remains a "patient" until discharged from medical care.

Patient
An individual who has been officially diagnosed with a health condition and is receiving formal medical care

Nonphysician clinicians may treat patients, but because they do not provide medical services, they are discouraged from using the term. For example, behavioral health counselors are likely to refer to their patients as "clients." Dependent practitioners, who work under the supervision of physicians (e.g., physical therapists), however, are likely to define their charges as patients.

Enrollees

Although health insurance plans have historically called their customers **enrollees**, use of this term has only recently become common among healthcare providers. However, with the ascendancy of managed care as a major force in healthcare, other healthcare organizations began to adopt this term. Thus, providers who contracted to provide services for members of a health plan began to think in terms of enrollees. This shift in nomenclature is significant because enrollees and patients have different attributes. Enrollees may also be referred to as *members, insureds,* or *covered lives.*

Enrollee
An individual who is enrolled in a health plan

Exhibit 2.3 discusses how different definitions of healthcare customers have implications for the operation of the system.

EXHIBIT 2.3
What's in
a Name:
Implications
of Redefining
the Patient

One of the developments in healthcare over the past couple of decades that has significant implications for marketing is the redefinition of health services users. The historical term *patient* is being replaced by the words *client*, *consumer*, and *customer*. Although the nomenclature changed in part to reflect the different parties that deal with the patient, this redefinition represents a paradigm shift in the health system's orientation toward the health services user.

Patient refers to a person who is formally under the care of a physician. Although other clinicians may also refer to their charges as patients, the term implies that a symptomatic person has been formally diagnosed as sick and now takes on a new set of attributes. Conceptually, a patient is more clearly differentiated from a nonpatient than, for example, a customer is from a noncustomer.

The patient role (also referred to as the "sick role"), like any social role, involves certain characteristics. Someone in this role is considered to be "abnormal" and thus different in important ways from other people. The patient role implies a degree of helplessness and a state of dependence on clinicians and health facilities. It also implies a condition of relative powerlessness and an inability to take an active part in the therapeutic process. A patient is also typically characterized by a relative lack of knowledge concerning the situation in question. The patient remains in this role until officially discharged by a physician.

A client is similar to a patient in many ways. In the healthcare context, a client is a patient of a nonphysician. Outside of healthcare, a client is someone who uses the services of a professional, and certain health professionals—such as mental health professionals, social workers, and other nonmedical personnel—may refer to their customers as clients.

The difference between patients and clients extends well beyond the different professionals involved. Clients have a more symmetrical power relationship with their service providers than patients do with their doctors. Clients are typically not thought of as being dependent to the extent that patients are, and clients can fire their providers much more readily than patients can fire their doctors. Thus, a client is theoretically less dependent, more involved in the decision-making process, and more knowledgeable about the issue at hand than a patient is. Ultimately, a client has more control over the situation than a patient does.

As healthcare became more marketing oriented, terms like *consumer* and *customer* were introduced. Although some purists may consider use of these terms a sacrilege, the fact is that—like it or not—patients are steadily taking on the characteristics of consumers and customers, not because of redefinition by marketers but because of the dramatic changes that have occurred in healthcare.

For the purposes of this text, a consumer is anyone who has the potential to purchase a healthcare good or service. In other industries, a consumer is often thought of as the end user of the product, but this is not necessarily a comfortable concept in healthcare. From a marketing perspective, anyone could be considered a consumer because nearly everyone is a potential user of health services. Whereas patients or clients are effectively under the direction, if not control, of health professionals, consumers are thought to independently determine the choices they make regarding health services. Thus, the consumer decision-making process is referred to more often than the patient decision-making process, which implies that the consumer is objectively evaluating health services options and making choices based on a variety of factors.

A customer, on the other hand, is a consumer who is currently using a good or service. For whatever reason, the customer has chosen to purchase a healthcare product. In many cases, this definition may be synonymous with the concept of patient, but from a marketing perspective, customers are thought of in different terms.

Unlike a patient (even if it is the same person), a customer is someone who is knowledgeable about the available options and has made a rational choice to consume particular goods or services. A customer is considered to be more independent and assertive than a patient and is likely to have expectations that differ from those of a patient. A patient might be concerned about humane treatment and effective outcomes, whereas a customer is also likely to expect fast and efficient service, convenient location, respectful treatment by practitioners, value for the money, and a meaningful role in the process.

This new *patient-customer* is having a major impact on the healthcare system, and the baby boom generation now coming to dominate the patient pool epitomizes the patient-customer. This person wants the outcomes of the healthcare system (as a patient does) as well as the benefits of being a customer. This development not only has implications for the delivery of care but also is important from a marketing perspective. Marketers solicit customers and patients in different ways. Customers and patients bring different traits to the examination room and use different criteria for measuring their satisfaction with services.

Healthcare marketers must be able to recognize the differences among the various users of health services and adapt marketing approaches accordingly. Clearly, the marketing approach, the message, the medium, and the means of evaluation will differ depending on whether the marketer is addressing patients, clients, consumers, or customers.

The Four Ps of Marketing

The **marketing mix** is the set of controllable variables that an organization involved in marketing uses to influence the target market. The mix includes product, price, place, and promotion. These four Ps have long been the basis for marketing strategy in other industries and are increasingly being considered by healthcare organizations. However, these aspects of the marketing mix do not necessarily have the same meaning for health professionals as they do for marketers in other industries.

Product

As discussed earlier, the product of healthcare represents what healthcare providers are marketing. Because it takes the form of ideas, goods, or services, product is difficult to precisely define in healthcare, which creates a challenge for healthcare marketers. For example, if a psychiatric problem is being treated with drugs (a good), the product is easy to specify (e.g., how many pills of how much dosage per day). If the same condition is being treated through counseling (a service), the description of the product is not as precise or standardized (e.g., an unpredictable number of counseling sessions).

In the past, healthcare providers seldom gave much thought to the product concept. A surgical procedure was considered just that and not something that had to be packaged. Today, however, the design of the product, its perceived attributes, and its packaging are all becoming more important concerns for healthcare providers and healthcare marketers.

Price

Price refers to the amount charged for a product, including the fees, charges, premium contributions, deductibles, copayments, and other out-of-pocket costs to consumers of health services. In economic terms, price is thought of in terms of an exchange. In other words, a healthcare provider offers a service in exchange for its customers' dollars. An employee paying an annual premium to a health plan, an insurance company reimbursing a physician's fee, or a consumer purchasing over-the-counter drugs are all exchanges involving a price. The price to the customer could also include the pain, discomfort, embarrassment, anxiety, frustration, and other emotional costs of dealing with providers, plans, and the disease or injury that prompted the experience. An obvious objective of marketing is to convince consumers that they will receive benefits for the price they pay.

Given the manner in which financing is structured in healthcare, price has not historically been a basis for competition. The issue of pricing for health services is a growing concern for marketers as the healthcare environment changes, and a number of factors are increasing the role of the pricing variable in developing a marketing strategy. For marketers, the challenge is understanding what a customer is willing to exchange for some want-satisfying good or service and developing a pricing approach compatible with the organization's goals and cost constraints.

Place

Place represents the manner in which goods or services are distributed for consumer use. Place relates to all factors of the transaction or relationship experience that make it easy, rather than difficult, for consumers to obtain an organization's products. The obvious factors of location and layout are included, and so are hours, access, obstacles, waits for appointments, claims payment, and so on. In most cases, negative place aspects of an encounter impose such costs as lost time, frustration in finding the service site, a parking fee, boredom, and other emotional burden. Positive place aspects usually nullify such costs. For example, when a physician offers early morning or evening hours, patients can obtain care on the way to or from work and thus avoid having to take time off from their jobs.

Place
The point of distribution for a healthcare product

In some cases, place factors may enhance perceptions of the product's quality, as when the physician's office or hospital is in a trendy location or on a campus that facilitates efficient treatment. Systems or health plans may speed up scheduling by allowing patients to make appointments via the Internet. The electronic storage of and online accessibility to medical records have added a different dimension to the concept of place. Allowing patients to sign up for health plans, check their status, and make benefit changes online at a work-site kiosk or at a home computer adds value to place.

Promotion

For many people, **promotion** has historically meant advertising, and advertising has meant marketing. Promotion includes any means of informing the marketplace that the organization has developed a response to meet its needs. Promotion involves a range of tactics involving publicity, advertising, and personal selling.

Promotion
Any means of informing the marketplace that the organization has developed a response to meet its needs

Promotion covers all forms of marketing communication and includes materials that deliver content in addition to those that foster transactions. For example, health plans can devise communications that help new members better understand their coverage, thereby enabling them to use their health plan more effectively. Providers can advise new patients on how to avoid place frustrations and costs, and address symptoms and concerns online before appointments to improve quality and patient satisfaction. The

Promotional mix
The combination of marketing techniques used to execute a marketing campaign

promotional mix describes the combination of techniques used by the marketer to achieve promotional goals.

Applying the Four Ps

Many observers find applying the traditional four Ps of the marketing mix to healthcare problematic. Some believe these dimensions of marketing are inappropriate for a service-oriented industry like healthcare. The uncomfortable fit between the four Ps of marketing and healthcare has even led some to pronounce the death of the four Ps and suggest their replacement with some other, more appropriate model for healthcare. Indeed, in today's competitive environment, some contend that additional Ps should be added to the list. Exhibit 2.4—written by Brian Tracy (2008)—presents the seven Ps, an update of the four Ps. These seven Ps may be more applicable or comprehensive for healthcare marketing purposes.

Other Marketing Processes

This section explains additional marketing concepts that are useful for readers to understand. Each of these concepts is addressed in greater detail later in the book.

Marketing Planning

Marketing planning
The development of a systematic process for promoting an organization, a good, or a service

Marketing planning may be defined as the development of a systematic process for promoting an organization, a service, or a product. This straightforward definition masks the wide variety of activities and potential complexity that characterize marketing planning. Marketing planning may be limited to a short-term promotional project or may be a component of a long-term strategic plan. It can focus alternatively on a product, a service, a program, or an organization. The marketing plan should summarize a company's marketing strategy and serve as a guide for all those involved in the company's marketing activities.

Of the various types of planning that could be carried out by a healthcare organization, marketing planning is most directly related to the customer. Marketing plans are, by definition, market driven, and they are single-minded in their focus on the customer. Whether the targeted customer is the patient, the referring physician, the employer, the health plan, or any number of other possibilities, the marketing plan is built around someone's needs. Although a consideration of internal factors is often pertinent (and **internal marketing** may be a component of many marketing plans), the marketing plan focuses on the characteristics of the external market with the objective of affecting one or more of these characteristics.

Internal marketing
The process of training and motivating customer service employees and support personnel to work as a team to generate customer satisfaction

Once you've developed your marketing strategy, there is a "Seven P Formula" you should use to continually evaluate and reevaluate your business activities. These seven are: product, price, promotion, place, packaging, positioning and people. As products, markets, customers and needs change rapidly, you must continually revisit these seven Ps to make sure you're on track and achieving the maximum results possible for you in today's marketplace.

Product

To begin with, develop the habit of looking at your product as though you were an outside marketing consultant brought in to help your company decide whether or not it's in the right business at this time. Ask critical questions such as, "Is your current product or service, or mix of products and services, appropriate and suitable for the market and the customers of today?"

Whenever you're having difficulty selling as much of your products or services as you'd like, you need to develop the habit of assessing your business honestly and asking, "Are these the right products or services for our customers today?"

Is there any product or service you're offering today that, knowing what you now know, you would not bring out again today? Compared to your competitors, is your product or service superior in some significant way to anything else available? If so, what is it? If not, could you develop an area of superiority? Should you be offering this product or service at all in the current marketplace?

Price

The second P in the formula is price. Develop the habit of continually examining and reexamining the prices of the products and services you sell to make sure they're still appropriate to the realities of the current market. Sometimes you need to lower your prices. At other times, it may be appropriate to raise your prices. Many companies have found that the profitability of certain products or services doesn't justify the amount of effort and resources that go into producing them. By raising their prices, they may lose a percentage of their customers, but the remaining percentage generates a profit on every sale. Could this be appropriate for you?

Sometimes you need to change your terms and conditions of sale. Sometimes, by spreading your price over a series of months or years, you can sell far more than you are today, and the interest you can charge

(continued)

EXHIBIT 2.4
The 7 Ps of Marketing
by Brian Tracy

will more than make up for the delay in cash receipts. Sometimes you can combine products and services together with special offers and special promotions. Sometimes you can include free additional items that cost you very little to produce but make your prices appear far more attractive to your customers.

In business, as in nature, whenever you experience resistance or frustration in any part of your sales or marketing activities, be open to revisiting that area. Be open to the possibility that your current pricing structure is not ideal for the current market. Be open to the need to revise your prices, if necessary, to remain competitive, to survive and thrive in a fast-changing marketplace.

Promotion

The third habit in marketing and sales is to think in terms of promotion all the time. Promotion includes all the ways you tell your customers about your products or services and how you then market and sell to them. Small changes in the way you promote and sell your products can lead to dramatic changes in your results. Even small changes in your advertising can lead immediately to higher sales. Experienced copy-writers can often increase the response rate from advertising by 500 percent by simply changing the headline on an advertisement.

Large and small companies in every industry continually experiment with different ways of advertising, promoting, and selling their products and services. And here is the rule: Whatever method of marketing and sales you're using today will, sooner or later, stop working. Sometimes it will stop working for reasons you know, and sometimes it will be for reasons you don't know. In either case, your methods of marketing and sales will eventually stop working, and you'll have to develop new sales, marketing and advertising approaches, offerings, and strategies.

Place

The fourth P in the marketing mix is the place where your product or service is actually sold. Develop the habit of reviewing and reflecting upon the exact location where the customer meets the salesperson. Sometimes a change in place can lead to a rapid increase in sales.

You can sell your product in many different places. Some companies use direct selling, sending their salespeople out to personally meet and talk with the prospect. Some sell by telemarketing. Some sell through catalogs or mail order. Some sell at trade shows or in retail establishments. Some sell in joint ventures with other similar products or services. Some companies use manufacturers' representatives or distributors. Many companies use a combination of two or more of these methods.

In each case, the entrepreneur must make the right choice about the very best location or place for the customer to receive essential buying information on the product or service needed to make a buying decision. What is yours? In what way should you change it? Where else could you offer your products or services?

Packaging

The fifth element in the marketing mix is the packaging. Develop the habit of standing back and looking at every visual element in the packaging of your product or service through the eyes of a critical prospect. Remember, people form their first impression about you within the first 30 seconds of seeing you or some element of your company. Small improvements in the packaging or external appearance of your product or service can often lead to completely different reactions from your customers.

Packaging refers to the way your product or service appears from the outside. Packaging also refers to your people and how they dress and groom. It refers to your offices, your waiting rooms, your brochures, your correspondence and every single visual element about your company. Everything counts. Everything helps or hurts. Everything affects your customer's confidence about dealing with you.

Positioning

The next P is positioning. You should develop the habit of thinking continually about how you are positioned in the hearts and minds of your customers. How do people think and talk about you when you're not present? How do people think and talk about your company? What positioning do you have in your market, in terms of the specific words people use when they describe you and your offerings to others?

In the famous book by Al Reis and Jack Trout, *Positioning*, the authors point out that how you are seen and thought about by your customers is the critical determinant of your success in a competitive marketplace. Attribution theory says that most customers think of you in terms of a single attribute, either positive or negative. Sometimes it's "service." Sometimes it's "excellence." Sometimes it's "quality engineering," as with Mercedes Benz. Sometimes it's "the ultimate driving machine," as with BMW. In every case, how deeply entrenched that attribute is in the minds of your customers and prospective customers

(continued)

determines how readily they'll buy your product or service and how much they'll pay.

Develop the habit of thinking about how you could improve your positioning. Begin by determining the position you'd like to have. If you could create the ideal impression in the hearts and minds of your customers, what would it be? What would you have to do in every customer interaction to get your customers to think and talk about you in that specific way? What changes do you need to make in the way you interact with customers today in order to be seen as the very best choice for your customers of tomorrow?

People

The final P of the marketing mix is people. Develop the habit of thinking in terms of the people inside and outside of your business who are responsible for every element of your sales and marketing strategy and activities.

It's amazing how many entrepreneurs and businesspeople will work extremely hard to think through every element of the marketing strategy and the marketing mix, and then pay little attention to the fact that every single decision and policy has to be carried out by a specific person in a specific way. Your ability to select, recruit, hire and retain the proper people, with the skills and abilities to do the job you need to have done, is more important than everything else put together.

In his best-selling book, *Good to Great*, Jim Collins discovered the most important factor applied by the best companies was that they first of all "got the right people on the bus, and the wrong people off the bus." Once these companies had hired the right people, the second step was to "get the right people in the right seats on the bus."

To be successful in business, you must develop the habit of thinking in terms of exactly who is going to carry out each task and responsibility. In many cases, it's not possible to move forward until you can attract and put the right person into the right position. Many of the best business plans ever developed sit on shelves today because the people who created them could not find the key people who could execute those plans.

Source: Tracy (2008). Used with permission from Brian Tracy International: www.brian tracy.com.

Marketing Management

Marketing management refers to the analysis, planning, implementation, and control of programs designed to build and maintain beneficial exchanges with targeted buyers for the purpose of achieving organizational objectives. The steps involved in the marketing management process include (1) analyzing marketing opportunities, (2) selecting target markets, (3) developing the marketing mix, and (4) managing the marketing effort.

Although marketing management is a well-defined function in most industries, it is still in its infancy in healthcare. The fragmented approach to much of the marketing that has taken place and the immature status of marketing in healthcare are reflected in the slow development of marketing management skills.

Marketing management
The analysis, planning, implementation, and control of marketing programs

Marketing Research

Marketing research is the function that links the consumer, customer, and public to the marketer through information. It is used to identify and define marketing opportunities and problems; to generate, refine, and evaluate marketing actions; to monitor marketing performance; and to improve understanding of the marketing process. Often used interchangeably with the term *market research*, it also encompasses product research, pricing research, promotional research, and distribution research. The marketing research process serves to identify the nature of the product or service, the characteristics of consumers, the size of the potential market, the nature of competitors, and any number of pieces essential to the marketing puzzle.

Marketing research
The collection of information for myriad marketing purposes, such as identifying opportunities and problems, evaluating actions, monitoring performance, and clarifying the process

Summary

As the healthcare industry has come to accept marketing as a legitimate function, health professionals have been exposed to a new vocabulary—the language of the marketer. Because health professionals hold various misconceptions about marketing, it is important to be on the same page when it comes to marketing terminology. Many marketing terms could be adopted by healthcare organizations unchanged, whereas others require modification based on the unique characteristics of healthcare.

Health professionals have many misperceptions about what marketing is and what its functions are. Marketing cannot be pigeonholed as advertising, direct mail, or any specific activity; it involves a whole range of activities—from conducting marketing research to evaluating a completed promotional campaign. Further, the functions of marketing are numerous and range from big-picture functions (such as determining the strategic direction of the health system) to highly focused functions (such as increasing participation in a patient-education class).

The healthcare industry presents a challenge in the application of marketing techniques. The concept of market does not exist in healthcare like it does it other industries, health professionals do not think in terms of products, and the nature of the customer is highly complex. A change of health professionals' mind-set is required for marketing to be effectively used within the healthcare arena.

The traditional four Ps of marketing—product, price, place, and promotion—have been adapted to healthcare, although not without some limitations. All four are somewhat problematic when applied to healthcare because of the peculiar characteristics of the industry. As a result, attempts have been made to modify these components of the marketing mix or replace them with concepts that are more suitable to the healthcare environment.

Key Points

- The field of marketing has its own vocabulary with which health professionals must become familiar.
- The healthcare field can adopt many marketing concepts directly from other industries, but others must be modified to address the uniqueness of healthcare.
- Marketing should be viewed in the broadest possible light—not simply as a set of marketing tools but as a contributor to organizational development.
- Marketing serves a number of functions in healthcare, and healthcare administrators should be sensitive to the implications marketing has for different levels of the organization.
- A wide range of marketing techniques are available to marketers, and their choice of technique depends on the circumstances.
- The traditional four Ps of the marketing mix—product, price, place, and promotion—can be applied to healthcare with modifications.
- Marketing involves so much more than promotions and must consider such processes as marketing research, marketing planning, and marketing management.

Discussion Questions

1. Why is it difficult to directly apply the marketing approaches used in other industries to healthcare?
2. Why do many health professionals have a misconception concerning the nature of marketing, and what are these misconceptions?
3. What is the distinction between goods and services, and what are the implications of these differences for healthcare?
4. What is the role of marketing as it relates to the various levels of the healthcare organization (e.g., senior managers versus product line managers)?
5. Which components of healthcare marketing have health professionals been comfortable with historically, and which techniques are gaining more acceptance today?
6. What factors have contributed to the conversion of the patient into a consumer, customer, or client, and what are the implications of this conversion for marketing?
7. What characteristics of healthcare make the four Ps of marketing difficult to apply directly to the healthcare organization?

Additional Resources

American Marketing Association: www.ama.org

Berkowitz, E. N. 2010. *Essentials of Healthcare Marketing,* 3rd ed. Sudbury, MA: Jones and Bartlett Learning.

MarketingProfs: www.marketingprofs.com

MARKETING AND THE HEALTHCARE ORGANIZATION

The notion of marketing as a corporate function was accepted by different healthcare organizations at different times. This chapter notes the factors that influenced that acceptance (continuing the historical discussion in Chapter 1) and addresses the unique healthcare attributes that call for healthcare organizations to tailor their marketing approaches. The marketing experiences and activities of various healthcare organizations are explored here as well.

Factors Affecting the Adoption of Healthcare Marketing

For-profit commercial businesses have led the way in carrying out formal marketing activities. From the start of the marketing era, these businesses employed the full range of marketing techniques, including advertising. The same was true of traditional businesses in healthcare, such as consumer products companies and retail-oriented organizations. As early as the 1950s, numerous healthcare brands had become household names as a result of aggressive marketing.

Marketers of consumer health products typically used the same techniques as did marketers of other types of products. However, some approaches unique to healthcare emerged. For example, insurance companies pioneered the concept of group sales, and pharmaceutical companies developed physician-oriented sales approaches. In general, however, the primarily nonprofit nature of the industry mitigated the widespread acceptance of marketing. Healthcare purists often equated marketing with advertising and considered it incompatible with the principles of a charitable organization. Charitable organizations were inherently conservative and generally thought that allocating resources for marketing purposes was in bad taste at best and unethical at worst.

Beginning in the 1970s, academic marketing experts asserted that marketing activities were common and acceptable among not-for-profit organizations (see, for example, Kotler 1975). Despite their assertion, health professionals as a group continued to resist the intrusion of formal marketing techniques. Further, as a practical matter, marketing was not a reimbursable expense for hospitals under the Medicare program. By the end of the 1970s, however, the mind-set of not-for-profit healthcare organizations began to change, giving rise to a new attitude toward business practices such as marketing. This section covers this evolution, while Exhibit 3.1 reviews some of the changes that occurred in not-for-profit healthcare organizations.

EXHIBIT 3.1
Putting the
Profit in the
Not-for-Profit
Organization

Many healthcare entities are chartered as not-for-profit organizations (NFPs). NFPs are typically conservative, particularly with regard to the expenditure of funds. They tend to restrict their spending to activities that directly relate to their mission. Historically, marketing activities have not been considered by NFPs as worthy uses of scarce organizational resources. Further, NFPs tended to view their goals as altruistic, setting them apart from their more avaricious for-profit kin. This stance fostered the perception that NFPs have nobler intentions than do for-profit healthcare organizations.

NFPs have historically eschewed the pursuit of profit as an activity that is beneath them, largely as a result of their lack of exposure to basic business practices. NFPs that have been exposed to standard business practices have resisted applying those practices, arguing that they are not in business but answering to a higher calling. During the 1980s, however, many NFPs in healthcare—particularly provider organizations—found that their world was changing and that they needed to rethink their stance on profit. The adage "no margin, no mission" was increasingly expressed during this period as NFPs began to realize the importance of profit for organizational survival. Although healthcare professionals are still loath to use the "p word," the pursuit of profit or net revenue under some other moniker came to be accepted. As a result of this new attitude, NFPs began to adopt many of the business practices of other industries and of the for-profit organizations that were prominent in healthcare at the time.

Marketing was one of the business practices that healthcare organizations came to accept. The margin necessary to support ongoing operations and continued development of the organization had to be nurtured, and the role of marketing in this process came to be recognized. If revenue was to flow to the bottom line, the organization had to increase customer traffic, sales volumes, market share, and all of the other indicators normally used in industry. Marketing was recognized as critical to the processes that would ultimately contribute to the bottom line. NFPs came to recognize the need to turn a profit and the importance of profitability to their continued viability and, ultimately, came to appreciate the contribution that marketing made in this regard.

The Growth in Competition

During the 1980s, healthcare providers were exposed to unprecedented competition on a number of fronts. For the first time, they were forced to profile their customers to determine their needs. They also had to develop a greater level of market intelligence to better understand their competitors.

A Shift in Emphasis

From Inpatient to Outpatient Care

At one time, medical care was synonymous with inpatient care, and hospitalization was often a prerequisite before insurance coverage kicked in. By the 1980s, however, numerous factors discouraged the use of inpatient care. The oupatient market was growing, physician referrals to inpatient care were being deemphasized, and consumerism was emerging as a force. Hospitals had to rapidly adjust to these market conditions and change their approach to marketing.

From Specialty to Primary Care

In the past, hospitals relied on the specialists on their medical staffs to admit patients and generate revenue. By the late 1980s, the use of specialists began to give way to the use of primary care physicians. Hospitals and health systems had to examine their referral patterns and began to actively court family practitioners, internists, and pediatricians. Marketers had to develop a means to showcase the primary care capabilities of their healthcare organizations to customers, consumers, and health plans. Today, although reimbursement still favors specialists, primary care physicians are seen as significant players in healthcare's future.

The Emergence of Employers as Major Customers

After World War II, employers began offering health insurance to their employees, passively footing the bill for their medical expenses. By the mid-1980s, employers were taking a more active role in managing their employees' health benefits. Suddenly, healthcare providers found they had a new customer with a set of needs different from that of other customers. Business coalitions formed to negotiate with healthcare providers from a position of strength, and the health benefit costs borne by employers became a major driver of healthcare reform.

The Increased Consumer Focus

Until the healthcare industry became market driven in the 1980s, patients' opinions were seldom considered important. All of a sudden, however, healthcare providers needed to know what the patient liked and did not like

Report card
A mechanism for comparing the performance and outcomes of providers and health plans

Need
A condition objectively determined as requiring a health service

Want
A consumer's desire (rather than a need) for a health service

about the services provided. Patient satisfaction surveys became commonplace, and **report cards** became a tool patients used to rate the performance of providers and health plans. Marketers had to not only identify the **needs** and **wants** of consumers but also recommend ways to improve customer satisfaction.

The Dominance of Managed Care

The emergence of managed care as a major force essentially changed the ground rules for healthcare providers. The patient had been transformed into an enrollee or a plan member. Instead of searching for sick patients who would require health services, marketers were encouraged to identify healthy persons who would not run up costs by using a lot of services. Healthcare providers participating in managed care plans had to shift their focus from treatment and cure to health maintenance. Managed care plans developed marketing expertise to capture the employer market, and managed care negotiations came to be considered by healthcare organizations as a marketing function.

The Changing Decision Maker

Before marketing took hold in healthcare, physicians made most of the clinical decisions and patients had limited control over their medical episodes. Later, health plans began exercising inordinate influence over the use of health services, directing their enrollees to specific provider networks. Consumerism, however, surged in the 1970s, 1980s, and 1990s and continues today. This has ushered a new set of decision makers and has forced healthcare organizations to research the characteristics of existing and potential customers and to determine their needs and wants.

Accommodating the Unique Attributes of Healthcare

The scope and nature of healthcare marketing had broadened considerably by the mid-1980s, and, like every industry did, healthcare modified its marketing approach to fit its particular needs. Some marketing techniques from other industries could be adopted without change, but many techniques were adapted for healthcare. At the same time, novel approaches were required to address the unique attributes of the healthcare industry.

Several healthcare attributes complicate marketing, the first of which are the multiple markets and/or consumer groups that healthcare organizations serve. A traditional business can focus its marketing on prospective customers in the general population, but healthcare marketers may have to consider physicians, nurses, patients, employee assistance personnel, managed care plans, and regulators as well. The marketing staff for a mental health or substance abuse program for adolescents, for example, might have to accommodate the needs of judges, probation officers, and social workers. Likewise, a marketer for a sports medicine program might have to consider employers, schools, and health plans among the potential customers—in addition to individuals.

Another attribute is that healthcare organizations have an opportunity to compete for employers' business and thus market to them accordingly. In the past, major employers were not considered to be an important market for healthcare organizations, although companies typically bore their employees' healthcare costs. Today, however, major employers often attempt to control rising healthcare costs by dealing directly with providers to meet their employees' healthcare needs.

Yet another unique healthcare attribute is that health insurance plans are likely to influence the medical facility choice of their members or enrollees. Although there may be allowances for using out-of-network practitioners (or the option of paying more out of pocket for that privilege), most health plans specify which facilities and practitioners their insured population can use. Healthcare organizations of all sizes spend an inordinate amount of time and effort negotiating contracts with health plans, and the more aggressive of these organizations see this situation as a marketing opportunity.

Organization-Specific Marketing Experiences and Activities

The many types of healthcare organizations are highly diverse, so marketing generalizations that would apply to all types cannot be made. To that end, this section addresses the specific marketing experiences and activities of a range of healthcare organizations, including providers, suppliers, consumer health product companies, pharmaceutical companies, insurance companies, and support services vendors.

Providers

Most people think about healthcare marketing campaigns as initiated by providers. The term **provider**, originally defined by the health insurance arena, refers to both health professionals (e.g., medical doctors, nurses, behavorial and mental health practitioners) and organizations that provide care and services to health plan members. The various categories of providers are described here.

Provider
A health professional or an organization that provides direct patient care or related support services

Hospitals

Hospitals are the most visible provider organizations, and their marketing activities are likely to be significant. Marketing by general hospitals can be traced back to the late 1970s, when a few hospitals hired marketers or established basic marketing departments. The real surge in marketing, however, occurred in the early to mid-1980s, when many hospitals became enamored with advertising. Ads for hospitals and their services flooded the print, radio, and TV media, and some hospitals advertised on billboards to reach the public. Although the ultimate benefit of these marketing expenditures was hard to determine, increased competition among providers during this period fueled the use of advertising. See Exhibit 3.2 for an example of hospital advertising.

By the 1990s, hospital administrators began to rethink their advertisement-focused marketing strategies. Advertising budgets—and, in some cases, marketing departments and personnel—were cut back. A balanced approach to marketing, which integrated advertising into public relations and communications activities and added direct sales capabilities, came to replace the former strategy. Hospitals adopted more contemporary forms of marketing by establishing marketing databases and call centers. Customer relationship marketing, direct-to-consumer marketing, and Internet marketing (then new to the scene) were also adopted in the 1990s. These trends demonstrated a shift from a sales approach to a relationship management approach to marketing.

Media advertising (print, TV, radio) was the approach of choice for cultivating the interest of the general public; specialty hospitals in particular attempted to maintain high visibility in their communities. National hospital and health system chains often conducted nationwide marketing campaigns supplemented by customized advertising in the local communities they served. Many of these chains employed sales forces that called on potential referrers of psychiatric or substance abuse patients. Public relations approaches, including holding open houses and disseminating feature stories, also were commonly used. A compelling website became customary for specialty hospitals, just as it did for other healthcare facilities. In fact, most hospitals subsequently took advantage of the electronic revolution. Driven by a variety of forces—including the implementation of the Affordable Care Act (ACA)—marketers recognized the need to better understand consumers and to have more direct interaction with existing and potential customers. Healthcare consumers quickly adopted social media, and the Web filled up with much information about health and healthcare. In the past few years, many providers and organizations have taken advantage of this new environment to help with communications, marketing, and healthcare initiatives.

Long-term care
Nonacute care provided for an extended period or, sometimes, until death

Nursing Homes and Assisted Living Facilities

The target market for nursing home care is much smaller than that for general hospital services, so marketing for these organizations is typically less visible and more subdued. Because their clientele need **long-term care**, nursing homes do not need as much patient volume as acute care and other

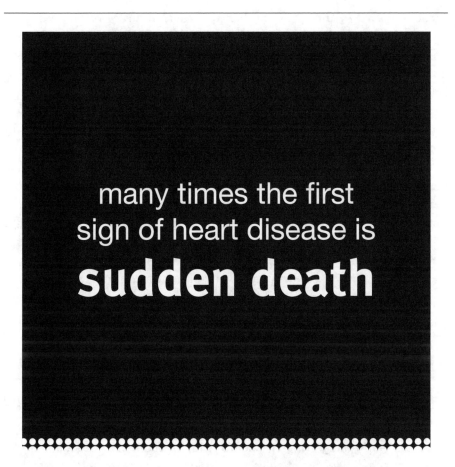

EXHIBIT 3.2
Sample Print
Advertisement

Heart disease can be scary. That's no excuse for ignoring it. Take charge of your heart health with your free online HeartAware assessment. We'll assess your risk and guide you to better health.

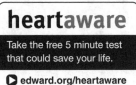

heartaware

Take the free 5 minute test that could save your life.

▶ edward.org/heartaware

EDWARD   **For people who don't like hospitals**

Source: Edward Hospital, Naperville, IL. Used with permission.

facilities do. Further, in this setting, someone other than the resident (end user of the service) may be involved in the admission decision, so the marketing activity must consider not only the prospective client but also his or her healthcare decision maker. Advertising tends to be the means used to remain top of mind and, where appropriate, to solidify relationships with referral agencies. **Word of mouth** is another important means of promoting nursing homes. Exhibit 3.3 describes research on the factors that contribute to positive nursing home recommendations; although the study was released in 2000, its findings are still cogent today. Additionally, websites such as www.aplaceformom.com are a modern way to connect those seeking nursing care with appropriate providers.

Assisted living facilities are more like nursing homes than hospitals in their approach to the market. They do not require a large volume of patients but a small number of qualified **prospects**. Typically, residents of assisted living facilities do not make the decision to enter the facility, so administrators gear the marketing efforts toward not only potential consumers but also their caregivers or decision makers. Although fewer nursing homes are being built, assisted living facilities continue to spring up around the country. Print and electronic media advertising is one important way that these facilities create and maintain positive publicity, and word-of-mouth endorsement is another way.

EXHIBIT 3.3
Nursing Home
Marketing:
What Are
Customers
Looking For?

As baby boomers age, the demand for nursing services is expected to increase. In preparation, healthcare marketers must develop a better understanding of the factors that influence choice of nursing home. Customers for nursing home services include not only residents but also third-party payers, employees, doctors, hospitals, and caregivers. In this era of the graying of America, with an enormous potential market for senior services of all sorts, keeping current customers satisfied is vital for positive word of mouth. It also is vital for nursing homes to recognize family and friends as customers who may generate positive word-of-mouth publicity. Both the resident and these proxies may be considered customers for nursing home services, so it is important to understand the needs of both groups. Meeting the needs of the resident is the organization's mission, but meeting the needs of the proxies may ensure that they continue to generate referrals to the business.

Data obtained from 2,709 residents living in 26 different nursing homes across the nation provide some insight into marketing issues. Of the residents surveyed, 71 percent were women. The average age of residents was 75 for males and 80 for females. Many of the residents were relatively new to their facility: 43 percent of the men had lived in the facility for less than one month, compared to 30 percent of the women. In addition, 21 percent of the female residents had been in the facility for more than three years, whereas only 12 percent of the male residents had been there that long. The reported health status of the residents (as measured on a 5-point scale, where 1 indicated "very poor" and 5 indicated "very good") did not vary by gender. Fifty-six percent of the residents were identified as having less than good health (fair, poor, or very poor ratings).

Survey administrators found that only 31 percent of the questionnaires were completed by residents. The others were completed by a family member other than a spouse (40 percent), a spouse (12 percent), some other person (10 percent), a legal guardian (4 percent), or a friend (3 percent). Completion of the questionnaire by a proxy was strongly associated with the resident's health.

The questions covered 39 service issues related to the nursing home experience. The questionnaire also contained a question to assess "positive word of mouth," which was defined as the "likelihood you would recommend the (facility) to others." Respondents reported that the nursing homes did well in the areas of courtesy and friendliness but not as well with noise, food, and responsiveness. The service variables with the lowest scores were noise level in and around the room, followed by variety of food selections and quality of the food. The highest marks were given to courtesy of the admitting staff, friendliness of nurses, and courtesy of the housekeeping staff. The issues found to require the greatest attention were those dealing with services provided by the aides (e.g., information from aides, assistance with meals, and response to the call button).

Interestingly, the satisfaction ratings differed depending on who was doing the rating. For example, residents were more positive about the aides and the facility than were family and friends. In fact, when the overall satisfaction scores were compared for each type of respondent, the residents gave the highest scores. Friends, family, and guardians gave lower scores than residents, although the difference between the scores the residents and other respondents gave was significant only where the other respondents were friends. Nevertheless, the likelihood of recommending the nursing home was higher among family members than among residents, and it was significantly higher among family members than among friends.

Fortunately for the facilities, the items with the lowest scores were not among those with the highest correlation to likelihood to recommend. Items that had the highest correlation to likelihood to recommend included respectful, dignified treatment and nurses' technical skill, ability to explain care, and friendliness—domains in which nursing

(continued)

facilities tend to score relatively well. Among the eight service domains, nursing was most strongly related to likelihood to recommend the facility. Experiences with dining and aides were also important predictors of likelihood to recommend. Admission issues, not surprisingly, influenced the families' and residents' likelihood to recommend, but not the other respondents' likelihood to recommend. Similarly, finance issues were strongly related to likelihood to recommend only for the residents and their legal guardians. When taken together, the service domains explained about 60 percent of the variation in likelihood to recommend.

Residents tended to give higher ratings than their proxies. This difference may indicate that residents are reluctant to criticize staff or service delivery processes on which they depend. In contrast, family members' responses were particularly critical of the aides and of housekeeping.

On the other hand, some of the score differences may stem from anxiety or guilt associated with placing a loved one in a nursing home. Family members want to be certain that the quality of care meets an appropriate standard. Clearly, there are many components to quality of care, and patient and family assessments are just one element. Nevertheless, these ratings can help organizations identify perceived strengths and weaknesses in service delivery and take corrective action to meet customer needs and manage word of mouth in the community.

The difficulty in identifying the customers for nursing home services creates special challenges in determining and meeting customer requirements. Should the facility operate with an eye to resident ratings or family ratings? Or should it attempt to meet the expectations of the respondents who gave the lowest scores, assuming that meeting the requirements of that group will exceed the requirements of the other groups? Nursing homes would be wise to collect data from all identified customers—patients and proxies—and make efforts to satisfy both. The net result would be not only more data from "other" consumers but potentially more data from the healthy residents whose voices previously have been lost to the proxy.

Irrespective of customer segment, the data suggest that nursing homes can maintain positive word of mouth by ensuring that nursing, aide services, and dining needs are met. Because the scores for nursing are already relatively high, the greatest opportunity appears to be in improving scores for aides and food quality.

Source: Adapted from Becker and Kaldenberg (2000).

Other Residential/Inpatient Facilities

Residential treatment centers operate their marketing in a manner similar to that of specialty hospitals. They tend to focus on ads for the general public and relationship building with potential referral agents. They often employ sales forces and may aggressively seek prospective customers.

As a group, inpatient facilities use public relations, advertising, and community outreach as their primary marketing techniques. Many use direct sales as well. Contemporary approaches—such as customer relationship management, database marketing, and Internet marketing—have become common. In the past ten years, provider organizations (especially hospitals) have focused on relationship development and harnessed sophisticated information technology–oriented tools. Marketers have turned to low-cost/high-exposure marketing techniques, such as Internet marketing (see also Chapter 11 for a discussion of social media marketing). See Case Study 3.1 for a discussion of some "offline" approaches.

Marketing by provider organizations is influenced by the unique characteristics of health services delivery. For example, hospitals generally do not attract customers directly; instead, they gain new customers when their medical staffs refer patients for admission. Similarly, many medical specialists do not accept customers directly but rely on **referrals** from primary care physicians and other specialists. Given that most people do not just walk into a specialist's office without a prior referral, advertising to the end user has limited value for many medical practices. These types of **referral relationships** typically do not exist in any other industry, and their presence complicates the marketing approach of provider organizations.

Ethical and regulatory considerations constrain the marketing activities of provider organizations. For the most part, it is inappropriate for healthcare providers to offer **incentives** to potential sources of business (as is typical practice in other industries). For example, it is unethical and even illegal for hospitals to give physicians bonuses for admitting patients.

Physicians and Other Clinicians

The marketing efforts of clinicians have, for the most part, lagged behind those of hospitals and other provider organizations. Many physicians did not face the same competitive situations that hospitals began facing in the 1980s. In addition, ethical constraints limited the amount of advertising considered acceptable by the medical profession. Individual physicians and professional medical associations were long hostile to the notion of formal marketing, although most doctors engaged in various forms of marketing to promote their practices.

Referral
The practice of one entity sending a customer to another entity for specialized or additional good or service

Referral relationship
An agreement between two or more entities that each will refer customers to the other

Incentive
An enticement offered to current or potential customers to achieve a desired result

CASE STUDY 3.1
Low-Intensity Marketing

Like many healthcare organizations, Yale–New Haven Hospital (YNHH) was being asked to do more with less when it came to marketing. Given its moderate advertising budget and the area's high media costs, YNHH had focused its advertising in the past on billboards, newspapers, and the Yellow Pages. Advertising via radio, television, and magazines was considered too expensive. From 1995 to 1999, the bulk of its advertising dollars went into three-quarter-page display ads in daily newspapers across Connecticut. These ads, developed through a lengthy review process with a traditional advertising agency, were ineffective in increasing consumer awareness because the limited budget prevented consistent exposure to the public.

To find a more effective yet inexpensive means of advertising, YNHH considered banner ads in newspapers. These ads are small strips that are 2 to 3 inches tall and range from 5 to 12 inches long. Usually one topic is covered per ad, and they may or may not include artwork. Banner ads are designed to pop out by using color and regular placement in the same place in the newspaper. They generally run on a daily basis and are placed at the top and bottom of the front page. The cost of the banner ad depends on its size and location. Most banner ads include a "call to action," giving the reader an opportunity to respond to the pitch.

As an experiment in early 1999, YNHH placed a half-inch by 12-inch strip ad at the bottom of the front page of the local newspaper twice a week. After monitoring the impact of the strips for a few months, there was no noticeable increase in calls to YNHH's call center for information or referral to a physician. A meeting was held with the local paper's sales executives to share the unfavorable results. The hospital informed the newspaper that it would cease running the banner ads if the newspaper did not develop a better approach. The paper came back with a new design that required discussions with and approval of the editorial side of the newspaper and major redesign of the paper's front page to develop space for a bigger ad at no additional cost.

YNHH expanded its banner ad initiative in the fall of 2000, and since then, more than 350 newspaper ads have been developed. Most of these ads promoted clinical programs such as heart, cancer, maternity, and diabetes, as well as ongoing clinical trials. Other ads were specific to the call center and promoted the physician referral program, the health information library, the nurse advice line, and the women's heart line. A third group of ads promoted consumer-oriented services, such as Web-based services, press conferences to announce newborn babies, and support groups. The final category of ads promoted general awareness of YNHH programs and announced special events, such as Nurses' Day.

Follow-up research indicated that the banner ad campaign was highly successful. Between the fall of 2000 and 2002, consumer awareness of YNHH in the southern Connecticut market increased from 29 percent to 49 percent. The proportion of consumers associating YNHH with state-of-the-art care increased from 22 percent to 40 percent. Because the hospital's marketing budget had declined 30 percent between 2000 and 2002, and there had been no increases in other marketing activity, the bulk of the change in consumers' attitudes and behaviors was attributed to the banner ads. In addition, 49 percent of the calls routed to the call center were generated by the banner ads during this period, and a large portion of follow-up calls for other services was stimulated by the banner ads. Evidence also suggested that callers who had found YNHH through the Yellow Pages often had been encouraged to seek them out after seeing the banner ads.

Although banner ads are not a panacea for marketing challenges, they have been generally beneficial to YNHH. They have generated considerable inquiries and have allowed the organization to spread its marketing budget much further than traditional advertising would have allowed. The volume of consumer interaction with the hospital has grown dramatically, and most of the increase in admissions during this period was attributed to the campaign. Furthermore, the banner ad campaign contributed substantially to the development of the YNHH customer database: As of 2003, 40,000 additional names had been added since the ads began running. These positive results were obtained at a time of declining newspaper readership. YNHH marketers found that their best customers were among the most loyal newspaper subscribers; with their inevitable health problems, older people were the last loyal customer group for this medium.

There is little downside to the use of banner ads as the focal point of a marketing campaign. Organizations must ensure, however, that they have the capability to respond to demand and must maintain a wide range of publications and other resource materials as references when responding to inquiries.

Source: Adapted from Gombeski and colleagues (2003).

(continued)

Case Study Discussion Questions

1. What prompted YNHH to rethink its use of banner ads in newspapers?
2. What changes were implemented to make the banner ads more effective?
3. What types of services appear to lend themselves to this type of advertising?
4. What was the impact of the new banner ads in terms of "traffic" generated for YNHH?
5. How could the declining importance of newspapers affect YNHH's reliance on this marketing technique?
6. What are the implications of the demographics of loyal newspaper subscribers for the use of this medium to reach healthcare consumers?
7. Are there more contemporary forms of media in which banner ads might be more effective?

Today, in contrast, increasing numbers of physicians and physician practices are using advertising to gain visibility and increase volume. These practices are often specialty groups that are trying to distinguish themselves from other specialists in their field. Physicians who offer elective procedures are involved even more heavily in advertising. Thus, ophthalmic surgeons who perform laser eye surgery and cosmetic surgeons, for example, are more likely than specialists who provide traditional services to advertise directly to consumers. Because insurance usually does not cover these services, these practitioners depend less on referrals from colleagues and more on direct solicitation of potential customers.

Physicians, in the past, emphasized networking and relationship development for marketing purposes. More recently, some have ventured into advertising, although much of the hard-sell advertising has been initiated by physicians involved in retail or elective aspects of healthcare. Physicians may send direct mail to reach selected audiences or to announce changes about their respective practices, and they are increasingly taking advantage of the Internet as a means of promoting their services and maintaining contact with their patients. In some markets, large physician groups are using managed care and health plan contracting as a means of market development.

The marketing level and approach clinicians carry out vary by profession and market. Among independent practitioners—such as dentists, podiatrists, and chiropractors—low-key advertising is a common technique to attract patients and maintain visibility. Some practitioners may rely on referral relationships, and others may use direct mail occasionally to contact prospects directly. Some of these practitioners have embraced Internet marketing.

Various types of alternative therapists employ a wide range of marketing techniques. Many advertise their services, often targeting select populations that are thought to be better prospects. An outreach approach is often important for alternative therapists who may have to educate the public about the forms of therapy or procedure they offer. Internet marketing has gained more traction among these unconventional providers than any other group.

Behavioral Health Providers

Behavioral health providers (e.g., psychiatrists, psychologists, licensed counselors and therapists) and their agencies take particular care when formulating and conveying their marketing message. For example, advertising for behavioral health programs (designed for patients with psychiatric and/or substance abuse issues) tends to be more sensitive to the audience and more subtle than the ads for other programs. Much of the marketing efforts for such programs center on behind-the-scenes relationship building, especially with private-pay patients.

Specialty Care Providers

Marketers for HIV/AIDS programs (and certain other specialized services) may face a number of challenges. First, for various reasons, individuals with HIV/AIDS may be difficult to identify and contact because they are not likely to want their condition broadcast. Second, they may be resistant to receiving unsolicited information from unknown parties. Third, they may have concerns about the confidentiality with which their stigmatized condition and personal information are handled by providers and/or marketers. Thus, marketers need to reach out to and attract those in need of services without inviting undue attention to the providers. Some organizations, for example, adopt generic names (e.g., Adult Special Services) or put up minimal signage to limit the potential for stigmatization of their current and prospective clients. Public service announcements and other forms of impersonal social marketing are often used to divert attention from individual sufferers and to minimize stigma. Brochures and other materials are given to physicians to encourage referrals of such patients.

Public Health Agencies

Most public health activities—such as monitoring air and water quality or inspecting sites where food is prepared—do not directly involve healthcare customers. But some activities—such as child immunization and nutritional counseling—do necessitate interacting with the public. Noncontroversial initiatives are typically promoted through word of mouth as well as via traditional information and referral channels. More controversial programs—such as family planning, teen pregnancy prevention, and sexually transmitted infection or disease (e.g., HIV/AIDS, HPV, genital herpes, chlamydia) intervention—require more aggressive yet more sensitive marketing approaches. Many public health agencies provide not only information but also some medical treatments and psychological counseling, and these services need to be promoted as well.

Public health agencies have relied on information and referral as well as public relations to publicize their services, and they have deployed community outreach programs to promote their work in local areas. In recent years, public health has taken on various conditions that are now thought to be public health issues, such as breastfeeding, obesity, and domestic violence. Public health agencies have become much more aggressive marketers and have integrated health communication into their marketing techniques. Myriad social marketing initiatives have been launched, many of which are coordinated by the Centers for Disease Control and Prevention or another federal agency. These include initiatives aimed to reduce the rates of sexually transmitted diseases and tuberculosis, for example, as well as nonclinical programs, such as nutritional counseling and family planning.

Suppliers

In healthcare, suppliers include a wide range of organizations that provide the goods and equipment to support the clinical, business, and other operations of a hospital, health system, physician practice, or another facility. Healthcare organizations use an extensive range of supplies, from office supplies (e.g., paper, pens, clipboards) to cloth products (e.g., linens, gowns) to medical disposables (e.g., gloves, syringes, gauze) to machinery (e.g., MRI, x-ray). In addition, facilities use patient care equipment (e.g., sterilizers, blood pressure machines, scales, stethoscopes, lab microscopes) and durable medical equipment (e.g., hospital beds, examination tables, wheelchairs). A large physician practice's vendor list may include several dozens of suppliers, and a hospital's list may go up to the hundreds. Healthcare organizations are the primary targets of the vendors of these supplies and equipment.

Supplies and equipment may be obtained directly from their manufacturers, but often they are obtained from distributors or vendors that handle a range of products. In either case, vendors are likely to advertise to their customers in trade publications read by hospital administrators, physicians and nurses, practice managers, and other personnel. Suppliers rely on sales representatives, who use the direct sales approach. They attend professional or association meetings that healthcare leaders, managers, and other facility decision makers as well as clinicians are likely to attend. They display and promote their products and talk to potential customers at healthcare exhibits.

Vendors that market medical supplies, biomedical equipment, and durable medical equipment operate in much the same manner as vendors in other industries. The primary difference is the logistics involved in connecting with a busy physician or the right administrator at a hospital or clinic to whom the vendor can make a presentation. The decision makers in other industries are often much more available and easier to identify. The types of marketing techniques healthcare suppliers generally use include direct sales, business-to-business marketing, advertising, and sales promotion. Suppliers also use the Internet for online marketing and promotion.

Consumer Health Product Companies

Although marketing by healthcare providers is still evolving, marketing by consumer health goods companies is a well-established phenomenon. Consumer health products have long been marketed to the American public; arguably, some of the best-known early consumer brands are associated with health-related products. Bayer, Johnson & Johnson, and Ex-Lax were household brand names before the modern healthcare system emerged in the United States.

Today, pharmacy shelves are filled with consumer health products, such as headache remedies, cold and cough medicines, adhesive bandages, heating pads, feminine hygiene products, and baby teething gels, among many other household and personal items. Household inventories may also include foot care, dental care, and eye care goods. Advances in home diagnosis, monitoring, and treatment have added kits and equipment to the consumer health options available. (Over-the-counter drugs are discussed later in the chapter.) Over-the-counter medicines and personal healthcare products are supplemented by a plethora of nutritional products, **cosmeceuticals** (such as anti-aging creams), and **nutraceuticals** (such as fish oil). These products bridge the gap between cosmetics and drugs and promise such results as younger skin, hair regrowth, or enhanced energy or immunity.

Complementary and alternative (or integrative) medicine and therapies (e.g., acupuncture, biofeedback, meditation, yoga and massage)—now widely accepted by American consumers—have also contributed to the rapid growth of consumer health products. A variety of natural products have entered the market, serving as alternatives or supplements to more conventional health goods and services.

The market for consumer health products in the United States is large and continues to expand, keeping pace with the population's more health conscious and do-it-yourself attitudes. The level of competition in this sector

Cosmeceuticals
Health or beauty products that combine the attributes of a cosmetic and a drug

Nutraceuticals
Food or dietary supplements that contain nutritional value and provide health benefits

is high and thus makes the use of aggressive marketing techniques essential to a consumer health product company's business strategy. In general, these products are marketed in a manner similar to the approach used for other, non-healthcare goods. Marketers rely heavily on media advertising (print and Internet) along with advertising inserts in popular publications. They also use such sales promotion techniques as discount coupons, rebates, and contests. They secure highly visible shelf space for in-store advertising.

Perhaps the most important development in marketing consumer health products has been the Internet as a marketplace for a wide range of products. For many marginal and new products, the Internet has become the primary promotional channel. In traditional mainstream marketplaces, these new products are shut out—for example, because of their lack of access to retail shelf space. But online, they can cater to a wider market that is receptive to innovation and to consumers who prefer to find and buy goods and services electronically.

Pharmaceutical Companies

Pharmaceutical manufacturing is an enormous and highly profitable industry in the United States. Sales of prescription drugs in 2012 were approximately $291 billion, accounting for 10 percent of annual healthcare expenditures in the United States (IMS Health 2013). Profits on pharmaceutical sales average 15 percent or three times the average for all industries. Despite its huge profit potential, the drug industry is highly risky and competitive. After receiving approval from the Food and Drug Administration, a new drug often faces stiff competition from other drugs already on the market and is granted patent protection for only a limited length of time.

Prescription drug use has grown dramatically since the research breakthroughs of the post–World War II period. The increased availability of more effective pharmaceuticals has shifted the therapeutic emphasis away from invasive procedures toward drug therapy. Patients today spend less time in the hospital and more time at the prescription counter. As a result, US healthcare expenditures, including expenditures on prescription drugs, are rising. However, the rate of the drug increase has slowed, with a 5 percent increase recoded between 2008 and 2012 (IMS Health 2013).

Because of the competitive nature of the industry and the pressure to recoup investments in research and development, the drug industry developed sophisticated, aggressive, and expensive marketing strategies. In 2012, approximately $27 billion was spent in the United States on pharmaceutical marketing (SK&A 2013). Marketing expenditures accounted for 30 percent or more of revenue; pharmaceutical companies spent more than half on "detailing" (direct physician contact) and $3.5 billion on advertising to consumers through TV, radio, magazines, newspapers, and outdoor bill-boards. They spent an additional $10 billion marketing to physicians through samples, meetings, and journal advertisements.

Medical Publications

One of the ways pharmaceutical companies promote themselves is through disseminating medical information in medical journals, industry-oriented newsletters/newspapers, research compendia, and other publications. They are heavy advertisers in medical journals (although many journals do not accept advertising). They sponsor research that generates articles submitted to—and they hope to be published in (if the findings are favorable)—medical journals. (Unfortunately, some drug manufacturers have been found guilty of paying medical scientists to write favorable reports on their drugs even when the research didn't support positive outcomes.)

Drug companies send doctors unsolicited "throwaway journals," which are typically newsletters or mini-newspapers containing summaries of research published in academic journals (which doctors may not have time to review). These throwaways may also take the form of trade journals in which the companies advertise or to which the medical professionals or researchers in their employ submit articles that promote their brand and products. Often, a company produces its own publication to serve as a "journalistic" format for its marketing efforts.

The volume of published medical information from pharmaceutical companies has mushroomed and has given doctors an alternative to the tedious process of sifting through the vast medical literature. By acting as information intermediaries, these companies help doctors save time and expense while maintaining some control over what doctors see and hear. This tactic used to be exclusively in print format but has now spread to the Internet.

Continuing Medical Education

Continuing medical education (CME) is one area of medical communication that is massively subsidized by the drug industry. Since the 1970s, physicians and other clinicians have been required to complete a minimum amount of accredited training each year to maintain their hospital privileges and professional certification. As a result, thousands of CME conferences are held each year. Drug companies participate as passive financial sponsors of CME conferences or as active partners in planning and staging these meetings. Most CME conferences now have pharmaceutical industry support; although some limitations have been placed on drug companies' influence, the conferences are still largely sponsored by these manufacturers.

Detailers and Physician Gifts

Field representatives (or "detailers") are a crucial link in the information chain between drug companies and clinicians. More than 30,000 detailers—one for every 20 American doctors—make tens of millions of office visits to doctors annually. They dispense promotional brochures and medical literature, speak with physicians and/or other staff about their products, and give them free samples. Physicians obtain much of their information about proprietary drugs in this way, making this activity—at least from the drug company's perspective—a successful marketing technique.

Gifts to physicians were a cornerstone of pharmaceutical marketing for many years. The most abundant category of gifts includes reminder items such as pens and notepads, which prominently display the name of a drug. Gifts are often offered to physicians in exchange for their attention to promotional material or presentations. "Drug lunches" in large hospitals and clinics are one such example, whereby the detailer buys lunch for an audience—usually medical students and junior physicians—and gives a presentation while they eat. Similarly, pharmaceutical companies sponsor dinner meetings during which representatives or other speakers tout the traits and benefits of their products. Physicians may offer testimonials regarding the merits of a drug, and they are often compensated for their time. Exorbitant gifts and cash payments of any amount were banned by the American Medical Association in 1990 and have been replaced with other gifts, such as medical textbooks and medical instruments. The length to which drug companies are allowed to go in marketing to doctors continues to be a source of controversy.

Mail Order, Direct to Consumer, Over the Counter, and Online Sales

Over the years, consumer, insurance, technology, medical innovation, and other trends in the US healthcare industry have changed the way prescription drugs are promoted, chosen, sold, and bought. Marketing techniques have rapidly adapted to each of these developments. The growth of managed care, for example, has had a profound effect on drug selection, with managers of both private and public health plans in a position to control billions of dollars of drug purchases each year. As a result, pharmaceutical marketers increased their attention toward wholesale purchasers, and physicians and consumers became secondary targets.

During the late 1970s and the 1980s, the relatively small industry of mail-order pharmacies grew dramatically, fueled by the greater pharmaceutical needs of an aging population and the cost advantages of the wholesale model. Because mail-order businesses sell drugs at lower costs than do many retail pharmacies, they obtain exclusive contracts to supply prescriptions to members of many managed care organizations. They also influence which drugs millions of people have access to. Thus, they have become targets for acquisition by pharmaceutical companies. By controlling the mail-order businesses, drug manufacturers can influence these pharmacies' recommendation patterns.

In the 1990s, the pharmaceutical industry introduced direct-to-consumer (DTC) marketing. While once they marketed almost exclusively to physicians, they now market directly to consumers. DTC advertising often prompts patients to seek treatment for previously untreated or undiagnosed conditions (e.g., low testosterone, dry eyes, shift work disorder); patients, in turn, pressure their physicians to prescribe drugs that they have seen in print ads or on TV commercials. A significant portion of the nearly $4 billion the pharmaceutical industry spends on consumer marketing consists of DTC advertising, and various surveys have found that these ads encourage patients to ask their doctors about a condition and its drug therapy and, to a lesser extent, about a specific drug (e.g., see ads for Viagra, Chantix, NuvaRing, Abilify, among countless others).

Generic drugs were yet another development that affected pharmaceutical marketing. These unbranded drugs are comparable (although not identical) in effectiveness to their brand-name, highly advertised counterparts but sell for a much lower price. Pharmacies can reduce prescription drug costs substantially through the substitution of generics. Pharmacists who counsel and educate patients at the point of care are primarily responsible for this phenomenon. Not surprisingly, pharmaceutical companies have sought to limit the presence of generic drugs that could be substituted for their name-brand prescriptions. Because of the lack of access to some medications and the generally high cost of prescribed drugs in the United States, many US patients cross the borders to Canada and Mexico to obtain what they need. In fact, drug manufacturers in those and other countries market both their brand-name and generic drugs to US consumers.

Many pharmaceuticals that do not require a prescription are sold over the counter (OTC). OTC drugs are promoted in a manner similar to that for consumer health products, but OTC medicines often have the power of pharmaceutical marketing behind them. Growth in the sales of OTC drugs has been boosted by the introduction of complementary and alternative therapies and natural products, which may not face the same advertising restrictions governing pharmaceutical marketers.

The past decade has seen the development and growth of prescription drug sales on the Internet; this commerce is carried out by mainstream pharmaceutical companies, mail-order pharmacies, and other entrepreneurs hoping to capture this lucrative market. Most online drug sellers are legitimate and adhere to ethical and professional guidelines, but some online drug distributors are less than wholesome: They sell prescription drugs without requiring a doctor's order from the buyers, and many (mostly based overseas) retailers are outright scammers. Online sales have significant implications for marketing. Because customers can easily access drug and related information on the Internet, the importance of and need for traditional marketing techniques are diminished.

Insurance Companies

Health insurance companies were among the earliest healthcare organizations to develop marketing strategies in the period after World War II. In the early days of health insurance, policies were generally sold to individuals or families, and health insurance plans were marketed in the same manner as other types of insurance. Health plans advertised their programs using a variety of techniques and marketed them out through a network of agents. Because health insurance was relatively novel until the 1960s, the marketing approach often involved educating the prospective customer.

By the 1960s, health insurance was predominantly sold wholesale through employers who purchased group plans on behalf of their employees. Group plans came to be the norm, and individual policies became increasingly uncommon. The spread and entrenchment of employer-based insurance was abetted by a substantially unionized workforce for whom health benefits became an almost inalienable right. Although group plans were advertised by insurance companies (e.g., through print, radio, TV, or billboards), they were primarily sold to large employers by sales forces representing a particular insurance company or brokers representing several health plans.

Managed Care and Defined Contribution Plans

During the last quarter of the twentieth century, alternative forms of financing for healthcare coverage were created for the purpose of competing with traditional indemnity insurance. In the 1970s, health maintenance organizations (HMOs) emerged as a form of prepaid insurance that minimized the fee-for-service aspect of reimbursement. HMOs and other alternatives to indemnity insurance came to be generically referred to as *managed care*.

Although a certain level of competition had always existed among health plans, the competition for enrollees was typically low key. The emergence of managed care incited much more intense competition with existing indemnity plans (and with each other). The marketing of managed care plans involved the same approaches used for group plans and individual plans. Legislation was passed that required employers to offer their employees a managed care plan, which meant employees were likely to have a choice between two or more plans. Thus, a managed care marketer's first task was to convince employers to offer his organization's plan to their employees. Subsequently, he had to encourage employees to choose his organization's plan over any others offered. Managed care plans began to offer special benefits to encourage enrollment and to retain employees once they were enrolled.

In the late 1990s, managed care enrollment leveled off, with at least half of all insured enrolled in some type of managed care plan. The defined contribution approach to health insurance benefits also emerged during this decade. Traditional insurance and managed care plans alike offered *defined benefits*, which meant the provisions of the plan were established up front and all enrollees received the same benefits regardless of their circumstances or preferences with defined contributions. Employees were given credit for a certain amount of insurance resources and could disburse these funds in the manner they saw fit by choosing options from a menu of benefits. The introduction of defined contribution plans made modification of existing marketing approaches necessary, as plans could now be customized for individual enrollees. The standardized approach to benefits that had become common gave way to a tailored approach. This development was propelled by health plans' use of the Internet to offer enrollees access to information on their benefits.

Self-Insurance, No Insurance, and Government-Sponsored Insurance

By the end of the 1990s, the conventional approach to group insurance had lost ground for various reasons. A growing number of employers were no longer offering insurance as a benefit, were cutting back their coverage, or were becoming "self-insured." In addition, a growing number of Americans were going without health insurance. This population came to include not only marginal participants in the economy but an increasing number of working-class and middle-class individuals who did not have access to group insurance. This state of affairs led to a revival of the individual insurance policy, a development driven by Internet marketing and distribution. Insurers began to offer health plans online, and they advertised this option through print and electronic media. Because they are national plans, they can enroll millions of individuals and thereby create a large enough pool of plan members to spread the risk. At some point in the past decade, the number of uninsured individuals and families in the Unites States totaled 47 million, by some estimates. With the passage of the ACA, this number has been reduced. (See the discussion on the ACA, how it has affected marketing, and how national plans have promoted the enrollment of group and individual members as well as the public at large.)

Another important aspect of health insurance involves government-sponsored insurance programs—namely, Medicare and Medicaid. There has been no competition among insurance plans for Medicare enrollees because US citizens and legal immigrants are automatically enrolled in the program when they reach age 65. Although alternatives to simple Medicare enrollment have been around since the 1970s, the federally approved (and subsidized) Medicare Advantage program was reorganized in 2003. Medicare Advantage plans are offered by private insurers to Medicare enrollees who seek additional coverage on top of Medicare benefits. Again, the federal government does not have to market Medicare because those eligible are automatically enrolled, but Medicare Advantage plans employ various marketing techniques to convince seniors that they are a more favorable option than traditional Medicare or competing Medicare Advantage plans. The introduction of the Medicare drug benefits program (Part D) required a social marketing effort to encourage Medicare beneficiaries to participate.

Medicaid enrollees sign up through their respective states on the basis of federally approved eligibility criteria. However, states have increasingly contracted out management of their Medicaid programs to private healthcare networks. Government agencies responsible for Medicaid programs have historically employed social marketing techniques to ensure that eligible individuals knew about these programs and the services they offer. In particular, new supplemental insurance programs, such as those for children, need to be promoted to those who can benefit from them.

Affordable Care Act

A major healthcare marketing effort in 2013 involved the national implementation of a key provision of the ACA: the signup for health insurance coverage to avoid a tax penalty. To facilitate this enrollment drive, the US Department of Health and Human Services (HHS) encouraged each state to set up its own health insurance exchange. Residents of states that did not set up an exchange could enroll through the federal exchange (www.healthcare .gov). States were offered incentives to expand their Medicaid coverage to low-income residents, although only half of the 50 states took advantage of this offer.

Given the politically driven controversy surrounding the ACA and its insurance coverage mandate, HHS embarked on a multipronged promotional effort. The effort included airing public service announcements on TV and radio, posting advertisements on popular websites, and engaging celebrity **campaign spokespersons**. Furthermore, HHS funded states to advertise their exchanges and contracted with various organizations to train and deploy "navigators" to assist people in the enrollment process.

Campaign spokesperson
An individual—typically well-known—who represents the organization's marketing campaign

Although the insurance coverage mandate met with immediate negative publicity upon its launch (because of persistent glitches in the federal exchange system that initially prevented people from completing their enrollment), it more than met its goal with 7.1 million signups by March 31, 2014. Whether the marketing efforts of HHS and its partner organizations contributed to ACA's enrollment success may be hard to determine, but it is safe to say that an overwhelming number of Americans saw, heard, or read the myriad announcements, reminders, and coverage related to this national campaign.

Support Services Vendors

Although hospitals and other facilities may provide many types of support services in-house, there have always been services that internal resources could not easily provide. Since the 1980s, healthcare organizations have been outsourcing an increasing number of services to specialized service providers.

Among the support services hospitals require are transcription services, billing and collections services, utilization review, recruitment and staffing services, hazardous waste disposal, laboratory services, and information technology. Information technology services have become particularly important as healthcare's dependence on technology has increased. In many cases, hospitals and other healthcare organizations have benefited from outsourcing these services.

Vendors that provide these services typically market via direct sales and often sponsor community events. They may also advertise in print or electronic media or use direct mail to maintain visibility. The Internet, too, has increasingly gained popularity as a vehicle for marketing a wide range of support services.

Summary

Healthcare's acceptance of marketing as a corporate function occurred at different times for different organizations. Even today, different healthcare organizations are at different stages of marketing maturity. For-profit healthcare businesses led the way in adopting formal marketing activities, while not-for-profit organizations were slow to do so. Although the scope of healthcare marketing had broadened considerably by the mid-1980s, few marketing techniques could be applied from other industries unchanged. Marketers had to develop novel approaches that took into consideration the unique attributes of the healthcare industry.

Hospitals' marketing activities are usually significant in scope, and other provider organizations (nursing homes, assisted living facilities, and other residential facilities) face their own marketing challenges. Most physicians have long engaged in informal types of marketing, although most were loath to advertise. Today, however, more physician practices are using advertising as a means of gaining visibility and attracting patients. Public health agencies promote activities—such as child immunizations and nutritional counseling—through traditional information and referral channels and through word of mouth and social marketing. Controversial programs—such as those dealing with family planning, teen pregnancy, and sexually transmitted infection or diseases—require aggressive yet sensitive approaches.

Supplier organizations typically engage marketing techniques in much the same manner as suppliers in other industries do, and consumer health products are marketed aggressively. Pharmaceutical companies allocate more of their budget to marketing than does any other type of healthcare organization. Health insurance companies were among the earliest healthcare organizations to employ marketing techniques. In the early days of health insurance, policies were generally sold to individuals or families, and health insurance plans were marketed in the same manner as other types of insurance. By the 1960s, health insurance was predominantly sold in wholesale fashion to employers on behalf of their employees. By the end of the 1990s, individual policies experienced a resurgence prompted in part by the ability to purchase insurance via the Internet. The 2010 passage and ongoing implementation of the ACA generated new opportunities and challenges for insurance companies.

Key Points

- Healthcare organizations adopted marketing practices at varying rates of speed, and the type of marketing technique chosen varies with the type of organization and its marketing maturity.
- For-profit entities like pharmaceutical, supplier, and insurance companies adopted marketing practices much faster than did organizations providing patient care.
- The nature of healthcare—and particularly the dominance of not-for-profit organizations—contributed to the slow adoption of marketing practices.
- Although organizations in other industries typically have one target audience, the constituents for healthcare services are multiple and varied.
- Historically, pharmaceutical companies' approach to marketing was unique in that they did not market directly to the end user but to an intermediary—the physician—who then prescribed the products to the patient.
- Every type of healthcare organization has unique marketing challenges and applies the techniques that are appropriate for its circumstances.

Discussion Questions

1. What are some factors that account for the different rates at which healthcare organizations have adopted marketing techniques?
2. How does the marketing of cardiology services by a hospital differ from the marketing of cosmetic surgery by a plastic surgeon?
3. In what ways are the approaches used by pharmaceutical companies to market prescription drugs unique to the healthcare industry?
4. In what ways does the marketing of individual health plans by insurance companies differ from the marketing of group insurance plans?
5. What marketing techniques were so routinely used by healthcare organizations that they were not recognized as marketing?
6. What role has technology played in the evolution of marketing in healthcare?
7. How has the healthcare industry progressed from an emphasis on sales to an emphasis on developing long-term customer relationships?

Additional Resources

Andreasen, A. R., and P. Kotler. 2007. *Strategic Marketing for Non-Profit Organizations*, 7th ed. Upper Saddle River, NJ: Prentice Hall.

Cellucci, L., C. Wiggins, and T. Farnsworth. 2014. *Healthcare Marketing: A Case Study Approach*. Chicago: Health Administration Press.

Thomas, R. K. 2008. "Marketing Your Healthcare Practice." Self-Study Course. Chicago: Health Administration Press.

———. 2007. *Health Services Marketing: A Guide for Practitioners*. New York: Springer.

Thomas, R. K., and M. Calhoun. 2007. *Marketing Matters: A Guide for Healthcare Executives*. Chicago: Health Administration Press.

HEALTHCARE MARKETS

All marketing efforts begin with an assessment of the market to be served. This assessment typically involves identifying potential customers and determining their characteristics. In healthcare, this task is a challenge because the markets for health services is different from any other markets. Marketers must define their customers, products, and marketing targets; understand customer decision making; and be knowledgeable about the sources of information consumers use. Healthcare has a bewildering variety of customers, providers, and payers with whom marketers must contend. These and other issues are discussed in Part II's chapters.

THE NATURE OF HEALTHCARE MARKETS

4

Marketing professionals in any industry must demonstrate an understanding of the market in which they operate. This issue is particularly important in healthcare because of the unique nature and variety of healthcare markets. This chapter discusses these unique characteristics, describes markets relevant to healthcare organizations, and reviews the various methods of defining markets and delineating market areas.

Marketing activities do not take place in a vacuum but are products of the sociocultural environment in which they occur. Understanding the intersection of healthcare and marketing requires understanding the societal framework in which both enterprises exist. For healthcare organizations to be successful in today's environment, they must develop an in-depth knowledge of their target population's social, political, and economic characteristics along with its lifestyles, attitudes, and other prominent traits. (These factors are discussed in more detail in Chapter 5.)

Although it is not possible to describe all of the social and health systems dimensions that are important in developing marketing initiatives, the key market dimensions are addressed in this chapter. Specifically, this chapter covers the types of markets for healthcare goods and services that have emerged and their implications for healthcare organizations.

Defining Markets

The establishment of a marketing function implies the existence of a *market*, which refers to both a marketplace and the potential customers—both individuals and organizations—for a good or service. This notion of a market has been expanded in healthcare. For healthcare marketers, a market is defined as a group of consumers who share some characteristics that affect their needs or wants and make them potential buyers of a healthcare product.

A market for healthcare goods or services can be delineated in a number of ways. The definition used depends on the purpose of the analysis, the product involved, the competitive environment, and the type of organization cultivating the market. Further, the nature of the market depends on the orientation of the organization involved in marketing. For example, the market for cardiac care may be identified as a five-county referral area, regardless of which providers offer cardiac care. In other words, everyone in that geographic area who potentially needs cardiac care constitutes the market. On the other hand, market may refer to the geographic area served by a particular healthcare organization—that is, Hospital X controls a five-county market area (regardless of the services it offers).

The term *market area* as used here is comparable to the term *service area* for all practical purposes. A service area identifies the geographic area served by not-for-profit organizations or the areas officially designated as the territory of a particular organization. For example, a health clinic that has been assigned a service area by a regulatory authority or a territory delimited on the basis of a health plan contract can constitute a service area. On the other hand, for-profit healthcare organizations, pharmaceutical companies, and distributors of consumer health products are more likely to be thought of as having market areas. As the healthcare industry has become more competitive and has come to accept marketing as a healthcare function, more and more healthcare organizations now frame their actions in terms of market areas.

Geographic unit
A physical area demarcated by defined boundaries and used as a basis for market analysis

Political or administrative unit
A bounded geographic area formally defined for administrative purposes, such as a state, county, municipality, or school district

Statistical unit
A bounded geographic area formally defined for data collection purposes, such as the geographic units developed by the Census Bureau

Functional unit
A bounded geographic area formally defined for the execution of some practical function, such as mail delivery

Geography

The first, and most common, method of defining a market is by geography. A *geographically based market* is delineated in terms of specified **geographic units**. Most market research, in fact, focuses on a census tract, zip code, or county (or a group of any of these units) as the basis for analysis. This type of market area is typically delineated in terms of the "official" boundaries of the geographic units chosen for analysis. Geographically based markets are popular because analysts and decision makers are familiar with established geographic boundaries, the de facto operating spheres of many organizations often correspond with specified geographic boundaries, and market data are typically collected and reported for established geographic units. Exhibit 4.1 describes the most common geographic units (**political or administrative units**, **statistical units**, and **functional units**) used by marketers.

In actuality, few markets (for healthcare or anything else) neatly follow the political/administrative, statistical, or functional boundaries. In fact, markets nearly always change faster than their formal boundaries do, and inevitably a mismatch occurs between a geographically defined market area and the actual market area. Furthermore, market areas are often gerrymandered to conform to geographic boundaries that represent a reasonable approximation of the service area under study, primarily because the available data are usually organized on the basis of these geographic units. In addition, a market is difficult to visualize unless it is considered in terms of concrete, recognized boundaries.

Nearly all healthcare marketing activities are linked to some geographic area. Public health agencies and community-based organizations typically have specific geographic areas over which they have authority or that they are designated to serve. Private-sector healthcare organizations typically plan for markets that are delineated on the basis of geography. For purposes of this discussion, the geographic units that healthcare marketers use can be divided into three major categories: political or administrative units, statistical units, and functional units.

Political or Administrative Units

Political or administrative divisions are the most commonly used geographic units in marketing. Many healthcare organizations have market areas that coincide with the political boundaries of cities, counties, or states. Standard political or administrative units are not only convenient for private-sector organizations to use in establishing their boundaries but also facilitate data collection because most statistics are compiled using these boundaries. The following political and administrative units are frequently used in marketing.

Nation

The nation (in this case, the United States) is defined by national boundaries. Although some national chains or consumer health product companies may be interested in data at the national level, few healthcare organizations operate in a national market. Nevertheless, statistics for the nation (e.g., mortality rates) are often important as a standard with which other levels of geography are compared.

States

States are major subnational political units. Data are typically available for 50 states, the District of Columbia, and several US territories. Because individual states are responsible for a broad range of administrative functions, states tend to be useful sources of social, demographic, economic, and environmental data. State agencies also are an important source of health-related data.

Counties

Counties (or, in some states, boroughs, townships, or parishes) are the primary units of local government. The nation is divided into more than 3,100 county units (including some cities that are politically designated

(continued)

EXHIBIT 4.1
Units of
Geography
in Healthcare
Marketing

as counties). The county is a critical unit for marketing, as many health-care organizations view their home county as their primary service area. States typically report most of their statistics at the county level, and the county health department is likely to be a major source of health data.

Cities

Cities are officially incorporated urban areas delineated by boundaries that may or may not coincide with other political boundaries. Although cities are typically contained within a particular county, many city boundaries extend across county lines. Because cities are incorporated according to the laws of the state in which they are located, there is lit-tle standardization with regard to boundary delineation. For this reason, cities are not useful units for market analyses. In many cases, however, certain city government agencies are involved in data collection activi-ties that may be useful to marketers.

Congressional Districts

Congressional districts are established locally and approved by the federal government. They are typically delineated by means of political compromise and do not correspond well with any other geographic unit. Although the **US Census Bureau** reports data for congressional districts, limited data are collected at the congressional district level. In addition, the boundaries tend to change over time, making these units not par-ticularly suitable for marketing purposes.

US Census Bureau
The federal agency responsible for the decennial census and other data collection activities

State Legislative Districts

State legislative districts have characteristics similar to those of con-gressional districts. They are drawn up by states primarily on the basis of political compromise. Although the Census Bureau reports data for state legislative districts, few data are collected specifically for these units. Further, their boundaries are subject to periodic change. For these reasons, they are not useful as units for purposes of healthcare marketing.

School Districts

School districts are established for the administration of local educa-tional systems. Such districts theoretically reflect the distribution of school-aged children in the population, but factors such as the migra-tion of students into and out of a district may play a role in determining the configuration of school districts in a community. Although school districts may be useful sources of data in developing population projections, few statistics are generated for this unit of geography, thereby limiting the usefulness of this source for marketing.

Statistical Units

Statistical areas are established to allow government agencies to collect and report data in an efficient and consistent manner. The guidelines for establishing most statistical units are promulgated by the federal government. The following are the most important statistical units in marketing.

Regions

The federal government establishes regions for statistical purposes by combining states into logical groupings. The Census Bureau has grouped the 50 states into four regions—Northeast, Midwest, South, and West—on the basis of geographic proximity and economic and social homogeneity. Although this unit is seldom used for marketing purposes, some federal health agencies report statistics at the regional level. (The term *regional* is alternatively used to refer to a group of counties or states delineated for some other purpose than data compilation [e.g., the Delta Regional Authority].)

Divisions

For statistical purposes, the federal government divides the nation's four regions into nine divisions. Each division includes several states, providing a finer breakdown of the nation's geography. Divisions are seldom used as a basis for health services marketing. The following list breaks down the nine census divisions by region.

Northeast Region
1. New England Division: Connecticut, Maine, Massachusetts, New Hampshire, Rhode Island, Vermont
2. Middle Atlantic Division: New Jersey, New York, Pennsylvania

Midwest Region
3. East North Central Division: Illinois, Indiana, Michigan, Ohio, Wisconsin
4. West North Central Division: Iowa, Kansas, Minnesota, Missouri, Nebraska, North Dakota, South Dakota

(continued)

South Region

5. South Atlantic Division: Delaware, District of Columbia, Florida, Georgia, Maryland, North Carolina, South Carolina, Virginia, West Virginia

6. East South Central Division: Alabama, Kentucky, Mississippi, Tennessee

7. West South Central Division: Arkansas, Louisiana, Oklahoma, Texas

West Region

8. Mountain Division: Arizona, Colorado, Idaho, Montana, Nevada, New Mexico, Utah, Wyoming

9. Pacific Division: Alaska, California, Hawaii, Oregon, Washington

Metropolitan Statistical Areas

The federal government delineates metropolitan statistical areas (MSAs) as a means of standardizing the boundaries of cities and urbanized areas. Because states have differing criteria for incorporating cities, the MSA concept provides a mechanism for creating comparable statistical areas. An MSA includes a central city, a central county, and any contiguous counties that are logically included in the urbanized area. Data available on MSAs are increasing, and this unit is often used to define market areas.

Census Tracts

Census tracts are small statistical subdivisions of a county established by the Census Bureau for data collection purposes. In theory, census tracts contain relatively homogeneous populations ranging in size from 1,500 to 8,000. For many purposes, the census tract is the ideal unit for compiling market data. It is large enough to be a meaningful geographic unit and small enough to contribute to a fine-grained view of larger areas. The Census Bureau collects extensive data at the census-tract level, and relatively current data are available through the American Community Survey. Limited health data are available at the census-tract level, although some government agencies do collect and report data for this unit of geography.

Census Block Groups

Census tracts are subdivided into census block groups that include approximately 1,000 residents. A tract is composed of a number of block groups, each containing several blocks. The block group provides an even finer picture of a community than does the tract level, although fewer data elements are likely to be compiled at the block-group level. Few health data are available at the level of the census block group. This is the smallest unit of census geography for which the American Community Survey reports data.

Census Blocks

Census block groups are subdivided into census blocks, the smallest unit of census geography. The term *block* comes from the four-sided shape formed from the perpendicular intersection of four streets, although some other visible feature (e.g., railroad track, stream) or invisible feature (e.g., city limits) sometimes serves as a boundary. Census blocks tend to be the most homogeneous of any unit of census geography, and the average block houses approximately 30 persons. Virtually no health data and only limited demographic data are available for census blocks.

Zip Code Tabulation Areas

Zip code tabulation areas (ZCTAs) were developed by the Census Bureau for tabulating summary statistics from the 2000 census. ZCTAs are generalized representations of US Postal Service zip code service areas. They are created by aggregating the Census 2000 blocks (whose addresses use a given zip code) into a ZCTA, and then that zip code is assigned a ZCTA code. These units approximate Postal Service five-digit zip codes found in a given area. The Census Bureau's intent was to create zip code–like areas that would remain more stable from **census** to census. Today, most population and housing data collected by the Census Bureau are available at the ZCTA level.

Census
A complete count of the people residing in a specific place at a specific time

Functional Units

Healthcare marketers use other geographic units that are often more suited to business development activities than are political or statistical units.

Zip Codes

Unlike the geographic units previously discussed, zip codes are not formal government entities. Their boundaries are set by the Postal Service and are subject to change as population shifts occur or the needs of the Postal Service dictate. This lack of stability means zip codes have

(continued)

limited value for historical analyses or for tracking phenomena over a long period. Further, zip codes seldom coincide with census tracts or other political or statistical boundaries, making the synthesis of data for various geographies extremely difficult. Zip codes tend to be much larger than census tracts, sometimes including tens of thousands of residents.

Nevertheless, the zip code is a useful unit for defining the market areas of smaller physician practices, smaller hospitals, and even specialty niches for larger health systems. **Commercial data vendors** compile a great deal of information at the zip-code level. More important, healthcare organizations typically acquire a zip code for virtually every consumer they come in contact with, making this unit an accessible geographic identifier linked to every customer record.

Commercial data vendor
A private organization that collects, compiles, analyzes, and disseminates data

Areas of Dominant Influence

Taken from media advertising, the **area of dominant influence** (ADI) refers to the geographic territory (typically a group of counties) over which a form of media (e.g., television, newspaper) maintains predominance. ADI is useful when healthcare marketers are interested in media promotions and want to determine the reach of a particular marketing campaign.

Area of dominant influence (ADI)
The geographic territory covered by a particular form of media

Natural Regions

Some areas are considered "natural" regions, as opposed to the official regions established by the Census Bureau. These natural regions are geographically based areas defined in terms of some unifying characteristic or characteristics. The two major examples are Appalachia (which includes parts of several states that share the Smoky Mountains and associated terrain) and the Mississippi River delta (which includes parts of several states that are in or adjacent to the floodplain of the Mississippi River). In both of these cases, the regions exhibit distinct physical features and cultures that set them apart from surrounding areas. Appalachian culture is built around coal mining and hardscrabble farming, while the Mississippi delta culture is built around "plantation" agriculture. The conditions of existence in both natural regions create a lifestyle with distinct characteristics. These two regions have been singled out by the federal government because of their high levels of poverty and lack of resources. Other less expansive natural regions might be identified across the country.

Population Segment

A second way of defining a market is in terms of a population segment or some component of the population. Marketers often report that the "market for Product X" is this or that market segment, and they are typically not referring to a geographically defined market area but to a more nebulous market defined in terms of demographics, psychographics, or some other population characteristic. Examples of markets defined in this manner include active seniors, women of childbearing age, and psychographically defined segments such as millennials.

Markets conceptualized in terms of population segments can be broad or narrow. For example, a market defined as "seniors" cuts a broad swath through the US population. On the other hand, a market defined as "seniors who require nursing home care" is a much narrower segment of the population. Similarly, the nature of the market could depend on whether one is speaking of a broad range of services (e.g., comprehensive inpatient services) or a narrowly defined individual service (e.g., outpatient eating disorder treatment).

Consumer Demand

A third way of delineating a market is from the perspective of the service itself; in other words, the market is defined by consumer **demand**. For example, healthcare organizations may seek to identify geographic areas that have large concentrations of potential patients for a particular service. Geographically defined and demographically defined markets start with the general characteristics of the population and work down to the population's specific healthcare needs, whereas demand-based markets start with a particular need or service and work backward to identify the relevant population of consumers. Examples of markets defined in this manner are populations in need of geriatric services or behavioral health services. A hospital may consider nearly the entire population in its defined service area as part of the market for hospital services, whereas a home health agency may envision a narrowly defined subsegment of the population as its potential market. Although markets defined according to consumer demand may coincide with established boundaries, they are just as likely to cut across geographic boundaries.

Demand
The extent to which a target population needs or wants a product or service

Opportunities

A fourth way of looking at markets is the existence of healthcare opportunities in a given area. A geographic area might be viewed with interest if there is a shortage of providers or lack of facilities in that area. An area characterized by a lack of competition is obviously attractive to an opportunistic organization. In other cases, the number of providers may be adequate, but their fragmentation may offer an opportunity for an organization that can appropriately package its services.

Areas (or populations) characterized by a high level of unmet health-care needs may present additional opportunities. An area (or a population) may appear to need a certain level or type of service, but, for whatever reason, the service is not available. For example, according to a demand model, a specified population should record a certain number of mammograms per year based on its size and composition. If the number of mammograms performed annually is significantly lower, this population may have an unmet need. Note that many unmet needs exist in populations with limited ability to pay for services. Depending on the type of organization performing the market research, these populations may or may not be appropriate target markets.

Similarly, opportunities may exist in areas where a gap analysis indicates a service shortfall or a mismatch between needs and services. The number of physicians or hospital beds that a given population can support is usually determined using various computer models. If the number of physicians and/or hospital beds located in the area falls below the expected number, there may be opportunities in that market.

Markets Without Walls

The fifth method of defining a market is embodied by the phrase "a market without walls." Certain markets are no longer defined by geographic units or population segments. For example, the markets for contact lenses, health food supplements, and certain home-testing products have become less dependent on location. These products may be purchased by mail order, through television shopping services, or via the Internet. In addition, the advent of telemedicine allows a specialist in one location to receive electronically transmitted test results for a patient in a different location. Patients and their doctors can interact via the Internet, thereby diminishing the importance of geographically defined markets.

Delineating Market Areas

Geographic Boundaries

If the market area is defined in geographic terms, the first step in developing an understanding of the market is delineating its boundaries. This defined geography then serves as the basis for profiling the market area population. (Note that not-for-profit healthcare organizations may refer to service area rather than market area, although the terms mean the same geography.) A number of methods can be used to specify the market area, and the method depends on the type of organization and the service involved.

Current Customer Distribution/Point of Origin

For a healthcare organization, the most direct means of delineating the market area is to determine the point of origin of current customers (e.g., by county, zip code, address). This information typically can be easily extracted from internal records and can be summarized at the appropriate level of geography; customer residences can be plotted on a map if desired to illustrate their spatial distribution. This exercise often allows the organization to infer additional information about their customers. It is not unusual, in fact, for an organization to be surprised by where their customers originate.

A growing number of healthcare providers are automating this process, either by purchasing mapping software or accessing online marketing systems that facilitate strategic marketing activities. The geographic area (e.g., zip code, county) from which a pre-specified percentage of customers are drawn may be designated as the provider's market area. As a rule of thumb, the area from which 75 to 80 percent of customers are drawn represents the core market area. (Although it may be worthwhile in some cases to target the area covered by 100 percent of the organization's customers, this is usually not very practical.)

Market areas can exist at different levels; for example, primary, secondary, and even tertiary market areas might be identified. The area that accounts for 60 percent of patients could be considered the primary market area, for example, and the area that accounts for the next 25 percent of patients might be considered the secondary service area. The area accounting for the remaining 15 percent of patients would be considered the tertiary market area. By taking this approach, the healthcare organization is able to develop a more refined view of the distribution of its customers. This information helps the marketer craft campaigns that address the respective needs of those in the primary, secondary, and tertiary markets.

Multiple market areas may exist for organizations that provide multiple services. Typically, the market area for general hospital services is likely to be different from that for facilities with more specialized offerings. Similarly, the market area for the hospital's obstetrics services may differ significantly in size and configuration from the market area for trauma care or orthopedic surgery. An urgent care center may be more dependent on residents who drive from other communities rather than on residents who live near the facility.

Delineating the market area in this manner assumes that customers are coming from their residences when they seek care. Although this assumption is correct more often than not, the location analysis should also account for customers who do not come from their residences but from other facilities (e.g., nursing homes) or from industrial or commercial sites (Pol and Thomas 2013). It is also important to consider the role of health insurance plans in steering customers to a facility. It may be that plan provisions require the use of network providers, which make customers' geographic origin a less relevant factor in delineating the market area.

Ideal Markets

In some situations, the existing market area may not match the organization's objectives. It could be that the characteristics of the residents in the existing market area have changed or that the organization's clientele may have moved away from the facility. The mobility of many US residents may mean that long-time customers have moved out of the service area and new potential customers have moved in. For example, a physician practice providing chronic care to the elderly may find that, over the years, the senior residents in the community have been replaced with young families who have limited or no need for the practice's services. In the case of an inner-city hospital whose clientele has moved to the suburbs but continues to patronize the facility, the question the provider must ask is, Is the existing market area appropriate to use as a framework for promoting services?

Prospective Markets

There may be times when it is necessary to delineate a market area for a service not yet offered. For a new service or a new location, data on customers' points of origin are, obviously, not yet available. One approach to work around that is to determine the maximum distance or driving time potential consumers would be willing to travel for a given health service. Computer software is available to perform this task, although in rapidly changing areas, driving times can become significantly different over a relatively short time.

Delineating prospective boundaries is much more difficult and usually requires the use of multiple techniques. One approach may be to determine the residential distribution of customers who use similar services. If another organization is offering the same or similar services, its market area boundaries might be used as a guide. Distance and/or driving-time data may be evaluated as well. However, a more indirect approach may be required because the service in question is new to the area. Data on the same service in a different market area may be available through professional networks. These data could help establish time/distance parameters. Surveys of potential consumers of these services (e.g., physicians and patients) may also provide valuable time/distance information. Case Study 4.1 describes an effort to capture an emerging market.

Once delineated, market area boundaries must be continually monitored for change. Traffic patterns and driving times change, and the entrance or exit of competition may significantly alter market area boundaries over a short time. Changes of taste and preference regarding physician services (e.g., increased interest in alternative therapies) or changes in patient type

CASE STUDY 4.1
Capturing an Emerging Market

The growing racial and ethnic diversity of the US population seems to overwhelm some healthcare providers. Health systems that are used to providing one-size-fits-all care are now faced with patient populations that are increasingly heterogeneous and whose members often have perspectives on healthcare different from those of the providers. However, if a provider can adapt to the needs of this growing market, a lot of opportunities will present themselves.

For example, promoting the opening of a birthing center to a community is challenging enough, but it becomes even more daunting when the residents speak 40 different languages. One hospital in an urban midwestern community not only took on this challenge but also turned it into one of the hospital's greatest marketing successes.

Thirteen hospitals within a ten-mile radius of the primary service area provided obstetrics services to the community. An estimated 24,274 women of childbearing age lived in the primary service area. Another 134,055 women of childbearing age lived in the secondary service area. A service area analysis identified the following ethnic breakdown for the population: 72.2 percent white (including 18.9 percent Hispanic), 11.2 percent Asian or Pacific Islander, 9.1 percent other, 7.0 percent African American, and 0.5 percent American Indian. The percentage of Asians in the service area was quadruple the state and national averages, and the percentage of Hispanics was double the state and national figures. The racial and ethnic breakdown, however, failed to convey the unique features of the service area. Among the white population, recent immigrants from the Middle East and Eastern Europe supplemented the Hispanic population. The Asian immigrants came predominantly from Korea, Pakistan, India, and the Philippines.

To more narrowly define the major ethnic breakdown of the childbearing market, obstetrics discharge data by physician were reviewed. Physicians were asked to identify the major ethnic and cultural groups of their patients. The following major groups using obstetrics services were identified: Indian, Pakistani, and Middle Eastern (29 percent); Korean (23 percent); Hispanic (13 percent); and Assyrian (6 percent). Research into cultural considerations for these groups identified a significant subgroup of Indian, Pakistani, and Middle Eastern patients who were Muslim. On the basis of this information, four target ethnic

(continued)

markets were defined: Korean, Middle Eastern, Muslim (Middle Eastern, Pakistani, and Indian), and Hispanic (Mexican, Puerto Rican, and Cuban).

To increase market share for obstetrics services at the hospital, marketing strategies were developed to raise awareness of the new family birthing center within these ethnic communities. To achieve this goal in a highly competitive market, the following objectives were adopted:

1. Differentiate services from those of competitors by means of
   - graphic images and color coding for directional signage in the facility;
   - multilingual and multicultural physicians (men and women), nursing staff, cultural liaisons, and interpreters;
   - culturally diverse artwork throughout the facility;
   - large state-of-the-art labor/delivery/recovery/postpartum rooms with hot tubs and space for family members;
   - ethnic menus, along with microwaves and refrigerators for patient use;
   - childbirth preparation classes taught in Spanish, Korean, Arabic, and Hindi by native speakers;
   - a family-centered program of care; and
   - superior quality measures.
2. Enhance the hospital's marketing presence through
   - creating a new maternity services brand for the hospital, featuring the graphic image of infant footprints;
   - aggressively marketing and promoting the new features and benefits of the hospital's maternity services; and
   - reinforcing the hospital's unique position as a provider of culturally sensitive, family-centered maternity care.
3. On the basis of these objectives, the following marketing initiatives were identified for the hospital:
   - Tailor market research to build knowledge and understanding of each ethnic group.
   - Implement culturally appropriate advertising campaigns for each targeted group, including native-language posters/fliers, newspaper ads, billboards, and radio ads.
   - Develop a comprehensive guide to hospital services in Spanish, Arabic, Hindi, and Korean.

- Launch aggressive media-relations efforts to promote the hospital's unique commitment to meeting the needs of its "neighborhood of nations."
- Implement a comprehensive community-relations program.
- Tailor a series of grand-opening events to each ethnic market, with ethnic menus, appropriate dignitaries, and entertainment.
- Develop a strong community presence for customized ethnic maternity services, with photos of the physical space and amenities in the hospital newsletter distributed to 125,000 households in the primary and secondary service areas.
- Distribute fliers to the religious institutions in the target market.

Source: Adapted from Noonan and Savolaine (2001).

Case Study Discussion Questions

1. What changes taking place in American society make a one-size-fits-all healthcare system obsolete?
2. What particular challenge did the community hospital face?
3. What marketing techniques were used to address the needs of a diverse population?
4. In what ways did the hospital disseminate its message to the community (rather than relying on impersonal advertising)?
5. What indicators could the hospital have used to evaluate the impact of these marketing efforts?

(e.g., increased demand for outpatient services) must also be monitored to determine their effect on market area boundaries. Exhibit 4.2 presents evidence of the existing geographic-based disparities in the use of health services.

Nongeographic Boundaries

Identifying non–geographically based markets involves a potentially more complicated process. Typically, these markets are defined in terms of size and composition, and the geographic area provides only the context. Thus, a national market would consider only the geographic boundaries of the United States as a framework within which to identify submarkets. An example would be the population of women who gave birth in the previous six months. With respect to a given service (e.g., mental health services for

EXHIBIT 4.2
Geographic
Variations in
Health Services
Utilization

Utilization
A measure of the
extent/level of
health services
use

Healthcare analysts and policymakers realized long ago that significant variation exists in the **utilization** of health services from community to community in the United States. As early as the 1970s, research revealed that the rate of procedures performed in different communities—even in adjacent states—varied to a degree not explained by population differences. The procedure rate could range from 10 percent of the patient population in some markets to 50 percent in others. These studies suggested that the volume of health services delivered was less a function of disease prevalence but more a reflection of the characteristics of the medical community and the practice patterns of local physicians.

One of the first studies to compare health services utilization was conducted by Wennberg, Freeman, and Culp (1987). This seminal study examined patterns of care in the cities of Boston and New Haven (Connecticut). Although the two cities were similar in terms of the factors that *should* determine the use of health services, they differed dramatically on almost every indicator of utilization. The hospital admission rate, for example, was nearly twice as high in Boston as it was in New Haven. Further, residents of Boston were much more likely to be hospitalized for various acute and chronic conditions than were residents of New Haven. The average annual per capita expenditure on healthcare in Boston was twice that of New Haven. However, the comparative utilization patterns were not always consistent. The rates of performance for certain procedures were much higher in Boston, but for others, they were much higher in New Haven. The findings from this study have subsequently been reinforced by numerous additional studies.

A number of factors account for these seemingly inexplicable differences. A major factor is the variation in physician practice patterns from community to community. In some communities, treating a problem with surgery is standard practice; in other communities, the standard calls for less invasive treatment. In some communities, conventional medical wisdom calls for hospitalization for certain diagnostic tests and procedures, whereas in others, handling such cases on an outpatient basis is customary.

Other factors contributing to different utilization rates include the relative supply of facilities and services. There is pressure, for example, to fill hospital beds if they are available and to use medical technology in which an organization has invested. In contrast to other industries, competition in healthcare often drives up both utilization levels and costs, thereby accounting for an additional degree of variation. Even the presence of a medical school may influence the level of utilization and the types of procedures performed. Increasingly, the level of managed care penetration is a significant factor influencing utilization rates.

Given these variations, how does an analyst determine the appropriate level of utilization? Is the reported level of utilization high or low? What should be realistically expected? Of course, one way to address this question is to use a standard rate of utilization, such as the rates developed by the National Center for Health Statistics. These rates provide useful benchmarks, but because most analyses focus on local markets, how appropriate are they for the market in question? There is no easy answer to this dilemma. The analyst must be able to gain enough knowledge about the local healthcare environment to make reasonable assessments about the appropriate level of utilization.

postpartum depression), the size of the **effective market** can be **estimated** at the national level.

When identifying market area boundaries on the basis of the location of non–geographically defined markets, the situation becomes more complicated. In an ideal world, the mere presence or absence of a target population (e.g., active seniors, women of childbearing age, Latinos, baby boomers) would be adequate. However, situations are seldom this clear-cut, and a non–geographically defined market is likely to be interspersed with populations that have other characteristics. In other words, marketers seldom find an either/or situation but find that market concentrations are more a matter of degree. Thus, measures of the concentration of the target population in a geographic area need to be developed.

The emphasis in data analysis may be placed on identifying areas with high or low concentrations of persons susceptible to certain illnesses or areas with shortages or surpluses of healthcare providers. For example, if a healthcare provider is interested in geographic areas with high concentrations of older persons, several procedures can be used. Suppose the larger market is a particular state, and the substate markets of interest are counties in that state. The goal is to identify the counties with the highest concentrations of persons aged 65 or older. The percentages of the population aged 65 to 74 and 75 or older is used as the basis for index construction. The indicator chosen depends on a number of factors, including the nature of the population, the type of service, and/or the marketing methodology being used. Ultimately, use of a methodology that combines both the number and percentage of seniors may be appropriate.

Effective market
The portion of the potential business within a market area believed to be suitable for cultivation

Estimate
The calculation of a figure in a current or past period using a statistical method

When viewing markets from a nongeographic perspective, a different identification strategy is used. The point of reference is a larger population, such as the United States or a region within the boundaries of the United States. The purpose of the exercise is to find concentrations of persons with certain characteristics in subgroups of the population. For example, if health insurance plans want to identify the segments of the population that had the highest rates of uninsureds, they might examine the composition of the nation's uninsured population.

An additional way of defining non–geographically based markets is in terms of consumer propensity to obtain a particular good or service. Market analysts in other industries have long identified population segments on the basis of their willingness, ability, and/or interest in a particular product. Although healthcare services cannot be viewed in exactly the same manner as these other products, there is increasing interest in identifying potential markets in terms of their propensity to be affected by a particular condition or to use/need a particular service. This approach is often based on demographic or psychographic profiling. If, for example, a propensity score of 100 indicates average use of a particular service, a score of 200 for a specific population segment suggests a propensity to use this service that is twice the average for the total population. On the other hand, a propensity score of 50 indicates a use rate that is half the average.

Profiling Markets

Primary data
Data generated directly through surveys, focus groups, observational methods, and other techniques

Once geographic boundaries for a market area or the parameters for a non–geographically defined market have been established, key attributes of the population within those boundaries can be specified. The development of a market profile involves collecting and analyzing detailed information about the market area(s) in question. Any and all characteristics relevant to service provision must be catalogued on the basis of whatever **primary data** and **secondary data** sources are available.

Market Size

Secondary data
Data collected through primary data collection and used for some other purpose, such as market research

Markets can be distinguished by several different dimensions. The first dimension is market size. *Size* here refers to the absolute number of potential consumers in a specific market area. The marketer typically begins by determining the total population within the market area. This figure indicates the universe of potential customers and must be refined to reflect the portion of the population relevant for the analysis. This refined assessment of the market would include only segments that represent prospective customers for the organization or its specific services.

Market Composition

The second dimension addressed in the profile is market **composition** or the makeup of the defined population. Composition is usually framed in terms of the number of persons in a particular area who have certain characteristics (i.e., demographic traits, socioeconomic attributes, psychographic profile). This profile should include characteristics such as marital status, household structure, educational level, and income. More detailed data on economic characteristics (e.g., labor force characteristics, housing values) may also be considered.

The demographic analysis is often accompanied by an assessment of the psychographic characteristics of the market area population. Information on the lifestyle categories of the target audience can be used to determine the likely health priorities and behavior of a population subgroup. Consumer attitudes are also likely to be considered as a component of **psychographic (or lifestyle) segmentation**. The attitudes of consumers in a market area have considerable influence on the demand for almost all types of health services.

During the profiling process, insurance coverage is typically assessed. The emphasis on insurance coverage varies depending on the nature of the organization. The payer mix of a market area and of an organization is a main consideration in the financial viability of the organization. The implementation of the Affordable Care Act (ACA) has had a major effect on patterns of health insurance coverage, and understanding the implications of this act for a defined market is essential.

Although many providers attempt to limit the number of self-pay patients they serve, there is a multibillion-dollar market for elective services that are not typically covered by insurance plans. The market for **vanity services**—such as facelifts, tummy tucks, and other cosmetic procedures—is primarily driven by patients who do not have insurance that covers these procedures. Another example is the **alternative therapy** industry, which emerged to challenge mainstream medicine and depends almost entirely on out-of-pocket expenditures by its customers.

Community type is also a consideration when collecting baseline data on the market. The dominant community type within the market area—whether urban, suburban, or rural—has important implications for health status and health behavior. Consumer attitudes are likely to differ between the various community types, and the existence of submarkets within the market area may be a complicating factor when developing a marketing plan. The service area for a hospital serving a major metropolitan area, for example, includes all three community types.

Composition
Characteristics exhibited by a population, such as demographics, lifestyle patterns, and payer categories

Psychographic (or lifestyle) segmentation
The process of subdividing a population into groups of like individuals on the basis of their psychographic designation

Vanity services
Health services, usually elective, intended to improve physical appearance or functioning

Alternative therapy
Therapeutic modalities used as alternatives or as complements to conventional allopathic medicine

Health Status

The health status of the market area population is the third dimension considered in a market profile. The level of morbidity in a population is a major concern for health services planners. **Incidence** and **prevalence** rates are likely to be important in the marketing analysis. The health status category includes measures of morbidity related to health status and disability indicators. To the extent possible, planners need to project future rates of incidence and prevalence to plan for anticipated developments in the medical arena.

The health status of the market area population defines the range of health service needs that is likely to exist. The services healthcare organizations provide are ideally designed to address the health problems that characterize the population of the market area. These health conditions should indicate the segments of the market to be targeted and the needs of the population the organization hopes to meet. For not-for-profit hospitals, a provision in the ACA mandates that a tax-exempt hospital periodically determine the unmet health needs of its service area.

A key objective in assessing health status is to determine the level of morbidity among the population of the market area. In particular, the amount of sickness in various categories (e.g., acute conditions, chronic conditions, reproductive health issues) must be determined. This allows researchers to profile the population in terms of the types of health conditions that are common. This provides not only a picture of health status for the target population but also a basis for calculating the organization's market share (in the absence of other market share data). Ultimately, these health conditions are converted into demand estimates for various types of services.

The primary challenge in determining health status is identifying and measuring the level of morbidity. Morbid conditions can be identified in a number of ways, and no single method adequately serves this purpose. The use of a variety of methods is required because, in the United States, no centralized registry of morbid conditions nor a systematic process exists for the comprehensive collection of morbidity data. Although the **Centers for Disease Control and Prevention (CDC)** has introduced the technological capability for reporting selected health conditions, no such mechanisms are available for the majority of health problems.

Health Services Demand

The fourth dimension involves translating health conditions affecting a population into demand for health services. The types of diseases and other health problems exhibited by the market area population should indicate the types of services needed. A market's need for childhood immunizations, for example, can be translated into demand for a specific number of health department clinics and clinic personnel. Similarly, the vanity service wants for

---

Incidence
The number of new cases of a disease, disability, or other health-related phenomenon in a population during a specified period; used to generate an incidence rate

Prevalence
The total number of cases of a disease, disability, or other health-related condition at a particular point in time; used to calculate a prevalence rate

Centers for Disease Control and Prevention (CDC)
The federal agency charged with monitoring morbidity and mortality in the United States

facelift or laser eye surgery, for example, can be translated into demand for plastic surgeons and ophthalmic surgeons.

In many cases, actual data on the market may not be available, and estimates of need must be calculated. Fortunately, a number of models have been developed for estimating and projecting the demand for a service using data on population characteristics and known utilization rates. These modeling techniques require an understanding of the service area and the manner in which these models operate. Modeled data are never as good as actual data, but the estimates generated by methodologically sound models are adequate for most purposes. In any case, modeled data must be used if the level of need is being projected for some future period.

Typically, the level of need is expressed in terms of a percentage of the population or a rate of some type. For example, calculations may reveal that 20 percent of the adult population is affected by a clinically identifiable emotional condition or that the crude birthrate is 15 births per 1,000 population. The most common measures of need would be the prevalence and incidence rates epidemiologists and public health officials use. These measures of the level of morbidity provide the baseline data on which the rest of the analysis depends.

Once the level of need has been determined for the defined market area, the number of potential cases in that area can be estimated. A high prevalence rate by itself does not ensure a meaningful market. Healthcare is a numbers game, and a critical mass is needed to support any service.

The extent to which the identified needs are being met is indicated, at least partially, by the health behavior of the market area population. Health behavior includes both formal utilization of health services and informal actions designed to prevent health problems and to maintain, enhance, or promote health. In terms of formal activities, potential indicators include hospital admissions, patient days, average lengths of stay, use of nonhospital facilities, physician office visits, visits to nonphysician practitioners, and drug use. In recent years, the use of freestanding medical facilities and alternative therapies has also become an important indicator.

Availability of Resources

The fifth dimension considers the availability of healthcare resources. Resources include existing healthcare personnel, facilities, and programs. The types of resources identified depend on the nature of the organization. A general hospital, for example, would want to determine the availability of resources comparable to its own—whether they are offered by a competing hospital or another healthcare organization. A medical specialty group, on the other hand, would be interested in the much narrower range of available resources in its specialty area.

Of the resources available to the community, healthcare organizations should hone in on those that are considered competition. In the past, hospitals knew other hospitals were their competitors, cardiologists knew other cardiologists were their competitors, and so forth. The environment has changed, and today, competition can take a number of forms. Many types of nonhospital organizations now compete with hospitals. These competitors are not always external to the hospital; in some cases, members of the hospital's own medical staff may set up rival services. The boundaries of specialty practice have become blurred as aggressive specialists seek to expand the range of services they offer. Purveyors of alternative therapies have also emerged to challenge mainstream physicians on many fronts.

In profiling the market area's resources and competition, considering the temporal dimension is also important. Whether determining the needs of the target market or identifying competing services, marketers must take the three time horizons—past, present, and future—into account. Although the current characteristics of the market area are a good starting point, historical trends must also be understood. Is the population growing or declining? Are the characteristics of the population today different from those five years ago? Is the number of competitors increasing? The most important time frame, however, is the future—whether two, five, or ten years down the road. The market area profile should project the future characteristics of the population, the future health services needs of that population, and likely future developments of competing organizations.

From Mass Market to Micromarket

When the healthcare industry first began to recognize the importance of marketing, the total population was considered the market for most services. Hospitals, for example, believed they provided all services to all people. They did not attempt to distinguish segments of the population and made only crude, geography-based distinctions between markets.

Media
Print or electronic modes of delivering a promotional message

Message
The information the marketer is trying to convey; the content of a promotional piece

Healthcare organizations operating in this mode typically take a mass marketing approach. *Mass marketing* involves developing generic messages and broadcasting them in a wide, untargeted manner to the entire service area. No attempt is made to target specific audiences, identify likely best customers, or tailor the message to a particular subgroup. This approach involves the use of mass **media** (e.g., newspaper, radio, television, Internet) to blanket the market area. The **message** has to be general, and it typically touts the merits of the organization rather than specific services.

As healthcare entered the marketing era, healthcare marketers adopted target marketing techniques. *Target marketing* involves the identification and subsequent cultivation of segments of the market area population that have certain attributes. These segments of the population may reside in a geographic area that is being emphasized, may be demographic or psychographic subsegments of the population, or may be individuals otherwise classified as prospective customers.

The intent of target marketing is to deliver a particular message to a particular audience to attract members of this segment of the population as customers. Target marketing is an efficient and cost-effective means of communicating a message to the target audience. By eliminating irrelevant segments of the population, marketing effort and expense are minimized. Target marketing, thus, offers the marketer more "bang for the buck." Although target marketing typically involves the use of traditional media, communication channels can be tailored to reach the target audience. Thus, wide-circulation newspapers and network television would be eschewed in favor of special-interest publications, radio stations appealing to specific audiences, and cable channels with certain viewer demographics.

In targeting audiences for specific goods and services, certain established rules should be applied. Target markets must be amenable to rating in terms of their potential, the markets must be realistic in size, the targeted customers must be reachable, and the targeted customers must have some minimum level of response potential. Assuming that the market is of adequate size, another consideration besides the potential number of cases is the geographic distribution of prospective customers within the market area. The importance of customer distribution varies with the type of service and the characteristics of the population. Some services are supported by a local population and others by a more far-flung population. On the other hand, some populations are much more mobile than others or are otherwise more or less sensitive to travel times and/or distances.

In recent years, many healthcare organizations have gone a step further and adopted a micromarketing approach. *Micromarketing* involves identifying and soliciting specific individuals or households. Identification of prospective customers at this level is usually not necessary to support healthcare marketing campaigns. However, in some situations, it may be more efficient and cost-effective to identify the individuals or households that are the best prospects for a particular service. For example, if an ophthalmic surgeon has determined that individuals with certain demographic and psychographic traits are better candidates for laser eye surgery than other consumers with other traits, the most effective approach may be narrow—contact people with those specific attributes directly through direct mail or telemarketing—rather than broad. Similarly, a hospital implementing a major donor drive may target only households that have the resources and propensity to make a substantial contribution.

Determining the Effectiveness of the Market

In healthcare, the potential market for a service may not correspond to the population that actually uses that service. Because the target population's level of need for a particular health service may or may not reflect its level of interest in that service, the best approach may be to determine the extent to which members of the target population want the service. Although conducting a preliminary analysis of the market area population and developing an estimate of the level of interest in a particular service may suffice, many situations require primary research. Ideally, no new program or service should be introduced without a consumer survey, and the newer the service or less familiar the market, the greater the need for primary research. Many new programs have failed because the target population's actual level of interest was much lower in reality than on paper.

Ascertaining the level of interest may be relatively straightforward. Market surveys often query consumers about their interest in the availability of a service and whether they would use the service if it were available. Healthcare marketers found early on, though, that these survey responses have to be carefully qualified. Typically, respondents express an interest in any new service that appears to benefit them specifically or the community generally. However, when their likelihood of using the service is qualified by introducing location or price considerations, the level of interest may change. For example, one survey found that a large portion of consumers in a target area were interested in a hospital-sponsored fitness program. When the likely location was disclosed, interest waned somewhat. It waned even further when the proposed fee schedule was introduced. Obviously, the more elective the service under consideration, the more important these qualifiers become. Factors such as payer mix and the existing competition must be taken into consideration in the determination of the effective market.

Payer mix
The combination of payment sources characterizing a population; the basis for payer segmentation

Payer
In healthcare, the individual or organization responsible for medical expenses

Reimbursement
In healthcare, compensation paid by a third-party payer to a provider or customer for the cost of services rendered/received

Payer Mix

A factor that has become increasingly important in developing a market profile is the consumer's ability to pay for health services. The analyst must determine the potential **payer mix** of the target population and estimate the expected level of **reimbursement** for a particular service. Given that different **payers** (e.g., commercial insurers, Medicare, Medicaid) offer different levels of reimbursement, the effective payer mix ultimately determines the actual level of payment.

The two bases for determining a target population's ability to pay are household income and type of health insurance coverage. For major health problems (i.e., problems requiring hospitalization or intensive services), the level of insurance coverage is the more important consideration. Employer-sponsored commercial insurance generally affords the highest level of reimbursement. Other forms of private insurance (e.g., Blue Cross) are also desirable. Although payments under Medicare and Medicaid are essentially guaranteed, reimbursement rates under these government insurance programs have historically been lower than those of commercial insurance plans. For elective services, the patient's income is usually more important than the type of insurance coverage.

In some areas, underinsurance is an issue, especially during an economic downturn. On the other hand, certain segments of the population may have insurance coverage, but copayment provisions, restrictions on benefits, and/or limitations on reimbursement may reduce the coverage's value. The emergence of managed care as a force in the market has obviously changed the playing field. Since the implementation of the ACA, millions of additional Americans have obtained health insurance. This development is affecting various market areas differently, so it is important to determine the extent to which a specific market has been affected by increased health plan enrollment—either through a health insurance exchange or Medicaid expansion.

Competition

The market potential for health services must be adjusted to take existing competitors into account. Except in rare cases where a market is not served at all, competitors in various guises inevitably exist. Indeed, the proliferation of competitors has been a major development in US healthcare. Some of these competitors may already be entrenched within the target area or population. Others may be just entering the market to challenge institutions that are already active there.

Regardless of the nature of the **competition**, the available market must be adjusted to account for it. A family practitioner opening an office in a community may face competition from other family practitioners, other primary care providers, public health clinics, urgent care centers, government-sponsored clinics, and even alternative therapists. A realistic assessment of the potential market must consider all of these factors.

Competition
The effort of two or more organizations acting independently to secure the business of the same customers

One method of assessing competition involves calculating the organization's market share and, if possible, the shares for each of its competitors. The numerator in these calculations is the number of cases recorded for the organization (or its competitors), and the denominator is the total instances of that phenomenon for the market area. Internal records on procedures, discharges, and/or diagnoses may serve as the numerators for market share calculations. Denominators may be derived from data made available in response to data reporting requirements. For example, hospital discharge data are often collected by state health departments and aggregated at geographic levels, such as the county level. A simple calculation divides the number of discharges from Hospital X in County Y by the total number of discharges in County Y. See Exhibit 4.3 for an example of a market share calculation.

In the absence of a clearinghouse for utilization data, another way to gather data for rate denominators is to generate estimates of the number of procedures and discharges using population and incidence information. For example, the number of diabetes cases in a market area can be estimated by multiplying national or regional incidence rates by population data specific to age or other enumerated factors known to differentiate the probability of a diabetes diagnosis. Estimates can be used as proxies for the actual data—when no market-specific count of procedures, discharges, or diagnoses is available that can serve as the market share denominator. Case Study 4.2 describes the steps involved in determining the effective market for a particular service.

The Changing Nature of Healthcare Markets

The healthcare arena used to be relatively stable and predictable—but not anymore. This dynamic must be considered because it has implications for identifying, profiling, and evaluating healthcare markets. Understanding the changes occurring in the healthcare market is necessary for effective decision making.

Several factors have contributed to the changing nature of healthcare markets. Many of these factors are inherent in the market areas themselves and are not directly health related. Market areas are constantly undergoing changes in demographic characteristics, population size, composition, and customer distribution; lifestyle changes have also become common.

The demand for services in a particular market or population segment may be influenced by a variety of factors, ranging from changing consumer

EXHIBIT 4.3
Calculating
Hospital Market
Shares for
Obstetrical
Admissions

Hospital	2013 OB Admissions	Market Share
Hospital X	200	14%
Hospital Y	400	29%
Hospital Z	600	43%
All Other	200	14%
Total	1,400	100%

CASE STUDY 4.2
Determining the Effective Market

Southern Health Systems (SHS), a fictional organization, established a satellite hospital in a growing suburban area ten years ago. Since then, the hospital has become relatively successful. It has attracted adequate medical staff and gradually increased its occupancy rate. At the time it opened, SHS was not authorized to offer labor-and-delivery services. Now, however, a significant market for maternity services has emerged, as the population has reached a critical mass and many young families have moved into the community.

In 2013, the SHS marketing staff was instructed to assess the situation and determine the current and future potential for maternity services within the market area. This assessment was needed if SHS decided to expand. Because the state requires a certificate of need to add any service, the organization needed the data to make a case for adding obstetrics beds. The SHS market analysts were cognizant of the need to not only identify the apparent potential for maternity services but also specify the effective demand.

As in any market research project, the analysts began by delineating the service area likely to be served by the proposed obstetrics program. Once satisfied that a defensible service area had been specified, the analysts profiled its population. They determined the size and characteristics of the current population and developed projections for the future that reflected anticipated changes in size and demographic characteristics.

According to the data available, the service area had approximately 42,000 residents. Estimates purchased from a demographic data vendor projected a population of 50,000 in ten years. The SHS analysts thought this figure represented the maximum population capacity of the area because virtually all available residential land would be built up by that time. The current demographic characteristics of the population were determined and projected ten years forward. The analysts focused on data on the population's age structure (especially the number of women in their childbearing years), marital status (unmarried suburban residents typically don't have children), and racial and ethnic composition. This latter attribute was considered important given the disparities in birth rates among the various racial and ethnic groups of the area. The psychographic (or lifestyle) characteristics of the population were

(continued)

also analyzed on the grounds that people in different lifestyle clusters exhibit different attitudes toward childbearing.

The analysts also researched the insurance coverage situation of the area. Because this information was not readily available, they had to conduct primary research. A **sample survey** of the area's households revealed that 75 percent of the population was covered by some form of commercial insurance. Small proportions were covered by Medicare, Medicaid, or military insurance, and a negligible number of residents were uninsured. The high level of insurance coverage was a positive finding.

Sample survey
The administration of a questionnaire to a segment of a target population that has been systematically selected

Satisfied that the number of women of childbearing age was adequate (23 percent of the population compared to 19 percent county-wide) and that a significant proportion of households were married couples with or without children (55 percent compared to 35 percent countywide), the analysts calculated current and anticipated levels of fertility for the population. Because detailed data were not available on the area population's fertility patterns, known figures for a similar population were applied.

The analysts calculated a proxy estimate of the birth rate for this population (15 births per 1,000 people), which turned out to be well above the county rate of 10 per 1,000. This estimate was not surprising, given that this population is skewed toward women of childbearing age. The general fertility rate also was calculated to determine the fertility rate for women of childbearing age (i.e., those aged 15–44), which turned out to be lower than that for the county overall (58 per 1,000 women aged 15–44 compared to 65 per 1,000). This calculation (rather than the crude birth rate) provided a more realistic view of the likely level of fertility for this population because it adjusted for the size of the childbearing-age population.

On the basis of these figures, the analysts estimated that the population would yield almost 700 births annually by the tenth year. Thus, 700 births became the base figure for calculating the effective market for obstetrics services. This figure was subsequently adjusted for various factors that were likely to affect its conversion into demand for SHS's proposed maternity services. One of the demographic factors that needed to be considered was the projected growth in the number of African Americans in the service area. Given the higher fertility rate for the African-American population, the anticipated number of births ten years out was adjusted to 750. However, psychographic data indicated that the career orientation of many of the area's women was likely to lower the potential number of births. Thus, the anticipated number of births was adjusted back down to 725.

A major consideration was the drag on potential demand represented by competition from other providers of obstetrics services. After all, this service would be new, and with the exception of existing patients of SHS facilities who might transfer their business to the satellite facility, SHS would have to cultivate a new set of obstetrics customers. Realistically, many, if not most, of the women of childbearing age in the community were likely to have existing relationships with obstetricians/gynecologists (OB/GYNs). These potential patients would have to be convinced to change to an OB/GYN affiliated with the new facility, or SHS would have to convince its existing OB/GYNs to join the staff of the new facility. Further, many potential customers would be constrained in their use of facilities by the health plans that cover their obstetrics care. Last, some of these potential maternity customers had already delivered children at another facility (or had otherwise positive experiences with a competing hospital) and would not be inclined to change hospitals without a good reason.

On the basis of their experiences elsewhere, the analysts believed the combined effect of these three factors (i.e., existing provider relationships, insurance steering, and previous experience) would reduce the potential market share to approximately 50 percent of the total in the short run, and SHS would grow this share to 60 percent over ten years. In the best of all worlds, the analysts believed a market share of 75–80 percent was the most they could ultimately hope for, so a 60 percent share in ten years was considered a reasonable estimate.

On the basis of adjustments necessitated by these facts, the analysts estimated that SHS would capture approximately 285 births during its first year of operation and approximately 420 births annually by the tenth year. Given that a minimum of 200 annual births was required to justify the cost of establishing the facility, the analysts concluded that the effective demand was adequate to support the proposed maternity service.

Case Study Discussion Questions

1. Why did the market analysts have to assess the size of the market before going forward with the development of a new obstetrics service?

(continued)

2. Why couldn't the analysts simply use the total population as the basis for determining the demand for obstetrics services?

3. To what extent might the lifestyle orientation of women in the market area influence their attitudes toward childbearing?

4. How important are the presence of other obstetrics service providers and the existing relationships between market area women and OB/GYN in determining the effective demand for obstetrics services?

5. What challenges do marketers face in introducing a new service to a market area, particularly a service as personal as obstetrics care?

preferences to newly introduced technology. National or regional trends related to service usage, especially in the consumption of elective services (e.g., liposuction), also contribute. Technological advances that make new procedures possible—and old procedures better—reshape the constellation of services offered and the way services are delivered (e.g., inpatient care versus outpatient care). Changing insurance arrangements could easily affect the level of demand for services in a specific market.

Another factor that contributes to changing markets is the fluid state of competition. Existing competitors are constantly changing locations, services, or marketing strategies. New competitors are continually entering the market, while other competitors are dropping out. This situation has been complicated by the emergence of national chains that may enter a market and, almost overnight, upset the competitive balance. National and state legislation that facilitate the creation of new partnerships (e.g., health alliances) or alter regulatory powers or procedures (e.g., for health maintenance organizations) reshape and, in some instances, create markets for services.

The ubiquity of change is one more reason to establish market research as an ongoing process rather than as an ad hoc activity. Identifying, profiling, and evaluating markets are not onetime activities to be returned to three, five, or ten years later. These three tasks should be an ongoing *process* used to continually search for market opportunities and reevaluate current strategies. Making these procedures routine, investing in the requisite hardware and software, and training personnel to perform these functions are essential tasks for nearly all health services providers. Case Study 4.3 describes the steps involved in identifying true market potential.

CASE STUDY 4.3
Is There Really a Market for It?

The primary objective in analyzing any market is to determine the potential demand for a good or service being offered to that market. The market analysis process typically determines the size and composition of the target market and profiles the identified area's demographic and socioeconomic characteristics. The market is also typically profiled in terms of health-related characteristics such as disease incidence, utilization rates, and referral patterns.

The initial market analysis attempts to estimate the market potential. The analyst will typically determine, for example, the age distribution, racial characteristics, and marital status of the target population along with such socioeconomic characteristics as income levels, workforce characteristics, and educational levels. Through this process, the analyst compiles all of the information necessary to determine the potential market for the goods or services being offered.

Years of experience with market analysis suggest that such characteristics need to be verified from as many perspectives as possible and interpreted on the basis of any information on the community that may have a bearing on the issue. An analyst must be able to read between the lines and capture the essence of the market, which may not be obvious from the raw data.

In some cases, especially when entering a new market, the analyst may have only secondary data. The analyst should verify this information through ground-level research using whatever means available—even primary research. In fact, the analyst may not be able to determine the effective level of demand in a market without surveying the residents.

A case in point involved a growing suburban area outside a medium-sized southern city. The community had all the earmarks of an up-and-coming suburb. Its population was growing rapidly, and an increasing number of upscale housing units were being constructed. Income levels were rising, and the socioeconomic status of the resident population was steadily increasing. An examination of the available data suggested a highly attractive market in terms of its demographics.

Analysis of the secondary data revealed that the market was composed of an upwardly mobile population with a moderately high level of ambulatory care needs. The population appeared to be ripe for innovative programs (e.g., freestanding birthing centers), progressive services (e.g., behavioral healthcare), and even trendy venues (e.g., fitness centers). In short, the community appeared to be a dream for marketers

(continued)

offering new services. Even better, virtually no competition had emerged in the community.

The analyst conducted a survey of community residents to confirm the conclusions drawn regarding the services this population would likely demand. The first clue that things were not as they seemed surfaced early in the interviewing process, when interviewers encountered high refusal rates and a generally hostile respondent population. Analysis of the survey data revealed that, contrary to the initial analysis, the population was anything but progressive. The residents of this suburb were traditional in their approach to healthcare and resistant to new or innovative services. They had little interest in such programs as women's services, fitness centers, and behavioral health programs, despite large numbers of residents who fit the profile for these services.

The high proportion of military personnel and retirees in the area also influenced the respondents' attitudes. These residents' situations were much different from those of typical suburban residents in that their military affiliation and retirement health plans influenced their health service utilization patterns.

Ultimately, the community was offered a basic package of primary care services. The gap between the residents' lifestyles and their socioeconomic status as well as the presence of a large military and retired population precluded the development of the types of services typically offered to a growing, upscale suburban population. Luckily for the hospital planning the services, its market analyst obtained the information necessary to prevent a serious strategic miscalculation based on the paper profile of the market area.

Case Study Discussion Questions

1. What characteristics of this fast-growing suburban population made hospital administrators envision a potential market?
2. When the suburb's population was initially examined, what types of services did the analyst think would appeal to the community?
3. What type of research was carried out to verify the conclusions based on secondary data for this population?
4. How did the findings from the consumer survey conflict with what was deduced from the secondary data?
5. What did the analyst discover about this population that discouraged the development of innovative health services?
6. Rather than cutting-edge services, what types of programs did the analyst conclude are more appropriate for this population?

Summary

An understanding of the market to be served is a critical requirement for marketing professionals in any industry. To appreciate the interface between healthcare and marketing, marketers must understand the societal framework in which both enterprises exist. Marketing professionals also must have a thorough knowledge of the social, political, and economic characteristics of the target population along with its lifestyles, attitudes, and other traits.

The market for healthcare goods and services can be delineated in a number of ways. Markets can be conceptualized on the basis of geographic scope, population characteristics, level of demand, and market potential. With the emergence of the Internet, markets without walls have also become common. The market area for an organization can be delineated in various ways, and the approach used depends on the circumstances. The geographic division used to define the market (e.g., zip code, county) depends on the characteristics of the organization and the type of services provided. Over time, healthcare marketers have moved away from a mass marketing approach to a target marketing or micromarketing approach in an effort to increase marketing precision.

Once defined, a market must be profiled in terms of its salient characteristics, including demographic and socioeconomic traits, psychographic or lifestyle attributes, health status, and patterns of health behavior. The population's ability to pay for care is an increasingly important consideration. Market characteristics are constantly changing, and market areas must be assessed in terms of past, present, and future traits.

A number of factors must be considered in determining the effective market for a healthcare organization. The total demand must be adjusted for such factors as ability to pay, consumer preferences, existing relationships, and presence of competitors. A distinction must also be made between consumer needs and wants when evaluating a potential market.

Key Points

- The decision to implement marketing implies that a market exists, but the word *market* has a different meaning in healthcare than it does in other industries.
- A healthcare market can be defined in a number of different ways.
- A number of geographic units may be used to delineate a healthcare market.
- Large healthcare organizations are likely to have a number of different markets to consider.

- Healthcare markets can be profiled in terms of their size, population composition, health status, and level of health services demand.
- Healthcare is unique in that not all people with a particular health condition are necessarily considered potential customers.
- Healthcare marketers must determine what portion of the total market represents the effective market for the organization's goods or services.
- Healthcare markets are often more dynamic than markets in other industries, as they must respond to developments in health conditions, treatment modalities, and reimbursement patterns.

Discussion Questions

1. What are some of the ways marketers define healthcare markets, and what determines how market delineation differs for various types of healthcare organizations?
2. What are some of the bases on which markets can be delineated, and what determines which approach is used?
3. How can a start-up organization delineate a market in which it has no history?
4. What determines the geographic division (e.g., county, zip code, census tract) at which a market area should be delineated?
5. Why is it sometimes difficult to delineate a market area using standard political or administrative boundaries?
6. How can marketers identify unmet healthcare needs that may indicate an untapped market?
7. To what extent has the Internet changed the way markets are organized?
8. What are the most salient demographic characteristics considered in profiling a population, and how may these traits differ according to the type of healthcare organization?
9. What arguments can be made for the use of psychographic analysis in healthcare marketing today?
10. Why is the ability to pay for healthcare an important factor to consider in a target market assessment?
11. What factors have prompted the transition from a mass marketing orientation to a target marketing orientation in healthcare?

Additional Resources

Dartmouth Atlas of Health Care, The. 2013. "Data by Region." www.dartmouth
    atlas.org/data/region/.
Pol, L. G., and R. K. Thomas. 1997. *Demography for Business Decision Making*. New
    York: Quorum.
US Census Bureau. 2012. "Guide to State and Local Census Geography." www
    .census.gov/geo/reference/geoguide.html.
———. 2012. *Statistical Abstract of the United States*. Washington, DC: Government
    Printing Office.

5

HEALTHCARE CONSUMERS AND CONSUMER BEHAVIOR

I n any industry, the goods and services offered reflect the needs, desires, and preferences of that industry's consumers. Although this generalization is true in healthcare to some extent, the industry defies this basic tenet in many ways. In healthcare, a distinction exists between patients, clients, consumers, and customers—although all of these terms are used at different times to define the purchasers and/or end users of healthcare goods and services. In this chapter, the different categories of people who consume health services and the implications of their attributes for marketing are discussed. The unusual nature of consumer behavior in healthcare is also described, along with the steps involved in the consumer decision-making process.

Who Are Healthcare Consumers?

Consumer, as the term is typically used in healthcare, refers to a person with the potential to consume a good or service. As noted in previous chapters, anyone who has a need or want—and presumably the ability to pay—for a product (a good or a service) can be considered a potential customer. According to this definition, the entire US population is a market for some type of healthcare good or service. Historically, healthcare organizations did not view consumers in this manner. The general assumption was that no one was a prospect for health services until that person became sick and sought care. Thus, healthcare providers made no attempt to develop relationships with nonpatients. Marketers in the consumer goods industries, on the other hand, have always pursued potential customers aggressively, assuming that nearly everyone has a need (or at least a want) that can be met.

How Healthcare Consumers Are Different from Other Consumers

Healthcare consumers differ from consumers of other products in a variety of ways. First, healthcare purchases are largely nondiscretionary in that serious consequences could result if no action is taken. Because of the nature of most healthcare episodes, the factors that drive healthcare consumption are different from those driving other purchases.

Second, a health professional typically orders services for the good of the patient. This is unique to healthcare in that goods or services are prescribed for the consumer and then the consumer is expected to comply with the prescribed treatment.

Third, healthcare consumers often do not know the price of the services they consume—and neither do those prescribing the service. This reflects the unusual financing arrangements in healthcare and the patient's lack of access to pricing information. Unlike the consumer behavior in other industries, the behavior of healthcare consumers is seldom affected by cost factors.

Fourth, healthcare consumers have little knowledge about the operation of the healthcare system and may have little or no direct experience with it. They have no basis in reality for evaluating the quality of the services they receive and must make judgments about their treatment on the basis of subjective criteria.

Fifth, most healthcare episodes have an emotional component not present in other consumer transactions. Medical care involves a certain level of anxiety for both the patient and his or her loved ones. As noted in Chapter 1, emotions like fear, pride, and vanity influence the behavior and decisions of patients and their families. Exhibit 5.1 presents the differences between healthcare consumers and other types of consumers.

How Healthcare Consumers Are Similar to Other Consumers

Although much has been made of the unique characteristics of healthcare consumers, they do share many similarities with consumers in other industries. Some healthcare episodes do involve emergency or life-threatening conditions, but most do not. Thus, most healthcare episodes compel the end user or those involved in the decision-making process to exercise some discretion. Further, many types of services are considered elective. Much like other consumers, healthcare consumers are likely to distinguish between needs and wants when consuming services. Clearly, most healthcare consumers would view angioplasty to correct a heart condition as a need but laser eye surgery to improve vision would be considered a want. The latter would typically be considered a **discretionary purchase**, whereas the former would be regarded as nondiscretionary.

Discretionary purchase
A purchase of a good or service that is elective rather than required

Healthcare consumers are like other consumers in that there is **elasticity** in the level of demand for healthcare goods and services. Years ago, the conventional wisdom was that the demand for health services was essentially inelastic; it was assumed that those who were sick consumed services and those who were well did not. Not only does this assumption reflect a dated notion of health and illness, but it also does not account for the vast number of elective services that are provided in healthcare. Today, the demand for

Elasticity
The tendency of demand to rise and fall in response to factors inside and outside the industry

EXHIBIT 5.1
Healthcare
Consumers
Versus Other
Consumers

Consumers of Health Services	Consumers of Other Services
Seldom determine their own need for services	Usually determine their own need for services
Seldom are the ultimate decision maker	Usually are the ultimate decision maker
Often make decisions subjectively	Usually make decisions objectively
Seldom have knowledge of the price	Always have knowledge of the price
Seldom make decisions based on price	Usually make decisions based on price
Are reimbursed by third party for most costs	Are rarely reimbursed by third party for costs
Usually make nondiscretionary purchases	Usually make discretionary purchases
Usually require a professional referral	Rarely require a professional referral
Have limited choices	Have unlimited choices
Have limited knowledge of service attributes	Have significant knowledge of service attributes
Have limited ability to judge quality of service	Are usually able to judge quality of service
Have limited ability to evaluate outcome	Are usually able to evaluate outcome
Have little recourse for unfavorable outcome	Have ample recourse for unfavorable outcome
Seldom are the ultimate targets for marketing	Always are the ultimate targets for marketing
Are not susceptible to standard marketing techniques	Are susceptible to standard marketing techniques

health services is seen as extremely elastic. The level of healthcare utilization is influenced by a wide range of factors independent of health status, including availability of services, access to health insurance, and physician practice patterns. Furthermore, the demand for health services can be manipulated—for example, by physicians who order greater or lesser amounts of a particular service or by marketing campaigns that make consumers aware of a service they did not know existed. Pharmaceutical advertising, for example, has convinced many consumers that they suffer from a condition they had never heard of before.

One final similarity relates to the ability to pay for services. Most patients pay for healthcare through some form of insurance. Those without insurance must pay out of pocket or resort to a healthcare *safety net* such as a public health clinic or charity hospital. Historically, healthcare was thought to be such a necessity that people found a way to pay for required services even if it meant going into debt. Many argued that community safety nets would ensure that all health problems were addressed in one way or another. Clearly, the ability to pay for care is a major consideration affecting the demand for healthcare goods and services. Admittedly, for elective procedures and other products not considered medically necessary, consumers may be unwilling to pay out of pocket and thus reduce the demand for services. During periods of economic prosperity, the volume of cosmetic surgery, laser eye surgery, and other vanity services increases; conversely, during periods of economic downturn, the volume of such discretionary expenditures decreases. Even medically necessary treatment may be cut back; for example, as a result of the Great Recession (2007–2009), the number of visits patients made to their physicians' offices decreased (AAFP 2009).

Since the emergence of modern medicine in the United States, the ability to pay for care has had implications for health services utilization. There are countless stories of patients who were unable to obtain care because they did not have the resources to pay for it. With physicians and hospitals demanding payment up front from people without insurance, the uninsured or those without financial means might be reluctant to seek treatment and even less likely to obtain care—even care considered medically necessary. (While the passage of the Affordable Care Act [ACA] could change this situation, it is too early to discern the law's impact on the uninsured and their behavior.) The inability to pay for healthcare is even more pronounced when prescription drugs are involved. A deathly ill patient can eventually be admitted to an emergency department, but necessary drugs cannot be obtained from a pharmacy without payment. Ultimately, healthcare consumers must weigh the economic implications of consuming goods and services just as consumers in any other industry must.

The Variety of Healthcare Customers

One important attribute of healthcare customers is their variety. The market for healthcare products includes not only individual consumers but also health professionals and health facilities. Although organizational needs may differ from individual needs, many of the same marketing issues pertain to both.

Individuals
Individual consumers fall into different categories, each with specific needs. In the eyes of the general public, the typical patient is someone requiring

life-saving services (first category). Life-threatening situations, however, are rare occurrences; when they do occur, their management requires dedicated personnel, equipment, and facilities. Most healthcare encounters involve a second category of individual consumers: people requiring routine services (those who present for treatment at a doctor's office, clinic, or therapy center). A third category includes customers who desire elective goods and services that are not considered medically necessary.

A fourth category includes those involved in self-care. Research has indicated that the prevalence of self-care is much greater than previously thought and that many people access the formal healthcare system only after they have exhausted other options. Thus, symptomatic individuals are likely to first self-diagnose (often with the aid of the Internet) and then self-medicate using a wide range of do-it-yourself remedies. Pharmacy shelves are stocked with products and devices for home testing and treatment, and the Internet has expanded the availability of and access to such products.

For these and other reasons, various terms are applied to today's purchasers and end users of healthcare products, and "patient" is giving way to other terms to better reflect the contemporary healthcare environment. Major terms were described in depth in Chapter 2, and Exhibit 5.2 summarizes them for the readers' reference. Note that these terms for individual customers are not mutually exclusive and that usage of each depends on the context. Someone who has become a psychiatric patient could just as easily be called a "client." This patient or client may also be referred to as the "end user" of the psychotherapy service and the "enrollee" if he or she is a member of the health plan that pays for the treatment. Overall, this patient is considered a "customer" of the psychiatric clinic or practice.

Health Professionals and Facilities

Numerous other customers—beyond individual patients—use a wide range of healthcare goods and services. Two major groups are health professionals and facilities.

Physicians

Physicians are thought of as providers of services, but they are also major consumers of healthcare goods and services. Hospitals ask physicians to join their medical staffs, and provider networks and health plans solicit the participation of physicians and other clinicians. Nursing homes, home health agencies, and hospices may depend on physicians for referrals; in turn, many physicians depend on referrals from other physicians.

Physicians are the customers of a variety of entities that provide **support services**, including billing and collection services, utilization review companies, medical supply distributors, biomedical equipment companies,

Support services
Nonclinical, operational activities that support the provision of medical care

EXHIBIT 5.2
A Typology
of Healthcare
Customer Terms

Term	Meaning	Determinant	Application
Patient	Person under the care of a healthcare provider	Formal diagnosis by a medical practitioner	Traditional term for a person receiving medical care
Client	Person who has a formal relationship with a healthcare provider	Entry into a therapeutic relationship with a provider (with or without a formal diagnosis)	Most often applied to relationships with nonphysician providers (e.g., mental health professionals)
End user	Person who receives a service or consumes a good	Receiver of the product, regardless of who orders it or pays for it	Used to distinguish between the person receiving the care and other parties (e.g., the party that pays the bill)
Enrollee	Person who is enrolled in a health plan or other group arrangement that finances healthcare	Formal membership by qualifying and paying a premium	Enrollment status determines covered services, copayments, and deductibles
Consumer	Anyone in the population who might use a health service	Inclusion in the population under consideration	Universe of potential customers to be targeted by marketers
Customer	Person who uses a service or purchases a good	Receiver of a good or service in exchange for something of value	Consumer who has been converted into a buyer of goods or services

and biohazard management companies. Physicians are customers of information technology vendors who sell or maintain practice management systems, imaging systems, and electronic patient record systems. Physicians have also traditionally been the primary customers of pharmaceutical companies.

Other Clinicians

Other clinicians—such as dentists, optometrists, podiatrists, chiropractors, mental health counselors, and other independent practitioners—have many of the same needs physicians have and are cultivated by similar marketing entities. These providers require supplies, equipment, billing and collections, information technology, and other services, just as physicians do.

Hospitals and Other Institutions

Hospitals and other provider institutions are customers of a wide range of healthcare-specific goods and services, in addition to users of the same consumer products as any other organization. These facilities or settings require medical supplies, biomedical equipment, and/or durable medical equipment (e.g., wheelchairs, hospital beds). They also need support services, including billing and collections, physician recruitment, and marketing. By providing food service, gift shops, and parking services, hospitals are customers of the suppliers for a spectrum of non-healthcare-related goods and services. Hospitals and other healthcare facilities are routine (and even heavy) users of office supplies, janitorial goods and services, computer software and hardware, and information technology vendors and consultants, among many other products and people.

Employers

Major employers are customers of health plans, managed care plans, providers, and provider networks. Most health plans are employer based, and competing health plans seek to contract with employers for the management of their employees' healthcare needs. Individual providers may seek to contract with employers that are self-insured or otherwise open to negotiated services. Employers are also customers of direct providers of care, including occupational health, employee assistance programs, fitness centers, and other services that healthcare organizations market directly to employers.

Others

Like companies in other industries, healthcare organizations have various other internal and external customers, including employees; the general public; the media; and federal, state, and local governments.

Every business should view the members of its workforce as its internal customers. In this regard, healthcare has generally lagged behind other industries. The mission, vision, values, goals, and objectives of the organization should be continually marketed to internal customers, and their input should be regularly solicited. The board of directors is another important group of internal customers. In most organizations, the board is charged with setting the enterprise's future direction and ensuring its progress toward this direction. This body also typically plays a critical role in determining the strategic direction of the organization.

The general public or the community is an external customer to be considered during strategy development and program implementation. It is important to create and sustain a positive public image and corporate goodwill. At some point, the organization may need to demonstrate or prove that it is a good community citizen. To justify their tax-exempt status, not-for-profits specifically are required to document and report the community benefit they provide to their public constituents.

The media, whether local or national, are yet another category of external customer that the organization must cultivate to ensure that its story is told—and told in the right manner. Long before hospitals, health systems, and other healthcare delivery practices had a formal marketing function, they had public relations departments that dealt with the media.

Many healthcare organizations have one or more branches of government as customers. Healthcare facilities and health professions are regulated by government agencies, so they often maintain a separate government-relations office to interface with these bodies. A not-for-profit's continued exemption from taxes depends on its good relationship with the appropriate government agency. The same goes for an organization located in an area where a certificate-of-need requirement exists.

Market segmentation
A process for grouping individuals or households who share similar characteristics for the purpose of target marketing

Segment
A component of a population or market defined on the basis of some characteristic relevant to marketers

Market Segmentation for Healthcare Products

In general, **market segmentation** is used to single out and call marketers' attention to certain segments of the population. Not every subgroup in a population qualifies as a target market, and certain rules of thumb help marketers identify a meaningful market **segment**. To be useful to a marketer, a segment should be

- *measurable* in that the data obtained on the segment's characteristics are accurate, complete, and detailed enough to allow for comparison, evaluation, and monitoring;
- *accessible* in that the segment can be reached by marketers effectively using standard marketing methods;

- *substantial* in that the segment is large enough to be considered for a dedicated marketing activity; and
- *meaningful* in that the segment includes consumers who have attributes relevant to the aims of the marketer.

Furthermore, a viable market segment should demonstrate a desire for the product being marketed and the ability to pay for it. Over the years, the growing emphasis on consumer engagement has raised marketers' sensitivity to the issue of consumers' readiness for change.

In healthcare, marketers implement market segmentation to better understand the unique traits of healthcare customers and the healthcare delivery environment as a whole. The common forms of market segmentation used are described in this section (and also considered in Chapter 4).

Demographic Segmentation

Market segmentation based on **demographics** is commonly used in consumer goods industries, and it is the best-known approach to identifying target markets. This type of segmentation defines demographically distinct subgroups on the basis of their need for various goods and services. The links between demographic characteristics and health status, health-related attitudes, and health behavior have been well established. For this reason, demographic segmentation is typically an early task in any marketing planning process.

Marketers typically segment the healthcare market in terms of age, sex, and race or **ethnicity**. Depending on the service to be offered, the market may be further segmented according to income level, educational level, or even marital status. The population may be further classified according to region of the country or type of community (e.g., rural, suburban, urban). Research has indicated, for example, that the demographic segment most likely to sign up for fitness programs includes affluent women between 35 and 40 years old living in suburban communities in the Midwest. (Chapter 7 provides additional detail on the demographic characteristics of healthcare populations.)

Demographics
The range of biosocial and sociocultural attributes of a population

Ethnicity
A common racial, national, tribal, religious, linguistic, or cultural trait or background of members of a population

Geographic Segmentation

An understanding of the spatial distribution of the target market has become increasingly important as a result of healthcare's reorientation toward the consumer. One of the implications of this trend has been an increased emphasis on the appropriate location of health facilities. A market-driven approach requires providers to take their services to consumers wherever they live, and major purchasers of healthcare products insist on convenient locations for their members or employees. Knowledge of the manner in which the patient

Geographic segmentation
A method of dividing a target audience on the basis of geographic location

population is distributed across the service area and an understanding of the links between **geographic segmentation** and other forms of segmentation are critical to the development of a marketing plan. (Geographic units used for geographic segmentation are described in Chapter 4.)

Marketers can segment the population in terms of geography in a number of ways. They can identify the geographic areas that constitute the market area for an organization (e.g., the zip codes from which a physician draws patients). They can segment the population by type of community—considering the area's rural, suburban, and urban residential components, for example, as separate markets. They can relate other variables (e.g., demographics, lifestyle) to particular geographic areas; for example, marketers commonly segment the market area geographically by income through identifying areas with low, medium, or high income levels. Exhibit 5.3 illustrates the geographic distribution of a demographic variable (race).

Psychographic Segmentation

Psychographics
The lifestyle characteristics of a population; see *lifestyle*

Lifestyle
The entirety of attitudes, preferences, and behaviors of an individual, a group, or a culture

For many types of goods and services, an understanding of the **psychographics** or **lifestyle** characteristics of the target population is essential. Lifestyle clusters in a population often transcend (or at least complement) that population's demographics. Most important, psychographics can be linked to the attitudes, perceptions, and expectations of the target population as well as to its propensity to purchase certain products. Although use of psychographic analysis in healthcare has lagged behind other industries, health professionals are finding a growing number of applications for this approach, and more healthcare data are being incorporated into psychographic segmentation systems.

Marketers can choose from a handful of different psychographic segmentation systems for use in partitioning the market area by lifestyle. For example, the MOSAIC system developed by Experian assigns one of 71 lifestyle clusters to most households in the United States. Knowing the assigned psychographic cluster of a household opens the door to a variety of other useful information in addition to available lifestyle attributes. Exhibit 5.4 graphically presents the psychographic breakdown of a market area by major lifestyle grouping.

Health Risk Segmentation

An approach to market segmentation unique to healthcare involves partitioning the population by level of health risk. This approach enables marketers to determine the type of health services most appropriate for a certain group and to craft the marketing message for those specific services. Health risk levels may be measured for a specific health condition (e.g., diabetes), a combination of conditions (e.g., obesity and hypertension), or a broad group of

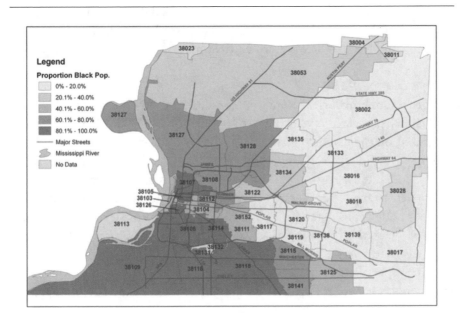

EXHIBIT 5.3
Distribution of the African-American Population, Memphis, Tennessee, 2010

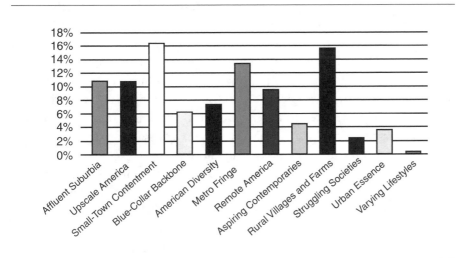

EXHIBIT 5.4
Market Segmentation by Lifestyle Group—Sample County

conditions (e.g., chronic disease). The risk level is quantified and presented numerically or, more commonly, ranked as low, moderate, or high.

From a marketing perspective, the level of risk affects the type of marketing message used and the timing of its delivery. Consumers with low risk need to receive information on prevention and health enhancement as well as the warning signs of health problems. Consumers with moderate risk need to be encouraged to take appropriate action and given related information.

Consumers with high risk need to be persuaded to take urgent action, informed of the types of healthcare goods and services available, and encouraged to comply with their prescribed treatment.

Usage Segmentation

Usage segmentation

A method of dividing a target audience on the basis of historical utilization of a product or an organization

Usage segmentation, a common approach in other industries, is now applied in healthcare. The market area population can be divided into categories based on the extent a particular service is used. In examining the use of **urgent care** clinics, for example, the population can be categorized as heavy users, moderate users, occasional users, and nonusers. This classification can be applied to many services but may be most useful for elective goods and services under consideration. Usage segmentation provides a basis for subsequent marketing planning that can be tailored, for example, to existing loyal customers versus noncustomers. Consumers' willingness to use certain services, especially elective procedures, often reflects the extent to which they are open to change. See Exhibit 5.5 for a discussion of the adoption process for new healthcare services.

Urgent care

Medical care for a condition that requires immediate attention but is not significant enough to warrant emergency care

Payer Segmentation

A form of market segmentation unique to healthcare involves targeting segments on the basis of their payer categories. The payer mix of the market area population has come to be one of the first considerations in profiling a target population. The existence of insurance coverage and the type of coverage available are major considerations in marketing most health services. Further, health plans cover some services and not others—an important consideration in marketing. For services routinely covered by insurance, a mass marketing approach may be appropriate. For elective services paid for out of pocket, a targeted marketing approach is typically more effective.

Market analysts typically categorize payers as follows: commercial insurers (sometimes managed care plans are a subcategory), Medicare, Medicaid, and other government programs (e.g., the military TRICARE). Those who are not covered by insurance and pay for health services out of pocket belong to a residual category referred to as the *uninsured*. Exhibit 5.6 illustrates the payer mix of a target market area.

Benefit Segmentation

Benefit segmentation

A method of dividing the target audience according to the benefits it seeks from a good or service

Different people buy the same or similar products for different reasons. **Benefit segmentation** is based on the idea that consumers can be grouped according to the principal benefit sought. The benefits consumers consider when making a purchase decision include quality, convenience, value, and ease of access. As healthcare has become more consumer driven, market researchers have sought to determine which buttons to push to make a

EXHIBIT 5.5
Who Adopts
Innovative
Services?

Despite their emphasis on research and innovation, healthcare organizations are relatively conservative. They adopt new techniques or treatment modalities only after extensive testing, and even then, practitioners may be reluctant to forsake tried-and-true procedures. Similarly, most healthcare customers tend to be conservative in their approach to care, preferring to stick with proven treatments rather than opt for more experimental approaches.

This perception of healthcare customers, however, masks the wide range of approaches to adopting health services. Baby boomers, for example, have been particularly open to innovative approaches. As a result, many novel health services have entered the market, including urgent care and alternative and complementary therapies. Clearly, some segments of society have a greater predilection for innovation than others.

Marketers have studied the process through which individuals come to adopt a new procedure or therapeutic modality, tracking progress from the point at which an individual first hears about an innovation to final adoption. In many ways, this process is similar to the consumer decision-making process. Various studies indicate that the consumer population can be grouped into five categories: innovators, early adopters, early majority, late majority, and laggards (Rogers 2003):

1. *Innovators* represent, on average, the first 2.5 percent of all those who adopt. They are eager to try new ideas and products. They have higher incomes, are better educated, and are more active outside their community than are noninnovators. They are less reliant on group norms, are more self-confident, and are more likely to obtain information from scientific sources and experts.

2. *Early adopters* represent, on average, the next 13.5 percent to adopt a product. They try the product early in its life cycle and—compared with innovators (who have a more cosmopolitan outlook)—are much more reliant on group norms and values and are more oriented to the local community. They are more likely to be opinion leaders because of their closer affiliation with groups. Because of its personal influence on others, this segment is regarded as the most important determinant of a new product's success.

3. *Early majority* members are the next 34 percent to adopt. They deliberate more carefully before adopting a new product; they

(continued)

collect more information and evaluate more options than early adopters do. Although slower to adopt, they are an important link in the diffusion process because they are positioned between the early and late adopters.

4. *Late majority* people are the next 34 percent to adopt. They are described as skeptics who eventually adopt an innovation because most of their friends have already done so. Subject to group norms, they adopt under the pressure to conform. They tend to be older, have below-average income and education, and rely primarily on word-of-mouth communication rather than mass-media messages.

5. *Laggards* are the final 16 percent to adopt. They are similar to innovators in their inattention to group norms. They are independent of the opinions of others and make decisions in terms of their past experiences. By the time they adopt an innovation, it has probably been superseded by something else. Laggards have the lowest socioeconomic status among all the adopter groups.

Healthcare marketers can improve their effectiveness by determining their product's level of innovation and using this information to target segments of the population most likely to adopt it. Efforts directed toward those who are least likely to adopt innovative goods or services are likely wasted.

Sources: Adapted from Assael (1992) and Rogers (2003).

product resonate with potential customers. The same service can be positioned in different ways, depending on the benefits sought by the target audience. Thus, the marketer might promote free, close-to-the-door parking to one segment, the quality of the staff to another segment, and competitive pricing to yet another segment. Exhibit 5.7 illustrates the results of a survey on benefits sought in a family practice clinic, and Exhibit 5.8 summarizes the different approaches to segmentation.

Consumer Behavior

Consumer behavior refers to a customer's pattern of consumption of goods and services. This pattern includes the factors that contribute to the behavior

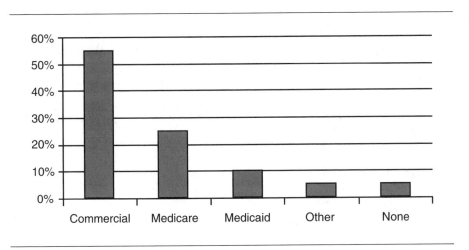

EXHIBIT 5.6
Payer Mix of a
Target Market

Attribute	Percentage of Respondents Seeking That Attribute
Convenient location	93
Extended hours	85
Same-day appointments	64
Free, nearby parking	63
Personal care manager	50
Online consultation	42
Low prices	31

Source: Thomas (2005).

EXHIBIT 5.7
Attributes
Sought in a
Family Practice
Center, Ranked
in Order of
Importance

and the processes that lead to a **purchase decision**. Because marketing is driven by consumer needs, an appreciation of the behavioral dimension of any target population is essential. Ultimately, consumer behavior is what a marketing campaign seeks to influence. While the behaviors of health professionals and healthcare organizations are equally important to understand, this discussion focuses on individual customers.

Purchase decision
A consumer's commitment to buy a good or to use a service

Healthcare consumers' decision criteria can be classified in the same manner as those of consumers in other industries. The factors that influence purchase decisions are technical, economic, social, and personal. Technical criteria include quality of care, clinical outcomes, the environment, and the amenities associated with health services. Economic criteria—perhaps the least relevant in healthcare—include the price of goods and services, the payment mechanism (e.g., insurance), and the perceived value of the service rendered. Social criteria include the status associated with the professional, the

EXHIBIT 5.8
Approaches
to Healthcare
Market
Segmentation

Basis for Segmentation	Focus	Example	Application
Demographic	Grouped by age, sex, race/ethnicity, and other demographic characteristics	Women of childbearing age	Conducting product development, target marketing
Geographic	Grouped by location, space, and other geographic dimensions	A fast-growing new suburb	Selecting a site
Psychographic	Grouped by a particular lifestyle	Generation X career women	Tailoring services or marketing messages to the lifestyle
Health risk	Grouped by level of health risks (low, moderate, and high)	Obese men, women, and children	Targeting for prevention messages and social marketing initiatives
Usage	Grouped by level of use (heavy users, moderate users, occasional users, and nonusers) of healthcare products	Single men who are heavy users of urgent care clinics	Tailoring marketing messages to level of usage
Payer	Grouped by payer/insurance categories (e.g., commercial, Medicare, Medicaid, other)	Medicare enrollees	Assessing the financial potential of a market segment
Benefit	Grouped by level of benefits desired	Consumers who demand speed and convenience	Determining the "hot buttons" of a targeted consumer group

facility, or the procedure performed as well as the influence of the consumer's social group. Personal criteria include the emotional aspects of the service, self-image issues, and even moral and ethical considerations.

Hierarchy of Healthcare Needs

It is traditional to think in terms of a **hierarchy of needs** in setting the context for analyzing consumer decision making. Most refer to the theory of motivation by psychologist Abraham Maslow (1970), who contended that the first order of need for human beings is physiological—that is, the need for food, water, air, shelter, sleep, sex, and warmth. Once these basic needs are met, individuals can begin to pursue safety and security needs, including freedom from threats and the establishment of security, order, and predictability in their lives. At this stage, health begins to emerge as a dimension of safety and security.

Hierarchy of needs
The prioritization of personal needs, which range from basic survival to self-actualization

With safety established, individuals can seek the next level in the hierarchy—social or companionship needs, which include friendship, affection, and a sense of belonging. Esteem or ego needs—such as self-respect, self-confidence, competence, achievement, independence, and prestige—are eventually added. Finally, at the top of the hierarchy is the need for self-actualization, which includes the fulfillment of personal potential through education, career development, and other goals. Only a few societies in the history of the world have achieved this top level.

The hierarchy level at which an individual or a population functions says a lot about its healthcare needs (and the approach a marketer should take). At the lower levels, survival needs dominate, whereby the population faces health threats from pathological agents and a danger-filled environment. At the higher levels, the threats common at the lower levels have been moderated and, rather than attempting to preserve life and limb, the population can focus on health maintenance and enhancement. At the highest level, the population's healthcare needs shift from life-saving procedures to public health considerations to self-actualization marked by such elective services as hair replacement, spa treatment, and cosmetic surgery.

From a marketing perspective, consumers who are at the basic survival level are likely to respond only to a marketing initiative that addresses their immediate healthcare needs. They are not going to respond to promotions for services that enhance their quality of life or require out-of-pocket expenditures (which explains the difficulty involved in convincing financially precarious people that they ought to invest in healthy lifestyles). As consumers progress up the hierarchy, they are more open to discretionary services and appreciate the importance of maintaining and enhancing their health status. At the self-actualization level, elective services like plastic surgery, breast implants, and teeth whitening become a means of raising status and enhancing self-esteem.

Ultimately, the types of healthcare products a person responds to, the communication method used to reach that person, and the message that resonates with that person reflect his or her position in the hierarchy-of-healthcare-needs model. Marketers are faced with the challenge of matching the product, medium, and message to the needs status of the target audience. Case Study 5.1 illustrates a marketing approach to a consumer behavior challenge.

Redefinition of the "Patient"

Of all the developments in healthcare during the 1980s and 1990s, perhaps the one with the most implications for healthcare marketing was the reconceptualization of the patient. (See Chapter 2 for further discussion.) By the end of the twentieth century, fewer health professionals were using the term *patient* because of its narrow connotation. Patients came to be referred to as *clients, customers, consumers,* or *enrollees.* The major consideration, regardless of the label applied, was the fact that clients, customers, consumers, and enrollees all had different characteristics from patients. While "patient" implies a dependent, submissive status, the other terms connote a more proactive involvement in the therapeutic process. Ultimately, this development made healthcare marketing more similar to the marketing activities of other industries, as the consumer of the product became—for the first time—the focus of the healthcare marketer. The emphasis healthcare marketers placed on consumer engagement in the early part of the twenty-first century reflects the growing need for marketing expertise.

CASE STUDY 5.1
Using Consumer Engagement to Encourage Wellness Behavior

Many companies have developed employee health management programs to control their healthcare costs and maintain a healthier, more productive workforce. They are encouraging employees to identify their health risks (by offerring health risk assessments) and, when appropriate, to take necessary actions to address those risks (by providing incentives to those who sign up for wellness classes, weight management programs, chronic disease management programs, and so forth). The benefits of participating in employee health programs are well documented and improve not only the health of the employee but also the company's bottom line.

Despite their known benefits, these programs have been challenging for employers to effectively implement. First, employees often resist health risk assessments. Employers can't mandate participation, so they offer incentives to do so—but even then, presentation rates for assessments are low. This resistance creates a problem because an assessment is typically required for placement in a wellness program. Second, and more significant, if and after health risks have been identified, many employees fail to commit to a wellness program. In the same way that incentives have little influence on participation in health risk assessments, incentives have a limited effect on continued use of fitness, chronic disease management, and other health and wellness programs.

Many observers contend that an organization's inability to generate the desired level of employee participation in internal health programs is a marketing problem. Many, if not most, people would be willing to undergo a health risk assessment if approached in an effective manner. Similarly, most people who realize they are at risk for a health problem would be willing to change their behavior under the right circumstances. Ultimately, the question is how to engage employees in a manner that elicits the desired results.

Heeding these facts, one company asked its marketing department to develop an approach that allowed it to target different groups of employees with a message that resonated with the employees' respective situations. The company believed that conveying the right message at the right time would go a long way toward engaging its workforce in its health improvement initiative.

To this end, the marketing department developed a questionnaire to be administered to all employees. Unlike the health risk assessment, the survey did not delve into the employees' detailed health conditions but asked only a few questions about their knowledge of health risks, their attitudes toward improving their health status, and the actions they were taking or were willing to take to improve their health. From the survey results, the marketers were able to group the workforce into four categories: (1) those who had limited knowledge of health issues and their own health status, (2) those who knew of their own health risks but were reluctant to take appropriate action, (3) those who were willing to take appropriate action but were not sure how to do it, and (4) those who were already involved in some type of wellness program.

(continued)

Armed with this information, the marketers developed a consumer engagement initiative that targeted the needs of each group but emphasized for all groups the core theme of living well. For the first group, the initiative focused on information dissemination to raise these employees' level of knowledge. The material created for the second group focused on changing these employees' attitudes and encouraging them to develop an appreciation of proactive measures. For the third group, the marketers cultivated these employees' awareness of available options and facilitated participation in those options. The marketing message for the fourth group was designed to reinforce existing desirable behavior. The overall intent was to progressively move employees in the first three categories to the fourth-category level using well-timed and stage-appropriate marketing messages.

After the consumer engagement initiative had operated for a year, a follow-up survey indicated these achievements: (1) the level of awareness of health risks among all employees had increased, (2) an increased number of health risk assessments had been performed, (3) a higher proportion of employees had signed up for company-sponsored wellness programs, and (4) the dropout rate for existing programs had decreased. Although the employer is still refining its employee health program, management concluded that a targeted consumer engagement approach influenced positive changes in knowledge, attitudes, and behavior among the respective employee groups. Although minor changes were made to make the program more attractive, the primary factor in its success was the implementation of an effective marketing initiative.

Case Study Discussion Questions

1. Why do employers think it is beneficial to assess their employees' health status and offer them health and wellness programs?
2. What factors prevent employees from reducing their health risks and taking steps to improve their health status?
3. What factors led the company to conclude that the ineffectiveness of the employee health program was a marketing issue?
4. Along what dimension(s) did the company marketers segment the employee population?
5. In what ways is this consumer engagement initiative an example of target marketing?
6. How was the effectiveness of this consumer engagement initiative evaluated?

Consumer Attitudes

Although patterns of consumer **attitudes** in US society tend to be complex, a new orientation toward healthcare clearly emerged during the second half of the twentieth century. As mentioned, when the "patient" transformed into the "customer," a new entity—one who had the combined expectations of a traditional patient and a contemporary customer—was created. This customer exhibited a new attitude, revealing the person to be more knowledgeable about the healthcare system; more open to innovative approaches; and more intent on playing an active role in the diagnostic, therapeutic, and health maintenance processes than any previous generations of consumers had been.

> **Attitude**
> A position a person has adopted in response to a theory, a belief, an object, an event, or another person

The new attitudes are fostered by baby boomers (and by extension successive groups of generation Xers and millennials), a cohort now facing the chronic conditions associated with middle and old age. Baby boomers have been influential in downplaying the importance of physicians and hospitals and have been the impetus for the rise of alternative therapy as a competitor to mainstream allopathic medicine.

Baby boomers favor a patient-centered approach to healthcare and are more likely to emphasize its nonmedical aspects. In general, they are less trusting of professionals and institutions and are control oriented to the point of stubbornness. They are more self-reliant, place greater value on self-care and home care, and are more outcomes oriented and cost sensitive. They pride themselves in getting results and extracting value for their expenditures. Although baby boomers began influencing the healthcare system in the 1980s by "voting with their feet" (i.e., switching to new types of providers), they have now assumed positions of power that have allowed them to shape the healthcare landscape.

To a certain extent, these new attitudes reflect the rise of consumerism that is affecting all segments of society. Seeing themselves as customers rather than patients pushed modern consumers to expect accurate and timely information, to demand participation in healthcare decisions that directly affect them and/or their loved ones, and to insist on receiving the highest-quality care possible. They want health services to be delivered close to their homes, involving minimal interruption to their family life and work schedules, and they want maximum value for their healthcare expenditures.

Consumer Decision Making

In healthcare, as previously noted, the end user of the product may not be the same person who makes the decision to purchase that product. Instead, another entity—a physician, a health plan representative, an employer, or a

Decision making
In healthcare,
the process of
determining the
need for a good or
service, evaluating
the available
options, and
making a choice

family member/guardian—may be responsible for this **decision making**, determining the what, why, who, where, when, and how much related to the service. As such, the marketer is challenged to identify the appropriate targets and the best placement for a promotional initiative.

Because the end user of a service may not be the ultimate target, healthcare marketers reach out to other categories of audiences. These audiences include the following:

- *Influencers.* Family members, counselors, and other health professionals who encourage consumers to use a particular good or service
- *Gatekeepers.* Primary care physicians, insurance plan personnel, discharge planners, and others responsible for channeling consumers into appropriate services
- *Decision makers.* Family members, primary care physicians, and caregivers who act directly on behalf of the end users
- *Buyers.* Employers, business coalitions, and other groups that might indirectly control the behavior of customers

The role of women in healthcare decision making illustrates the importance of understanding parties other than the end user. Data on health services utilization indicate that women use a disproportionate share of healthcare resources (NCHS 2009). Further, women generally make most of the healthcare decisions for their children and often for their husbands. They are also likely to be involved in decision making for their parents, siblings, and other dependent family members. Women consume at least half of the personal health services in the United States, and they account for more than 80 percent of the decisions to purchase healthcare goods or use healthcare services (HCPro 2007).

Steps in Healthcare Decision Making

A basic understanding of the decision-making process consumers go through when purchasing goods and services is important for marketing planning purposes. The decision-making steps are an amalgam of approaches adapted for the healthcare environment and should be taken into consideration when developing a marketing plan (Berkowitz and Hillestad 2012). The approach marketers take depends on what step the consumer is in.

1. *Problem recognition.* The consumer acknowledges a problem or need. The marketer's task is to identify the circumstances or stimuli that triggered the need and to use this knowledge to develop marketing strategies that spark consumer interest.

2. *Information search.* The consumer is interested enough in the problem to search for more information about it. The similarities and differences in information-gathering approaches between healthcare customers and other consumers are discussed in Exhibit 5.9.

3. *Initial awareness.* The consumer is exposed for the first time to the goods or services being marketed. This step could occur during the information-search step, alerting the consumer to the various options for addressing the problem.

4. *Knowledge emergence.* The consumer begins to understand the available goods or services and their potential advantages and disadvantages.

5. *Alternative evaluation.* The consumer evaluates all of the available options to make a rational, informed decision. The consumer may rule out some goods or services at this point to pare down the choices.

6. *Contract assessment.* The consumer considers whether his or her insurance plan covers the options being weighed or if the service provider accepts his or her insurance. The decision stops here for options that conflict with the customer's insurance plan.

7. *Preference assignment.* The consumer develops a preference for a good or service over another (e.g., a podiatrist vs. an orthopedic surgeon) or for one provider over the others (e.g., podiatrist A vs. podiatrist B or C).

8. *Purchase decision.* The consumer (or someone else) selects, among his or her preferences, the good or service to be purchased or used.

9. *Product usage.* The consumer buys the good or uses the service. This step could be as simple as applying the product acquired at a pharmacy or a medical supply store or as complex as undergoing a heart transplant.

10. *Post-purchase behavior.* The consumer, along with family members and other parties involved, assesses whether the purchase is satisfactory. If satisfied, he or she becomes an advocate for the product or service (or, if dissatisfied, a detractor).

EXHIBIT 5.9
Information
Search by
Healthcare
Consumers

The information search process, historically carried out by healthcare consumers, differed considerably from the process followed by consumers in other industries. In healthcare, lack of information was typical, and the structure of the healthcare delivery system was (and still is) complicated—even for seasoned health professionals. Accurate and updated information and data on provider and organizational quality, value, outcomes, and other indicators—which cannot be fully conveyed by promotional material—were not often easily accessible to the public.

(continued)

Faced with this lack of information, where did the healthcare consumer turn?

Healthcare consumers have turned to two primary sources of information—one informal and one formal. The informal and primary source comprises family members, friends, relatives, neighbors, coworkers, and associates on social networks (e.g., Facebook, Twitter). These sources offer insights based on their own experiences, word of mouth, and other information they have gathered. The formal and secondary source includes physicians, other clinicians, and healthcare personnel. Because of their position in the organization and the training and knowledge they have, these sources can give authoritative advice and point the consumer to more resources.

Information from these two major sources can be supplemented by reports, findings, and announcements from the media. Historically, magazines, newspapers, books, and even newsletters as well as radio and television programs and news were the primary print and electronic media sources. These sources of information continue to be important today.

With the introduction of Medicare and Medicaid in the 1960s and the emergence of managed care in the 1980s, healthcare consumers turned to their health plans as a source of information on providers (mostly in response to the restrictions health plans imposed on the use of practitioners, facilities, and programs). Managed care plans have been particularly aggressive in establishing call centers and encouraging their enrollees to seek information before making health-related decisions.

In the 1990s, the Internet came to the fore and since then has become a major source of information for all consumers (there are purportedly more websites related to healthcare than any other topic). Most healthcare consumers with Internet access have, at some point, researched online a medical condition, a healthcare service or facility, or a clinician or provider organization. Today's consumers are increasingly armed with Internet-generated information and questions when they visit their doctors. Although the information and data available on the Internet are not always reliable (nor their quality high), they do jump-start the consumer's research. The Internet—whether social media, online newspapers, healthcare blogs, healthcare association and provider websites, or private or governmental quality rating and reporting systems—has progressively narrowed the gap between how healthcare customers and other consumers search for product information.

In addition to these decision-making process steps, marketers must consider in their marketing planning how consumers decide to change their behavior when they are ready. Exhibit 5.10 describes the five stages of behavioral change.

Summary

Although the consumer is the primary concern of almost every industry, only in recent years has healthcare come to think in terms of consumers rather than patients. Most healthcare providers in the past gave no thought to consumers until they entered the system as patients. The pre-patient and post-patient phases were neglected, and healthy people were not considered candidates for health services.

Marketers in any field spend much of their time trying to get potential customers to change their knowledge, attitudes, and behavior patterns. In healthcare, these efforts may involve educating customers to persuade them to switch to the service being marketed, to adjust their attitudes toward a particular provider, or to encourage them to change their lifestyles to improve their health. For this reason, marketers strive to understand the factors that cause individuals to modify their behavior.

One classic approach to understanding was developed by Prochaska, Norcross, and DiClemente (1995). Through their study of initiatives aimed at changing behaviors that are detrimental to health (e.g., smoking), they developed a model, which marketers could easily apply to promotional purposes, of how an individual goes through five stages when dealing with change:

1. *Pre-contemplation.* The individual has not yet thought about taking action. For example, this individual could have a healthcare condition but is unaware of it (e.g., high cholesterol).
2. *Contemplation.* The individual becomes aware of the problem and is considering doing something about it. For example, the individual with high cholesterol found out about this condition at a health fair.
3. *Preparation.* The individual has decided to start taking steps toward addressing the problem. For example, the person has

(continued)

EXHIBIT 5.10
A Stages-of-Change Approach to Market Assessment

become convinced that some action is required and begins to examine options to lower his or her cholesterol.

4. *Action.* The individual proactively faces the problem with whatever resources are available. For example, the person with high cholesterol visits a primary care physician or a nutritional counselor.

5. *Maintenance.* The individual continues the course of treatment that has been prescribed. The person with high cholesterol, for example, regularly eats a low-fat diet and takes prescribed medication.

Marketers target groups of people at various stages of this change model. The stage that a target population occupies is the stage at which the marketing technique will be focused. For example, individuals in the pre-contemplation stage clearly need awareness and information, so the marketer will use educational approaches to reach this audience and get them to move to the next stage. The marketer can tailor this approach depending on the stage being targeted.

As healthcare became more market driven, the importance of the consumer was increasingly recognized. Healthcare organizations redefined patients as customers and came to appreciate the variety of customers they serve. Today, healthcare constituents take the form of consumers, customers, clients, patients, and enrollees, all of which have unique characteristics. Other customers to be cultivated by healthcare organizations may include employers, board members, government agencies, the press/media, and the general public.

Because of the unique characteristics of the healthcare industry, healthcare consumers are different from consumers in other industries. At the same time, however, these two types of consumers share some common characteristics. To reach the massive healthcare market efficiently, marketers can segment the population on the basis of demographics, geographic, psychographics, health risks, usage, payers, and benefits.

Along with healthcare's increased emphasis on the consumer came increased attention to consumer behavior. Healthcare consumers generally follow the same steps as other consumers when making purchase decisions; they begin by recognizing a need and end with an assessment of their purchase. However, healthcare consumers' purchasing behaviors are influenced by aspects unique to healthcare that do not concern consumers of other products.

Key Points

- Healthcare providers were not used to thinking of patients as consumers. Redefining the patient as a consumer has encouraged wider use of marketing in healthcare.
- Marketers should be sensitive to the ways healthcare consumers differ from consumers of other products. At the same time, healthcare consumers share many of the attributes of consumers of other products.
- Although the patient is typically thought of as the primary consumer of health services, large healthcare organizations often have a wide variety of customers to satisfy.
- Users of health services are called by different terms, depending on the context (e.g., patient, client, customer, consumer, enrollee, end user).
- Healthcare organizations themselves (e.g., hospitals, physician practices) are customers for a wide range of goods and services.
- The healthcare market can be segmented in a number of ways— demographics, geographic, psychographics, health risks, usage, payers, and benefits.
- The consumer decision-making process for healthcare is similar in most ways to the process for other goods or services.
- Healthcare consumers seek information from a variety of sources, and the Internet has become a very important resource.
- The consumer decision-making process in healthcare is different in that someone other than the end user may make the decision and/or pay for the services.
- The consumer decision-making process is influenced by an individual's readiness to change and willingness to innovate.

Discussion Questions

1. Why is everyone in society arguably considered a potential consumer of health services?
2. Why didn't the healthcare industry historically view customers or patients as consumers?

3. In what ways are healthcare consumers different from consumers of other goods and services?

4. In what ways are healthcare consumers similar to consumers of other goods and services?

5. How can one distinguish between the different varieties of healthcare customers (e.g., patients, clients, end users, enrollees)?

6. What are some examples of institutional customers for healthcare goods and services?

7. Why do healthcare organizations often have a much wider range of customers than do organizations in other industries?

8. What are some of the dimensions along which the market for health services can be segmented?

9. What are the major steps in the decision-making process for healthcare consumers, and how do these steps differ from those in other industries?

Additional Resources

Keckley, P. H., and S. Coughlin. 2012. *2012 Survey of U.S. Health Care Consumers: Five-Year Look Back.* http://dupress.com/articles/2012-survey-of-u-s-health-care-consumers-five-year-look-back/.

Pinnell, J. 2003. "Improving Healthcare Marketing Through Market Segmentation and Targeting." www.warc.com/fulltext/ESOMAR/78785.htm.

Prochaska, J. O., J. C. Norcross, and C. C. DiClemente. 1994. *Changing for Good: The Revolutionary Program That Explains the Six Stages of Change and Teaches You How to Free Yourself from Bad Habits.* New York: William Morrow.

HEALTHCARE PRODUCTS

I n developing a marketing initiative, a marketer's first task is to understand the product to be promoted. In healthcare, the product may be something as simple as a bottle of aspirin or as complex as heart transplant surgery. Whether simple or complex, the product must be conceptualized in a manner conducive to effective promotion. This chapter addresses the issues involved in defining the product to be marketed. The implications of defining the product in various ways are reviewed, and the emerging retail aspect of healthcare is discussed.

For purposes of this discussion, the normally interchangeable terms *goods* and *services* are considered as two types of product. Unlike marketers in other industries, who tend to promote clearly defined products, healthcare marketers expend a great deal of effort determining exactly what they are marketing.

The first questions a marketer is likely to ask in developing a marketing initiative are (1) What is the product? and (2) How is it being sold? In most other industries, the answers would be straightforward and relatively easy to provide because the product is its reason for existence; an executive who cannot specify his or her company's product is not likely to succeed in today's environment. The situation is not so simple in healthcare, as health professionals do not think in terms of products. A health professional's response to "What is your product?" may be along the lines of "quality care," "improved health," or "treatment and cure." Although these answers sound great, they are not helpful to a marketer.

Product Mix

An organization's *product mix* refers to the combination of goods, services, and ideas that it promotes to consumers. Large healthcare organizations, like hospitals, offer a wide range of goods and services. They perform hundreds of intangible services and procedures and dispense or sell hundreds of tangible goods (e.g., drugs, supplies, equipment) in the course of normal operations. At the same time, they often promote ideas to plant a particular perception in the consumer's mind. The organization's brand image, for example, is an idea that can be promoted through marketing. Quality care, professionalism, value, or other subjective but desirable attributes may also be promoted. Ultimately, the product mix determines the focus of marketing activities.

Goods Versus Services

The purchase of goods tends to involve a single episode, whereas the purchase of services may be an ongoing process. Although healthcare is generally perceived as a service, the sale of goods is ubiquitous in the industry—goods that range from consumer health products to pharmaceuticals to home-testing kits to durable medical equipment. A physical examination, a flu shot, and open-heart surgery are all examples of health services. Most people would recognize each of these activities as a service, but the nature of services is often difficult to describe.

The primary distinction between goods and services is their tangibility—the extent to which the product can be examined, touched, or experienced before purchase. Second, goods and services can be distinguished by their durability. Services tend to be consumed at the time they are administered (e.g., immunization), whereas goods tend to last for an indefinite time (e.g., a blood-pressure monitoring device). These distinctions clearly determine the marketing strategy developed for each category.

Healthcare is unlike other industries in that the various stakeholders of the same service tend to have diverging perceptions, depending on the role they play in the service rendered. In the case of childbirth, for example, the mother may see it as a natural experience, the physician could view it as a medical episode, and the hospital administrator could regard it as an accounting event. Alternatively, the mother could see it as a unitary episode, the physician as a series of discrete activities, and the administrator as a group of billable and nonbillable items; the healthcare marketer might view it as yet something else. The marketer's task is to conceptualize the product and package it appropriately—that is, present the service in a manner to which the consumer can relate.

Consumer Goods Versus Industrial Goods

Goods can be classified by their users and buyers. *Consumer goods* are purchased by the end user of the items. In most industries, these items are divided into three categories: (1) convenience goods, (2) shopping goods, and (3) specialty goods.

Convenience good
A product consumers purchase frequently without forethought

Convenience goods are those that people purchase regularly and as needed, such as cold or headache remedies, dental floss, and tissues. Because the consumer engages in little deliberation when purchasing such items, name recognition and product distribution are critical concerns for the marketer. The manufacturers of over-the-counter drugs, for example, expend considerable effort in establishing brand identity and prominently displaying their product in retail outlets.

Shopping goods are products that require the consumer to search for and compare competing brands on attributes such as price, style, or features. Fitness equipment, computers, and cameras are common examples of shopping goods. Marketers of shopping goods must differentiate their brand from the competitors' brands by emphasizing features that are important to their customers. Salespeople often play a major role in helping consumers learn about alternative brands.

Specialty goods are specific items a consumer seeks. Often, the consumer is loyal to a particular brand and will go to great lengths to find that brand among a multitude of others. Common specialty items include exclusive brands of jewelry, perfume, or electronic equipment as well as one-of-a-kind or imported food or drink. Few goods in healthcare are included in the specialty category.

Industrial goods are products purchased for use in the manufacture of other products, which will at some point be purchased by the ultimate consumer. (Note the distinction between consumer goods for personal use and goods purchased for professional or institutional use.) Industrial products are stratified into two broad levels. **Production goods** are those that are made into a final product; raw materials (such as the chemicals of a prescription drug) fit into this category. **Support goods** are those used to enable the production of goods or provision of services. Examples include a computed tomography (CT) scanner, an examination table, and the printer used to generate patient bills.

Nondurable Versus Durable Goods

A **nondurable good** is a product that should be consumed within a defined time frame (e.g., unprocessed or fresh foods, drugs, bandages). A **durable good** is a product that lasts for an extended period (e.g., hospital beds, wheelchairs, computer hardware).

The differences between goods and services and between nondurable and durable goods are important considerations in any marketing initiative. Nondurable products are often heavily advertised because they are perishable and are purchased frequently. Marketers prominently display them in stores to directly sell them to consumers. Durable products usually cost more than nondurable products and are often more complicated to use. For these products, a personal sales approach is often used to answer questions and explain the intricacies of the product.

Product or Service Lines

In the 1980s, following the lead of other industries, healthcare organizations began to develop *product* or *service lines*. Most industries have product lines, but in healthcare, the term **service lines** is more in keeping with the mission of healthcare providers. To establish service lines, a hospital's programs are

---

Shopping good
A product consumers compare to competing brands (on price, style, and features) before purchasing

Specialty good
A product—often expensive—that carries a brand name

Production good
A product or raw material used to produce other goods

Support good
A product used to supply or support the provision of goods and services

Nondurable good
A product used once or a few times and then disposed of

Durable good
A product used repeatedly over an extended period

Service line
A bundle of unique, related services

organized into vertical groupings centered on specific clinical areas. Specialty areas frequently selected for service lines include women's services, cancer care, cardiology, orthopedics, and pediatrics. Each service line is considered semiautonomous, and the service line manager is charged with the vertical integration of the relevant clinical services and necessary support functions. Thus, the service line administrator has broad control over the range of activities (including marketing) that support the service line.

Packaging
The presentation of the physical attributes or the positioning of a good or service

Some observers contend that service lines are little more than a **packaging** of services for marketing purposes. Although there are certainly cases in which the service line relates more to packaging than substance, in most cases a certain level of reorganization occurs around the specific clinical area. See Exhibit 6.1 for a discussion of the service line approach.

Ways to Conceptualize Products

A marketer must be able to conceptualize the products offered by the health-care organization. That is, the marketing approach must reflect the nature and complexity of the product, and the marketer must understand who uses the product and how they use it. This section discusses the differences between various product categories.

Level of Care

Primary care
Basic, routine health services, including preventive care

Primary care refers to basic health services (i.e., general examination or physical, taking medical history, physician consultation, preventive services) and the treatment of minor, nonurgent problems. Primary care may involve some self-care and the services of a nonphysician health professional (e.g., pharmacist); for some ethnic groups, primary care could involve a folk healer.

Formal primary care services are generally provided by physicians who have been trained in family practice, general internal medicine, obstetrics/gynecology, and pediatrics. These practitioners are typically community based (rather than hospital based), rely on direct first contact with patients rather than referrals from other physicians, and provide continuous rather than episodic care. Physician extenders, such as nurse practitioners and physician assistants, are taking on a growing responsibility for primary care. In the mental health system, psychologists and other types of counselors provide the primary level of care. Medical specialists may also provide some primary care.

Primary care is generally delivered in a physician's office or in some type of clinic. Hospital outpatient departments, urgent care centers, neighborhood clinics, and other ambulatory care facilities also provide primary care services. For certain segments of the population, the hospital emergency department is a source of primary care. In addition, the home has become a

EXHIBIT 6.1
Healthcare
Service Lines
and Marketing

Since the 1980s, many hospitals have adopted the service line management concept long established in other industries. Service line management appeared attractive to hospitals looking for ways to become more agile, move closer to their customers, strengthen relationships with physicians, become more profitable, and move beyond cost cutting and reengineering to develop more innovative and effective ways of serving their patients (Ireland 2003).

A service line is a tightly integrated, overlapping network of semi-autonomous clinical services and a business enterprise that bundles needed resources to provide specialized, focused care and value to a patient population. The most common service lines include cardiovascular services, orthopedics, rehabilitation, women's services, children's services, and oncology services. Service lines can be virtual in that all components may not be under one roof; some services are horizontal and cross departments and disciplines. A service line may be created around a business that is already well established, or the concept may be used to focus on a new service or niche.

The product line concept was developed by organizations in other industries—most notably Procter & Gamble, General Electric, and General Motors—to decentralize decision making; make strategic planning more effective; improve cost management and productivity; improve communication and collaboration; and, most important, help its product line management teams better understand the needs of their customers. The product line management concept emerged in the healthcare industry in the 1980s as an organizational effort to deal with prospective reimbursement, a tight economic environment, declining revenues, and intense competition—all of which drove the need for improving the way hospitals did business. In healthcare, this concept has probably been carried furthest by pharmaceutical companies that organize their business enterprise by product lines.

Many of the gains from service line management were erased with the emergence of managed care and other innovative financing structures in the late 1980s. Although many hospitals maintained their service line orientation throughout the 1990s, the concept was latent and reemerged only around 1997, when hospitals began to renew their patient focus. This revitalized service line management model defines a hospital's clinical services; allocates organizational resources—human, financial, and strategic—to these service lines; and clearly assigns accountability for performance to a service line leader.

(continued)

This service line platform integrates clinical and support services on a matrix management grid to create horizontal integration of clinical services along a traditional continuum of care along with the vertical integration of support services. Also built into this platform are education and wellness programs, retail models, business development tactics, and a strong focus on physician relationships—all with an increased emphasis on creating enhanced quality and value for patients.

Because the service line is sensitive to its costs and operational dynamics, its customers, and its competition, hospitals and health systems are able to decentralize accountability for strategic, operational, and financial performance from the corporate or executive office to the clinical service line. This shift in accountability to the service line maximizes hospital capacity by focusing on the best use of space and resources and provides more flexibility in managing growth.

Whether the service line concept is an effective approach to healthcare strategy development is still open to debate, and little hard evidence of the merits of this approach exists. Service line management does facilitate the marketing of services in many ways, and the close relationship between operations and marketing that can develop is an advantage.

Around 2005 another wave of interest in service line management in healthcare emerged (Litch 2007). This renewed interest reflected a growing emphasis on quality control, integrated services, and physician collaboration. From a marketing perspective, the growing need to establish an advantageous market position appeared to drive the revival.

The significance of service lines to customers is not clear. Ideally, service lines are designed to address consumer needs, but most consumers probably think about healthcare as a continuum of services that extend across clinical lines, not in terms of vertical silos of care. As service lines become more entrenched in healthcare, a better understanding of their meaning for consumers should be established.

common site for the provision of primary care. This trend has been driven by the financial pressures on inpatient care, changing consumer preferences, and improved home care technology. Case Study 6.1 addresses the marketing of primary care services for an urgent care center.

Emergency care
Emergency treatment or services in response to an urgent medical need

In terms of hospital services, primary care refers to services that can be provided at a general hospital. Hospital primary care typically includes routine medical and surgical procedures, diagnostic tests, and obstetrics services as well as **emergency care** (although not major trauma) and many outpatient services. Hospital-based primary care tends to be unspecialized and requires a relatively low level of technological sophistication.

Secondary care involves a higher degree of specialization and technological sophistication than primary care because of the increased severity of the health problems encountered. Physician care is provided by more highly trained practitioners, such as specialized surgeons (e.g., urologists, ophthalmologists) and specialized internists (e.g., cardiologists, oncologists). Problems requiring more specialized skills and more sophisticated biomedical equipment are included in this category. Although much of the care is still provided in a physician's office or clinic, these specialists tend to spend a large share of their time in the hospital setting. Secondary hospitals are capable of providing more complex technological backup, physician specialist support, and ancillary services than are primary care hospitals. These facilities can handle moderately complex surgical and medical cases and serve as referral centers for primary care facilities.

> **Secondary care** Services for conditions that are moderately complex and need a moderate level of resources and skills

CASE STUDY 6.1
Marketing an Urgent Care Center

During the 1980s, some enterprising healthcare professionals believed that an alternative to the traditional physician's office was needed. While they conceded that many patients desired a long-term relationship with a physician and were willing to accept the deficiencies of the typical physician practice to obtain it, they also thought there was a significant portion of the population that did not have an established physician relationship but occasionally required some type of care. Some of these consumers were new to the community and had not found a regular physician, while others had become disillusioned with their physician but had not yet found a replacement. Still others were dissatisfied with the conditions under which care had to be obtained—long waits for an appointment, long waits in the waiting room, short time (often only five minutes) spent with the doctor, and a big bill afterwards. Out of this frustrating situation, the urgent care center was born.

The concept behind urgent care centers was to develop conveniently located (i.e., in the community) walk-in clinics staffed by the same types of physicians encountered in a doctor's office. Each center would offer basic services only and refer patients with anything more than a minor condition to another facility. Although the center would accept insurance, it would charge a low fee to attract patients without insurance and

(continued)

patients with insurance who were turned off by their regular physicians. The center would not maintain medical records beyond the basics, assuming most visits were one-time events. They would have the advantage of quick service with none of the hassle associated with a typical physician's office.

Convinced there was a demand for this type of service in a highly mobile, convenience-oriented society, physician entrepreneurs in a mid-sized city in the South set out to establish a network of seven urgent care centers at strategically located sites. They chose fairly new suburban areas close to high-traffic commercial and retail centers, believing that these locations would attract the customers they were seeking. Having taken something of a location gamble, they faced the challenge of marketing the new concept. They brought in marketers to survey consumers to determine the best prospects for urgent care centers.

Upon reviewing the surveys, the physicians developed a fairly clear idea of their prospective customers. The best prospects were 25- to 40-year-old men and women who were highly mobile (often new to the community), fairly well educated, and more often than not in a two-income family without children. Whites appeared to be more open to the idea than nonwhites. Those in the middle- to upper-middle-class income categories were great prospects; the more affluent were not attracted, and the downscale populations were intimidated by this practice model and concerned about having to pay cash upfront. In terms of lifestyle, the survey showed that those who were progressive, innovative, highly mobile, and more focused on the present than the future were more likely to use the service.

This information confirmed the developers' intuition about locating the centers in newly emerging affluent suburbs, and they set out to market this service to the target population. Taking advantage of various sources of data, the developers were able to target the households that displayed the desired characteristics within a five-mile radius of each site. Of the seven urgent care centers established, five were successful and two significantly underperformed. The only discernable differences between the successful and unsuccessful ones were the lower visibility and lower drive-by traffic characterizing the latter.

The developers' ability to target the most likely prospects helped them launch a successful promotional campaign that quickly resulted in a high volume of business. Without knowledge of the most likely prospects, the marketers' efforts would have been ineffective and the growth of the urgent care center clientele would have been much slower.

Case Study Discussion Questions

1. What factors encouraged the entrepreneurs to develop an alternative to the traditional source of primary care?
2. What characteristics did the urgent care center concept have that might make it unattractive to mainstream healthcare consumers?
3. What assumptions did the developers make at the outset about the demand for such a service and the type of consumers who might use it?
4. From their market research, did the developers find that the urgent care center model would appeal to the general population or that some segments of the population would find it more attractive than others?
5. What was the profile of the best prospects for utilization of an urgent care center?
6. How did knowledge of the characteristics of the best prospects contribute to an effective marketing campaign?
7. Given the characteristics of the best prospects, what attributes of the urgent care centers should be highlighted in promotional material?

Tertiary care addresses the most complex of surgical and medical conditions. The practitioners tend to be subspecialists housed in highly complex and technologically advanced facilities. Complex procedures, such as emergency care for a heart attack and reconstructive surgery, are performed at facilities that provide extensive support services in the form of personnel and technology. Tertiary care cases are usually handled by a team of medical and/or surgical specialists who are supported by the hospital's radiology, pathology, and anesthesiology physician staff. Tertiary care is generally provided at a few centers that serve large geographic areas. Single hospitals are often not sufficient for the provision of tertiary care; a medical center may be required. These centers typically support functions not directly related to patient care, such as teaching and research.

> **Tertiary care**
> Services for conditions that are highly complex (or serious) and need specialized clinicians, equipment, and facilities

Some procedures performed at tertiary facilities may be considered **quaternary care**. Organ transplantation—especially involving vital organs such as the heart, lungs, and pancreas—is one example of quaternary care. Complicated trauma cases are another example. This level of care is restricted to major medical centers, often in medical school settings. These procedures require the most sophisticated equipment and are often performed in association with research activities.

> **Quaternary care**
> Specialized services provided in large medical centers for complex conditions

The level of care plays an important role in determining the type of marketing technique to use. Consumers often have more discretion in decisions about primary care than about specialized forms of care. They can typically choose their primary care physician (although their insurance plan may limit their choices), and they can obtain primary care through urgent care centers or emergency departments if the situation warrants. However, specialists—especially those involved in tertiary or quaternary care—are more difficult to access. Specialists typically require a referral from another physician or health professional, and insurance plans are reluctant to reimburse for the services of a specialist if the proper procedures have not been followed.

Because of these factors, consumers are a more viable marketing target for primary care services than for more specialized services. Marketing tertiary or quaternary care to the general public is not likely to be effective because someone other than the patient typically makes the treatment decision. Nevertheless, consumers need to be made aware of all available services, even if they cannot access them directly. See Exhibit 6.2 for a graphic depiction of the levels of healthcare.

Level of Urgency

Health problems are generally classified as routine, urgent, or emergent. Routine health problems make up the bulk of primary care episodes, and many, if not most, urgent care episodes involve routine care that is provided during off-hours. Emergency care typically involves at least secondary care, if not tertiary or quaternary care.

Although marketing can influence the use of all three categories of care, some are more amenable to marketing than others. In general, routine care—such as primary care—allows the most discretion by the consumer. Therefore, marketing for routine care is relatively straightforward and typically focuses on promoting available services directly to potential customers.

In some ways, potential urgent care patients may be more amenable to marketing than even routine care patients. Potential customers of urgent care centers may not have a regular source of care and are thus likely to be responsive to marketing messages when the need for care arises. Marketing for urgent care is not as straightforward, however, as that for routine care. Although most consumers will need urgent care at one time or another, its unpredictable nature and the many segments of the population that prefer more traditional primary care services pose a challenge for healthcare marketers. A marketer charged with promoting an urgent care center must be aware of the attributes that lead consumers to choose an urgent care center rather than their private practitioner or a hospital emergency department.

Emergency services are perhaps the most difficult to market effectively to the general population. Emergency department use is a rare event and

Procedures	Location	Practitioner
	Quaternary Care	
Organ transplantation, complex trauma	Multi-institution medical centers	Teams of super-specialist physicians
	Tertiary Care	
Specialized surgery, complex medical cases	Large-scale comprehensive hospitals with extensive technological support	Physician subspecialists
	Secondary Care	
Moderately complex medical and surgical cases	Moderate-scale hospitals, some freestanding surgery and diagnostic centers	Physician specialists
	Primary Care	
Routine care, standard tests, simple surgery, prevention, counseling	General hospitals, clinics, physicians' offices, urgent care centers, counseling centers	Primary care physicians, extenders

EXHIBIT 6.2

Levels of Healthcare in the United States

↑

Complexity

Severity

Specialization

Source: Adapted from Pol and Thomas (2013).

decisions about emergency care are often made under duress. In situations where people choose the hospital emergency department, their physician's affiliations and/or health plan restrictions are likely to be considerations. If, for example, a patient is taken to an emergency department at a hospital not in her network, she would have to be transferred to an in-network facility for her insurance to cover the charges. The marketer's approach to the general public might include promoting the quality of the organization's emergency services and promising a high level of patient satisfaction.

In most cases, someone other than the patient is likely to make the choice about emergency care when the need arises. For serious conditions, emergency medical technicians will make the decision on the basis of the proximity of an emergency department or the type of emergency services required. Thus, emergency services may be more appropriately marketed to ambulance companies, emergency medical technicians, police dispatchers, and other decision makers rather than to the general public.

Inpatient Versus Outpatient Care

Inpatient care
Medical care provided by a hospital to patients who are admitted for at least one night

Inpatient care requires at least an overnight stay and is typically provided in hospitals. **Outpatient** (or ambulatory) **care** includes less than 24 hours' stay in a health facility. Outpatient services typically allow more consumer discretion than do inpatient services. Consumers may present themselves for many outpatient services without a prior relationship or even an appointment. The use of inpatient services requires at minimum a referral and/or admission by a physician, and possibly authorization by the patient's health insurance plan. While the general public can be directly targeted for outpatient care, the marketing approach for inpatient care should focus on establishing and cultivating a loyal medical staff and negotiating favorable contracts with health plans.

Outpatient care
Medical care provided outside a hospital or an inpatient facility; also known as *ambulatory care*

Medical Versus Surgical Services

Medical procedures involve treatments based primarily on drug therapy, and surgical procedures are therapies that primarily involve surgery of some type. Of course, when any surgery is performed, some drugs are administered, and when drug therapy is administered, some surgical procedures, however minor, may be required.

These two approaches to care are obviously different and are implemented by different specialists. Medical therapy is typically carried out by internists and internal medicine specialists (e.g., nephrologists, gastroenterologists), and surgery is performed by general surgeons or surgical specialists (e.g., ophthalmic surgeons, orthopedic surgeons). Although risk is inherent in both types of therapies, the general public usually attributes greater risk to surgical procedures. In either case, the marketer must emphasize the benefits and minimize the risks of the procedures involved.

Diagnosis Versus Treatment

Diagnostic procedures are used to assess health status and to test for the presence of a pathological condition. Treatments (or therapeutic procedures) are used to treat a condition once it has been diagnosed. Many diagnostic procedures are routine and administered at regular intervals to asymptomatic individuals; these procedures are usually referred to as *screening tests*. Tests administered in response to observed symptoms are usually referred to as *diagnostic tests*. For example, there are screening mammograms and diagnostic mammograms. This distinction is important because the same test might be marketed in a different manner according to its use. Clearly, the approach to marketing differs on the basis of whether the product is a diagnosis or a treatment. With diagnostic procedures, the emphasis is on prevention and early detection, and the intent is to maintain health. With treatment procedures, the emphasis is on treatment and cure, and the intent is to restore health.

Clinical Versus Nonclinical Services

Clinical services involve the administration of a formal medical procedure. Examinations, diagnostic tests, and therapeutic procedures administered by a clinical practitioner are examples of clinical services.

Healthcare providers have added a number of nonclinical services to complement their clinical services. Some hospitals, for example, provide valet parking, food services for nonpatients, and senior discount programs. In addition, some practitioners link their patients to support groups, while others offer childcare or transportation. As noted in Chapter 10, some healthcare organizations have even launched concierge services.

Obviously, nonclinical amenities are marketed differently from clinical services. Although clinical care may seem to be the most important (they generate the most revenue), consumers are more likely to evaluate their experiences on the basis of the nonclinical aspects. Thus, marketers need to give nonclinical services adequate attention.

Elective Versus Nonelective Procedures

Nonelective procedures are those considered medically necessary, although they do not always deal with life-threatening conditions. **Elective procedures**, on the other hand, are those that patients voluntarily choose to undergo, such as a nontherapeutic abortion, laser eye surgery, face-lifts, and hair transplantation. Some surgery (e.g., for tennis elbow) might not be considered medically necessary and thus be classified as elective. Nonelective services are considered nondiscretionary, while elective services are considered discretionary.

Nonelective procedure
A clinical service considered medically necessary

Elective procedure
A clinical service not considered medically necessary and obtained at the discretion of the customer

Although elective and nonelective procedures may be marketed in much the same manner, there are significant differences to note. For one thing, the decision maker is likely to be different. Nonelective surgery is generally prescribed by a medical practitioner and, being medically necessary, is covered under a health insurance plan. On the other hand, the decision to undergo an elective procedure is generally made by the patient, perhaps on the advice of a medical practitioner. Because of their elective nature, these procedures are typically not covered by insurance. For these reasons, marketers have to promote nonelective procedures and elective procedures differently. For nonelective procedures, demand cannot be influenced by marketing to as great an extent. Thus, the emphasis must be on influencing the choice of provider when a condition arises. On the other hand, a hospital seeking patients for nonelective procedures may target its marketing toward admitting and referring physicians to channel referrals into its system.

The marketing of elective procedures has a lot in common with the marketing of nonmedical services. Providers of these services are much more prone to advertise their services and often compete on the same basis as providers of other types of services. Thus, eye surgeons and plastic surgeons may advertise their low prices, convenient locations, and efficient customer service. In addition, creating demand for these services may be possible. Most balding men probably suffered in silence with their hair loss until they saw promotions for a hair restoration clinic; this introduction of a new service essentially established a market where one did not exist before.

Life cycle
The maturation of a population, a product, or an industry from birth to death

One additional way to categorize products is in terms of their point in the product **life cycle**. A product may be in the introductory, growth, maturity, or decline stage. A product's position in the life cycle is significant in that it shapes the marketing strategy that should be pursued. An innovative service is likely to be marketed differently, for example, from a mature service. Exhibit 6.3 describes the product life cycle and its implications for marketing.

Common Healthcare Products

This section elaborates on the types of products in either goods or services categories and the types of healthcare organizations that provide them. The marketing team generally focuses its campaign on a specific service rather than the organization in general, so it is critical for marketers to understand how to classify healthcare products.

Categories of Goods

As mentioned earlier, healthcare organizations and providers sell a significant number of goods. For example, hospitals not only provide their patients with medication, food, home monitoring kits, and sundry supplies but also sell to patients and others crutches, braces, prosthetics, and other durable goods. They may also sell goods through a gift shop, a resource library, or another retail-type enterprise. Some hospital service line extensions may sell goods on a retail basis. For example, the fitness center might sell nutritional supplements, athletic attire, and exercise equipment, while the cardiac rehabilitation program may sell DVDs, books, and other resources and tools. Exhibit 6.4 describes the emergence of retail medicine.

Other types of institutions providing inpatient care may sell similar goods, although none is likely to match the range a hospital offers. Nursing homes, residential treatment centers, and assisted living centers typically

EXHIBIT 6.3
The Product
Life Cycle

Healthcare products, like other products, experience a natural life cycle that comprises four stages: introduction, growth, maturity, and decline. Marketers need to understand these four stages to craft an effective marketing strategy. If an organization is primarily involved in providing inpatient services, for example, marketers need to recognize where inpatient services can be placed in the life cycle. Or, if a marketing plan is being developed for a specific procedure, the marketer must determine where that procedure resides in the life cycle.

The first stage in the product's life cycle is the **introductory** (or market development) **stage**. A new product is likely to be innovative, so most of the marketing effort is directed toward creating awareness and cultivating the **early adopters** in the market. At this stage, there are relatively few competitors and products are not yet standardized. The market is relatively easy to enter because the established players are few, although in healthcare, regulatory requirements often must be met (such as Food and Drug Administration approval). New pharmaceuticals are one example of a healthcare product subject to regulation.

At the **growth stage**, the product has become established and the market has accepted it. Expansion is rapid, as new customers are attracted and more competitors enter the arena. Products become increasingly standardized, although enhancements may continue to contribute to product evolution. Marketing planning at this stage emphasizes differentiation of the organization, product, or service. The rapid growth of cosmetic surgery during the 1990s is an example of this type of expansion.

By the **maturity stage**, the product has matured, most of the potential customers have been captured, and growth is beginning to taper off. Because few new customers are available, competition for existing customers increases. Product features and pricing are highly standardized, and little differentiation remains between competitors. The number of competitors decreases as consolidation occurs, and it becomes increasingly difficult for new players to enter the market. Marketing activities emphasize retaining existing customers and/or capturing customers from competitors. Traditional hospital inpatient services are an example of a product that has reached the maturity stage.

When a product reaches maturity, it must adapt to its new state to remain viable. At this point, three strategies may be used to stretch the lifespan of the product: (1) modify the product, (2) modify the market, or (3) reposition the product. Hospitals have used all of these strategies by

(continued)

Introductory stage
The first phase of a product's life cycle in which the product or industry is launched

Early adopter
An individual or a group willing to try new products and services before they are accepted by the general public

Growth stage
The second phase of a product's life cycle in which the product or industry gains dominance in the market

Maturity stage
The third phase of a product's life cycle in which the product or industry reaches its apex and ceases to grow

Decline stage
The fourth phase of a product's life cycle in which the product or industry decreases in importance and is supplanted by another

adding goods and/or services to their existing product mix, promoting their services to new markets, and shifting some services from the inpatient to the outpatient setting.

In the **decline stage**, the number of customers decreases as consumers substitute new products or services. Typically, a shakeout occurs among industry players as the dominant competitors squeeze out the less entrenched and as other competitors adopt a different strategic direction. Competition among the remaining players for existing customers becomes even more heated. Because no innovations are being introduced and the customer base cannot be expanded, the remaining competitors tend to emphasize cost reduction to maintain profitability.

The role of marketing changes depending on the product's stage in the life cycle. The stage influences the packaging of products, the promotional techniques, the approaches to competitors, and the relationships with other organizations.

During the introductory stage—when the product represents an innovation—the marketer's primary task is to educate consumers about the product while facilitating a first-to-market approach. During the growth stage, marketers focus on differentiating the product from those of competitors by capitalizing on its attributes and penetrating new markets. During the maturity stage, the role of marketing shifts dramatically. There are few new customers for the product, so marketers focus on retaining existing customers and capturing customers from competitors. Market consolidation is likely to occur at this stage, and the marketer may be involved in enhancing the organization's image during this period of turmoil. During the decline stage, the marketer must focus on maintaining current customers and presenting the product in creative new ways to extend its life span.

provide supplies, medication, food, and other nondurable goods to their patients or residents. Some of these goods are considered part and parcel of the room charge or surgical fee, and others are itemized on the patient's bill.

Many of the same procedures performed on hospital patients are carried out in physicians' offices, so physicians provide many of the same goods, such as wound dressings, casts, disposable supplies, and medications. These goods are typically not itemized separately but are included in the overall cost of the professional services. Some physicians have become increasingly involved in the retail aspect of healthcare, offering their patients a range of related goods. For example, a cardiologist may sell exercise DVDs,

The concept of *retail medicine*—or healthcare available to the masses outside the traditional institutional setting—is a relatively new **niche** in the elective outpatient healthcare marketplace. Retail medicine is a collection of unique, personalized products and services that help patients manage their healthcare. Patients often pay for these products and services out of pocket rather than through their insurance company. In its broadest sense, retail medicine includes a range of activities, from selling products in physicians' offices, clinics, and hospitals to establishing comprehensive body imaging centers. Some of the more common goods and services sold include dietary supplements, wellness programs, cosmetic medical products and services, and diagnostic and imaging tests (Woods 2007). By the turn of the twenty-first century, retail medicine had gathered significant momentum as entrepreneurs sought to profit from high consumer demand that traditional medicine had failed to meet (Pyrek 2002).

Aging baby boomers—the vast majority of whom consume retail medicine—are more concerned about their health than were any previous American generations and, as a result, are driving a lot of the interest in retail medicine. In addition, retail medicine introduced to the healthcare community new buzzwords and phrases, including *medical entrepreneurs*, who market their services to consumers known as the *worried well* and the *worried wealthy*.

One trend in retail medicine was the development of walk-in primary care clinics in nontraditional settings. Many large retail stores added primary care services to supplement the existing optometry and dental services on site. For example, the Walgreen's drug store chain introduced Take Care Clinics, in-store walk-in clinics that are staffed by nurse practitioners and that cater to customers who are not interested in long-term physician relationships, have an immediate healthcare need, and may not have the insurance to cover a more expensive visit to a traditional healthcare setting (Take Care Health Services 2009a). By 2009, Take Care Clinics were operating in 340 Walgreen's pharmacies and Take Care Health had become the nation's leading provider of workplace-based healthcare services. These services include on-site health, wellness, and fitness centers; on-site pharmacies; and health promotion and disease management programs. Take Care Health Employer Solutions operates nearly 370 workplace health centers and pharmacies for 180 clients in 45 states as well as in Washington, DC, and Guam (Take Care Health Services 2009b). Similarly, CVS/Caremark,

(continued)

EXHIBIT 6.4
The Emergence of Retail Medicine

Niche
A segment of a market that can be carved out because of the uniqueness of the target population, the geographic area, or the product being promoted

---

Walgreen's primary pharmacy competitor, opened up Minute Clinics on site. A number of other retail medicine chains installed primary care outlets in shopping malls and in big-box stores like Wal-Mart and Target. Even some hospital systems set up branded clinics in retail stores in their market areas. This trend continues today: 1,350 clinics were operating in retail establishments in 2013 (Gardner 2013).

Another trend was the full-body scan, which medical entrepreneurs purport to reveal abnormalities in the body—ranging from tumors and gallstones to clogged arteries to cancer—so that they can be addressed before they become life threatening. Such scans promise to detect latent signs of medical conditions as well.

Other examples of retail medicine include healthcare organizations building fitness and wellness programs and opening them up to the general public and providers selling consumer goods related to their specialty straight out of their offices. Obstetrician and pediatrician practices, for example, might sell books or DVDs on childbirth and parenting, or dermatologists may peddle a line of products for skin care, sun protection, and hair growth.

---

educational CDs, heart-healthy cookbooks, or medical alert wristbands. Although these retail activities are not endorsed by the American Medical Association, they have become entrenched in a number of medical practices.

Among other independent practitioners, some sell numerous goods and others sell relatively few. A major part of an optometrist's business (and, to a lesser extent, an ophthalmologist's) is the sale of eyeglasses and contact lenses. Likewise, although dentists and dental specialists primarily provide services, a considerable portion of their revenue may be derived from the sale of dentures, braces, and even high-end toothbrushes.

Categories of Services

The primary function of a healthcare provider is to offer services aimed at addressing a particular healthcare need. A hospital's fee schedule, for example, includes thousands of individual services. It is not practical to itemize all of these services; therefore, only the major categories are noted in this section.

One way of looking at these services is in terms of clinical areas. Services may be classified as obstetrics, pediatrics, cardiac, oncology, orthopedics, and so forth. The services provided to obstetric patients, for example, are grouped together, as are those in the other clinical categories. Medicare's prospective payment system recognized these categories and made them the industry standard. Various clinical support services, such as radiology and laboratory services, are generally provided independent of a particular specialty and serve patients in all of the clinical categories.

Another way of classifying the services provided by hospitals (and certain other facilities) is to distinguish between facility-based services and professional services. Items associated with a hospital stay include the room, nursing services, technical services, and some overhead. Charges for these and other services are bundled in the per diem room rate, but services that involve variable costs (e.g., breathing treatments) may be charged separately—as part of the facility fee. Hospital-based physicians (e.g., radiologists, anesthesiologists, hospitalists) also submit separate bills, which may be combined with the facility charges. Attending and consulting physicians typically bill separately for their professional fees because they are not employed by the hospital.

The services a hospital provides may be divided into diagnostic and therapeutic categories involving different **coding systems**. Routine diagnostic procedures (e.g., x-rays, blood tests, urinalyses) and specialized diagnostic tests (e.g., mammograms, CT scans, bone density tests) are offered in the hospital setting. Hospitals, out of all healthcare organizations, typically provide the widest array of diagnostic capabilities; other clinicians offer few diagnostic tests that are not available in hospitals.

Coding system
A structure for classifying and recording medical diagnoses, procedures, and other events

Therapeutic procedures account for the widest range of treatments provided in hospitals. They take the form of the simplest treatments, such as administration of medication or intravenous fluids, as well as most complex procedures, such as open heart surgery and organ transplantation. As noted earlier, these procedures are typically grouped into clinical categories and supervised by administrators dedicated to that clinical sphere.

It is impossible to develop an understanding of the bewildering range of diagnostic and therapeutic services without a working knowledge of the manner in which conditions and procedures are classified. Marketers need to have at least a basic knowledge of the classification or coding systems used in healthcare. Exhibit 6.5 provides an overview of these systems.

Hospitals provide another distinct category of services: emergency care. The emergency department is designed to handle cases urgent enough that they cannot be processed through normal admission procedures. Theoretically, this department handles serious injuries and health conditions that require immediate attention. Emergency departments are staffed with physicians and nurses trained in emergency medicine and are backed up by a full range of hospital personnel. Emergency departments maintain or have access to diagnostic equipment that expeditiously determines a patient's condition. Services provided in the emergency department are charged separately from those for inpatients. Like inpatients, emergency patients are charged both a facility fee and a professional fee.

EXHIBIT 6.5
Coding
Systems in
Healthcare

The following is a brief introduction to the common classification or coding systems used in healthcare. Additional research into each is recommended for marketers or anyone seeking a more comprehensive discussion.

International Classification of Diseases

International Classification of Diseases (ICD) The standard coding system medical practitioners use to classify diseases

The most widely recognized disease classification system is the **International Classification of Diseases (ICD)** developed by the World Health Organization. The ICD is used to classify medical conditions and procedures that occur in hospitals and certain other healthcare settings. The ICD-9 classification system (still in use in the United States) includes two components: diagnoses and procedures. A set of codes is assigned to each component. These codes are detailed enough that fine distinctions can be made among different diagnoses and procedures. (A different system is used for recording procedures in physicians' offices and other outpatient settings.)

The diagnoses component comprises 17 disease and injury categories and 2 supplementary classifications. In each category, major specific conditions are listed in detail. A three-digit number is assigned to the major subdivisions in each of the 17 categories. These three-digit numbers are extended by another digit to indicate a subcategory within the larger category (to add clinical detail or isolate terms for clinical accuracy). A fifth digit is sometimes added to specify factors further associated with the diagnosis. For example, in the ICD-9, Hodgkin's disease—a form of malignant neoplasm or cancer—is coded 201. Hodgkin's sarcoma, a particular type of Hodgkin's disease, is coded 201.2. If the Hodgkin's sarcoma affects the lymph nodes of the neck, it is coded 201.21.

Current Procedural Terminology

Current procedural terminology (CPT) The coding system used to classify medical procedures for record-keeping purposes

Although the ICD focuses on procedures performed under the auspices of a hospital or clinic, the **current procedural terminology (CPT)** system relates exclusively to procedures and services performed by physicians. Physician-provided procedures and services are divided into five categories: medicine, anesthesiology, surgery, radiology, and pathology and laboratory services. In the fourth edition of this classification system—CPT-4—each procedure and service is identified by a five-digit code.

Examples of coded procedures include surgical operations, office visits, and x-ray readings. The provider determines the most accurate descriptor from the CPT guidebook and assigns that code to the procedure. Modifiers may also be appended to the five-digit identifying code.

Modifiers may indicate situations in which an adjunctive service was performed. Approximately 7,000 variations of procedures and services are catalogued.

Another set of codes has been developed to supplement the CPT codes. The Healthcare Common Procedure Coding System (or HCPCS), administered by the Centers for Medicare & Medicaid Services (CMS), lists services provided by physicians and other providers that are not covered under the CPT coding scheme. This includes certain physician services and nonphysician services, such as ambulance, physical therapy, and durable medical equipment rental.

Diagnosis-Related Groups

In an attempt to contain costs under the Medicare program, the federal government introduced a prospective payment system (PPS) as the basis for reimbursement for health services provided to Medicare beneficiaries. PPS limits the amount of reimbursement for services provided to each category of patient on the basis of rates determined by CMS.

The basis for prospective payment is the **diagnosis-related group (DRG)**. Using the patient's primary diagnosis as the starting point, CMS has developed a mechanism that assigns every hospital patient to one of more than 700 DRGs. The idea is to link payment to the consumption of resources, assuming that a patient's diagnosis is the best predictor of resource utilization. To refine the more than 700 diagnostic categories, the primary diagnosis is modified by such factors as coexisting diagnoses, the presence of complications, the patient's age, and the usual length of hospital stay. For situations in which DRGs represent too fine a distinction among conditions, the nearly 1,000 DRGs have been grouped into 23 major diagnostic categories based on the different body systems and other factors.

Diagnosis-related group (DRG)
The coding system used to classify inpatient diagnoses and procedures

Although introduced for use in federal healthcare programs, the DRG system was quickly adopted by other health plans as a basis for reimbursement. This system has become the standard classification scheme for hospitalized patients in the United States and has been adopted by other countries around the world.

Ambulatory Payment Classification

In response to rising outpatient costs, CMS developed a system for the outpatient environment called the *ambulatory payment classification (APC)*. Like the DRG, the APC focuses on the facility component of healthcare costs and not on physician charges. The basis for the fee is

(continued)

the patient visit rather than the entire episode of care, as in the case of DRGs. APC-specific diagnosis codes have been developed, and CPT codes continue to be used to classify procedures and ancillary services. Introduced in August 2000, APC codes are now widely used in outpatient facilities.

Diagnostic and Statistical Manual

The definitive reference on the classification of mental disorders is the **Diagnostic and Statistical Manual (DSM),** which is currently in its fifth edition (DSM-V). Published by the American Psychiatric Association, the DSM remains the last word on mental disease classification despite long-standing criticism of its scheme. Its 18 major categories of mental illness and more than 450 identified mental conditions are considered exhaustive.

The DSM is derived in part from the ICD. Like the ICD, it is structured around five-digit codes. The fourth digit indicates the variety of the disorder under discussion, and the fifth digit refers to any special consideration related to the case. Unlike the other classification systems discussed, the DSM contains detailed descriptions of the disorders categorized therein and thus serves as a very useful reference.

Diagnostic and Statistical Manual (DSM)
The coding system used to classify behavioral health problems

Hospitals are likely to offer spin-off services related to their inpatient activities. For example, many hospitals have established occupational health programs and sports medicine programs to serve their patients and the community. Some hospitals offer home health, rehabilitation, and hospice programs as extensions of their core activities. These programs may contain some unique services, but they—for the most part—are repackaged from existing services. For example, a fitness program targeting the hospital's employees and community residents might combine existing services, such as physical examinations, stress testing, cardiac rehabilitation services, and recreational therapy; the services might be provided by nonmedical fitness personnel such as personal trainers and aerobics instructors.

Other categories of services that hospitals are likely to offer include prevention, education, and community outreach programs. Health educators may teach prevention to patients while they are hospitalized or may provide educational programs outside the hospital to patients or the general public. Nurses may provide educational services to postsurgical and obstetric patients, and nutritionists may offer guidance to a wide range of patient types. Some of these prevention and education services are built into the facility fee; others are billed separately to the patient. Community outreach programs involve information and referral, health education, and wellness training generally geared toward the general public. They could also include home visits by hospital staff for purposes of monitoring health problems.

Categories of Settings and Providers

Earlier chapters have enumerated the various practitioners and providers in healthcare, and that information is reviewed here to put it in the context of the healthcare product. No other institutional setting provides the range of services that a general hospital does, although some specialty hospitals may provide unique services. General hospitals offer the full range of services considered under primary, secondary, and tertiary care. Only the most advanced general hospitals, however, provide the most complex tertiary and quaternary care. Specialty hospitals may be dedicated to a particular population (e.g., women, children) or to a specific condition (e.g., substance abuse, mental illness). In the case of the former, services similar to those provided in a general hospital are likely to be offered, although the emphasis is on specialized services for the population in question. On the other hand, a psychiatric hospital is likely to provide services not found in other clinical settings.

Hospitals provide support services of which patients are seldom aware, such as janitorial, landscaping, and parking services. Even less obvious, hospitals provide such services as medical records management, information systems operation, research services, and marketing services. Fees for these services are bundled into per diem or overhead charges.

Other facilities that house patients on an inpatient basis include nursing homes and residential treatment centers. Assisted living facilities may also provide health services. The term *nursing home* is a misnomer in that nursing homes typically provide a limited amount of medical care. Most of the services provided in a nursing home are custodial and involve the personal care of residents. As required, nursing personnel administer medication, monitor chronic conditions, and provide other forms of routine care. Physicians are on call but are not typically in residence. Unlike charges for hospital services, the charges for most services provided to nursing home residents are included in the monthly fee. Nonroutine health services are usually covered by a third-party payer, such as private insurance, Medicare, or Medicaid.

Residential treatment centers provide a narrower range of services than do hospitals but a broader range than do nursing homes. Unlike nursing homes, they are involved in the active treatment of most of their residents. Facilities for treating addictions or mental disorders, for example, provide services that are usually folded into the per diem charges of the treatment center.

Physicians are the most common type of practitioner the public encounters when seeking health services. The range of services physicians provide varies with the specialty involved, although most specialists provide a core group of routine medical procedures and diagnostic tests such as x-rays, blood tests, and urinalyses. Primary care physicians (i.e., family practitioners, obstetricians/gynecologists, pediatricians, general internists) provide the bulk of routine care and, increasingly, are taking on the management of chronic patients. Specialists, as the term implies, focus on particular health problems. Patients are typically referred to specialists by their primary care physician, although some patients, depending on the health problem, may go straight to a specialist.

The services offered by nonphysician practitioners vary depending on the profession. For example, optometrists offer vision exams and a limited range of eye-related therapies, chiropractors perform examinations and provide a narrow range of procedures aimed at spinal manipulation, and podiatrists perform examinations and offer a range of medical and surgical procedures for the treatment of foot problems.

The services of various mental health or behavioral health professionals are focused on the treatment of emotional and mental disorders, including counseling, psychotherapy, and drug therapy. The range of conditions for which treatment is available has expanded over time; mental health professionals may also treat such conditions as substance abuse, eating disorders, and Alzheimer's disease. Mental health services generally have been viewed separately from the treatment of physical health problems. This separation prompted the creation of a disease classification system unique to the mental health field. (See Exhibit 6.5 for a discussion of the DSM classification system.) The most serious mental disorders are likely to be treated by a psychiatrist—a medical doctor with specialized training in mental disorders.

Alternative (or complementary) therapy practitioners offer services that take diverse therapeutic approaches to health problems. This category includes practitioners of acupuncture, massage therapy, homeopathy, naturopathy, and other nonmainstream therapies. The use of alternative therapies has grown in popularity, and many insurance plans now cover alternative therapy interventions. Many of these services are still considered elective, however, so they must be paid for out of pocket. Alternative therapists have been some of the more aggressive marketers among health professionals. Their efforts have raised consumers' awareness of—and created niche markets for—alternative products.

One other category of service providers that should be considered in this context involves social service organizations. Although most of these organizations do not provide medical care, many do perform services that are health related and are often reimbursable by third-party payers. For example, agencies addressing HIV/AIDS issues may provide diagnostic tests for HIV, and a family planning agency might provide physical examinations and perform clinical procedures. As the definition of health expands, the boundaries between healthcare providers and social service agencies can be expected to blur.

Summary

The first task of any marketer is to develop an understanding of the products being marketed. The healthcare industry, however, is not used to thinking in terms of products, and marketers often have to help health professionals define the goods and services they are offering to their customers. The complexity of the product mix in healthcare creates a challenge for marketers. Because of this complexity, healthcare organizations often market ideas, concepts, or images in addition to discrete goods and services.

Healthcare marketers must be able to distinguish between the variety of goods and services offered, recognize the relationship between various products and the relevant market segment, and develop marketing initiatives accordingly. Healthcare is complicated in that products may reflect different levels of patient need, different clinical settings, and varying clinical skills. The marketing approach will be dictated, for example, by whether the treatment is routine or urgent, is elective or medically necessary, or is performed in an inpatient or outpatient setting. Some healthcare organizations have adopted service line management to help organize the management of various types of care.

The operation of the healthcare system is complicated by a diversity of practitioners who provide an overwhelming variety of services. Physicians, other clinicians, and auxiliary personnel all provide care. In the hospital setting, the types of service providers are even more diverse. Traditional practitioners have also been joined by alternative therapists, further complicating the picture. Practitioners use a bewildering array of coding systems with which the marketer must become familiar. Furthermore, healthcare is provided in numerous settings, including clinicians' offices, community clinics, mental health centers, hospitals, nursing homes, and residential treatment centers.

Key Points

- The healthcare field is characterized by a bewildering array of goods and services, resulting in a complex product mix.
- The product offered in healthcare varies with the type of practitioner and healthcare setting, and healthcare organizations use complicated coding systems to classify their products.

- Many goods and services in healthcare are marketed to the end user (typically the patient), but institutional customers in healthcare, such as clinics and hospitals, are also major purchasers of goods and services.
- Health professionals have not traditionally thought in terms of products, and marketers have to help them define what they are trying to market.
- The delivery of services in healthcare—and the marketing thereof—is complicated in that consumers may be characterized by differing levels of need, problems with differing levels of urgency, and a wide range of health conditions.
- Healthcare products are dispensed by a great diversity of practitioners in a wide variety of settings.

Discussion Questions

1. Why were healthcare organizations not concerned about carefully defining their products in the past?
2. What makes healthcare products difficult to clearly define?
3. What are the distinctions between healthcare goods and services, and what are the implications of these distinctions for marketing?
4. How do the challenges involved in marketing health services to consumers differ from the challenges involved in marketing products to healthcare organizations?
5. In what ways is the complexity of the product mix of large healthcare organizations a challenge for marketers?
6. Given the complexity of a hospital's service offerings, what dangers exist with regard to marketing services at cross-purposes (e.g., simultaneously marketing the urgent care center and the emergency department, or the outpatient mental health center and the psychiatric ward)?
7. What is service line management, and what are the pros and cons of using a service line management approach in healthcare?

Additional Resources

American Medical Association retail store: https://commerce.ama-assn.org/store /catalog/categoryDetail.jsp?category_id=cat1150004&navAction=jump.
American Psychiatric Assocation. 2013. *Diagnostic and Statistical Manual,* 5th ed. Washington, DC: American Psychiatric Publishing.

Centers for Medicare & Medicaid Services: www.cms.gov.

Freedonia Group. 2008. *Cosmetic Surgery Products to 2012.* Cleveland, OH: Freedonia Group.

Kalorama Information. 2007. *Retail Clinics: The Emerging Market for Convenience and In-Store Healthcare.* Rockville, MD: Kalorama Information.

Synovitz, L. B., and K. L. Larson. 2012. *Complementary and Alternative Medicine for Health Professionals.* Sudbury, MA: Jones and Bartlett Learning.

FACTORS IN HEALTH SERVICES UTILIZATION

The decision to offer a health service is generally predicated on the presumed level of demand for that service. Once it is offered, virtually all decisions related to its continued provision become a function of demand. For this reason, healthcare marketers spend a great deal of time and effort determining current and future levels of demand for aggregate or specific services offered by their organization. Calculating demand is challenging —particularly in healthcare—and requires an understanding of the many factors that influence the ultimate utilization of health services.

These factors have become increasingly complex, and past utilization patterns are seldom predictive of future demand. The demographic, socioeconomic, and psychographic attributes of a population all play important roles. At the same time, managed care arrangements and financing trends artificially influence demand. These developments have made projecting demand for health services an increasingly challenging task at a time when the ability to do so is critical to the survival of most healthcare organizations.

Conceptualizing Demand

In the context of health services, *demand* is an imprecise concept. The term is often used interchangeably with other terms, and no one definition is universally accepted. Because it is so vague and used in so many different ways, demand is difficult to define operationally. Part of this dilemma stems from a lack of agreement regarding *who* the customer for health services is.

Customer identification is seldom an issue in other industries, but it is a paramount concern in healthcare. Typically, the end user (usually the patient) is the primary customer and his or her demand is thought of as consumer demand. However, there are other customers—such as physicians, health insurance plans, and employers—that are equally (if not more) influential in determining demand. For a health plan, the customer may be the manager of an employer-sponsored benefits package. For a medical supply or equipment company, the customer may be a retail distributor. As previously noted, demand in healthcare may not be generated directly by the end user but by an intermediary. Thus, physicians may determine patient demand for hospital care and pharmaceuticals, insurance companies may dictate the demand for services because of the treatments they cover, and so forth.

Creating demand—perhaps where none existed before—is an important function for marketers. Artificially building demand may seem inappropriate, but it can legitimately be used in many situations, including when introducing a new drug or treatment for a recently discovered disease. Exhibit 7.1 illustrates this process.

Perhaps the best way to approach the demand concept is to examine its component parts. From a marketing perspective, demand can be conceptualized as the ultimate result of the combined effect of (1) healthcare needs, (2) healthcare wants, (3) recommended standards for healthcare, and (4) utilization patterns (Thomas 2003a).

Healthcare Needs

Healthcare needs (the first component of demand) can be defined in terms of the overall health status of a population or, more specifically, in terms of the number of health conditions among the population that require medical treatment. These conditions are those that an objective evaluation—for example, a physical examination—would uncover. The services required to address these conditions might be considered *absolute needs,* which exist without the influence of any other factors. These epidemiologically based needs that a team of health professionals would identify in a sweep through a community are thought to reflect the true prevalence of illness in the population. All things being equal, the absolute level of need should not vary much from population to population.

On the basis of its characteristics, a population can be expected to experience various health conditions. However, the existence of clinically identified health problems—at least in contemporary societies—does not translate directly into demand. In fact, the mismatch between identified needs and the ultimate utilization of services is substantial. Many conditions go untreated (indeed, even undiagnosed) for various reasons. Many other conditions for which treatment is obtained would not be considered as absolute needs using objective criteria. For example, no team of epidemiologists assessing the healthcare needs of a community is likely to identify sagging facial skin as a health problem. Yet tens of thousands of facelifts are performed in the United States every year by medical doctors. Thus, demand for a health service might exist even though no clinical need exists for the service.

Healthcare Wants

Healthcare wants (the second component of demand) arise from a population's wishes or desires for health services. Unlike needs, however, wants would not necessarily be uncovered by a sweep of public health investigators

EXHIBIT 7.1
Creating
Demand for
a Healthcare
Product

Healthcare products are generally introduced to a market in response to a demonstrated demand, and providers develop their products in response to an established health condition or other perceived need. However, it is not unusual for healthcare organizations to proactively identify new conditions to which their existing product can be applied; they then call on their marketers to create demand for that product. Pharmaceutical companies, for example, have been particularly aggressive in their attempts to define new health conditions that could benefit from one of their existing products, and they subsequently promote that product to consumers and physicians who write prescriptions. To create demand, however, an organization must demonstrate to the public and the medical community that (1) an identifiable health problem exists and (2) the company has a product that can treat that problem.

Marketers create demand for a healthcare product in several ways, including classifying ordinary processes or ailments of life as medical problems, portraying mild symptoms as portents of a serious disease, defining personal or social problems as medical problems, conceptualizing risks as diseases, and maximizing disease prevalence estimates to enhance the perceived size of a medical problem. A key strategy of pharmaceutical companies has been to target the news media with stories designed to create awareness of a condition or disease and draw attention to the latest treatment. Company-sponsored advisory boards often supply the "experts" for these stories, consumer groups provide the "victims," and public relations companies provide media outlets with a positive spin on the latest medical "breakthrough."

For example, on the basis of research conducted in Australia, analysts identified a concerted effort by a pharmaceutical company to generate demand for a product it developed to treat irritable bowel syndrome (IBS). IBS is considered a common functional disorder and a "diagnosis of exclusion" covering a range of symptom severity. Without question, many people with the condition are severely disabled by their symptoms, but the arrival of new drugs for IBS prompted drug manufacturers to change the way the world thought about IBS.

In this case, a communications company was engaged to formulate a medical education program to promote the perception of IBS as a "credible, common, and concrete disease." The educational program was part of a leading manufacturer's marketing strategy for a drug specifically for IBS. The key aim of the campaign was to establish in the minds of physicians that IBS was a significant and discrete disease state. Further,

(continued)

the campaign sought to convince consumers that IBS was a recognized medical disorder for which there was a new, clinically proven therapy.

The process for generating demand involved establishing an advisory board to provide key parties with current opinions about gastroenterology and best practice guidelines for diagnosing and managing IBS. In addition, the board produced a newsletter in the prelaunch period to "establish the market" and convince medical specialists of the condition's seriousness and credibility. This newsletter was accompanied by a series of advertorials published in medical journals and distributed to general practitioners by pharmaceutical sales personnel. Other groups targeted with promotional material included pharmacists, nurses, and patients.

Although portrayed by the pharmaceutical company as a medical education plan, the campaign was intended ultimately to create demand for a drug it was selling. This marketing strategy has become common among pharmaceutical companies and adopted by other healthcare organizations.

Source: Adapted from Moynihan, Heath, and Henry (2002).

through a community. Desired services are determined less by the absolute needs of a population than by the factors that influence the consumption of nonhealthcare goods and services. Many services that are consumed are considered medically unnecessary or elective and thus are wants, not needs. Tummy tucks and laser eye surgery are examples of such services.

Healthcare wants are determined less by the level of biological morbidity in the population and more by nonmedical factors. Wants may be determined by personal traits, such as fear and vanity; by social characteristics, such as group pressure and family influence; or by cultural factors, such as societal trends. For this reason, the level of wants is likely to be elastic and more susceptible to the influence of marketers. The US healthcare system has evolved to accommodate the wants of the consumer, and many healthcare organizations cater to people desiring elective services that might be considered medically unnecessary.

The type of organization and the services it offers dictate whether needs or wants are the main consideration in marketing efforts. For example, a clinic for persons with HIV/AIDS deals with basic needs, and few elective procedures are relevant to the treatment of that disease. On the other hand, a plastic surgeon specializing in body sculpting is likely to focus on the want-driven demand generated by those motivated by vanity (see Exhibit 7.2 for a discussion of marketing approaches for an elective procedure). At the same time, if a plastic surgeon also maintains a reconstructive surgery practice for trauma victims, then both wants and needs would be addressed.

Recommended Standards for Healthcare

Recommended standards for the provision of services make up the third component of demand. It primarily involves diagnostic procedures and disease management activities recommended for patients who display certain symptoms or are at risk for a specified health problem.

The medical community has developed recommendations for how often diagnostic tests should be performed, the circumstances under which a medical procedure should be performed, and the implementation of certain treatment plans for patients. These standards differ on the basis of health condition, age group, population segment, health risk, and so forth. For example, the American Cancer Society (2013) recommends an annual mammogram for all women starting at age 40 (despite a 2014 research finding, published in the *British Medical Journal*, that annual mammograms may not be more efficacious in saving lives than are self-exams) and a prostate exam for all men beginning at age 50—but at age 45 for men who have a family history of prostate cancer. The National Cholesterol Education Program recommends cholesterol testing starting at age 20 every five years or more frequently if other risk factors are present; similarly, the US Preventive Services

With the resurgence of consumerism driven by baby boomers, the emphasis on alternative therapies, and the wellness and fitness movement, consumers have started making more of the decisions regarding health services. As they have assumed a greater role in decision making, consumers have become an increasingly important target for healthcare marketers.
 	
   One area ripe for the application of direct marketing methods is elective surgery. *Elective procedures*—that is, those not considered medically necessary and thus not reimbursable through health insurance plans—constitute a significant proportion of the procedures performed by medical practitioners. Procedures from elective knee surgery to laser eye correction to facelifts are included in this category. These procedures are elective in that the consumer, not the physician or health plan, usually chooses to undergo them.
 	
   Candidates for many types of elective surgeries are characterized by a particular profile and do not represent a cross-section of the
<div align="right">*(continued)*</div>
	EXHIBIT 7.2
	Marketing an Elective Procedure: The Case of Laser Eye Surgery

population. The most effective approach to developing a consumer profile involves gathering patient data that specify the characteristics of the best prospects for the service. Aggregate data on the patients obtaining facelifts or elective knee surgery, for example, could be used to identify others in the population who have the same characteristics. Even better, however, are actual names and addresses of patients who have obtained these services. This information can be used to link the patients to various consumer databases to develop a more in-depth profile of the typical candidate for a procedure. Thus, patients for a particular service can be profiled in terms of their demographic characteristics, lifestyle orientation, and consumer behavior, among other characteristics.

Laser eye surgery has grown in popularity as new techniques have been perfected and outcomes improved. This procedure is almost always elective, requires out-of-pocket expenditures by the patient, can be expensive, and appeals disproportionately to certain segments of the population. Interest in laser eye surgery is particularly high today, spurred by burgeoning worldwide demand.

To support the development of a marketing campaign, researchers obtained patient data from a successful laser surgery clinic. Names and addresses were requested for those who had undergone the procedure; those who had presented themselves for surgery but turned out to be clinically ineligible; and those who had indicated an interest in laser eye surgery at some point but, as far as could be determined, had never undergone the procedure. The analysis involved approximately 700 laser eye surgery patients (and medically ineligible prospective customers) and another 1,200 prospective customers who had inquired about the surgery but never followed through. In addition, a random sample of 1,000 consumers was drawn from the zip codes associated with the patient/prospect sample.

Researchers gathered the data necessary for the analysis by matching the compiled names and addresses to the consumer data maintained by Experian Marketing Services. The data obtained from Experian included the following:

- *Individual-level data*, such as age, marital status, and gender
- *Household-level data*, such as home ownership, estimated household income, and presence of children
- *Geographically based data*, such as the median household income of the census block group in which the consumer lived, the racial

and ethnic profile of the block group, the median home value, and the MOSAIC lifestyle cluster assigned to each household (which is discussed later in Exhibit 7.3)

To ensure that the patient sample and the random sample represented the same underlying population, any consumer whose zip code fell outside the primary area served by the ophthalmic surgery practice was removed from the research database.

When the characteristics of the patients, prospects, and matched general population were compared, significant differences were found in the demographics and household characteristics of the three groups. Differences were found in age, gender, race, marital status, income levels, and rates of home ownership. When the groups were compared on the basis of MOSAIC lifestyle clusters, four of the clusters—typically assigned to neighborhoods of low socioeconomic status—were determined to be negatively associated with interest in laser eye surgery. From these comparative data, a logistic regression model was derived to predict the probability that a given consumer would fit the profile of previous laser eye surgery patients. The **predictive model** ultimately chosen demonstrated reasonable predictive validity. Overall, 63 percent of the sample was correctly classified as either a patient or nonpatient. Although a logistic regression model yields both false positives and false negatives, the overall result—with 60 percent of the positives correctly classified and 66 percent of the negatives correctly classified—indicated that this model could be used to significantly increase the probability of identifying prospects for laser eye surgery within a defined population. In the final analysis, the characteristics that had the most predictive power (in no particular order) were race, age, gender, marital status, and income. Although these factors all contributed to a person's likelihood of pursuing laser eye surgery, certain occupational statuses and lifestyle categories reduced a person's likelihood of becoming a patient.

The ability to predict classification of an individual as a patient versus a nonpatient was improved dramatically by using this model. Careful use of the model as a basis for identifying targets for direct mail (i.e., targeting those who fall into the top three deciles of customer potential) would increase the hit rate significantly and could drive up marketing effectiveness by 300 percent. As a result, the bottom-line impact on an ophthalmic surgery practice could be significant.

Predictive model
A statistical method for identifying and quantifying the likely future need for health services on the basis of known utilization patterns for a defined population

---

Source: Adapted from Barber, Thomas, and Huang (2001).

Task Force recommends cholesterol testing as early as age 20, especially for people with cardiovascular risks (WebMD 2011).

As health professionals and providers have become more attuned to disease prevention and health maintenance, the number of guidelines and recommendations has increased along with the number of diagnostic and screening procedures available. Many of these standards serve a public health purpose, so they may be promoted through social marketing efforts by the American Cancer Society, the American Heart Association, and other public and private groups. The rise in the number of physician-ordered or recommended diagnostic tests may also reflect the practice of *defensive medicine*, a high-cost trend of overtesting and overtreating patients so that the physician can avoid malpractice liability.

Utilization Patterns

The fourth component of demand is the utilization of health services, ideally the end result of the effect of the first three components. The amount of services consumed is frequently used as a proxy measure for demand because utilization rates can be calculated for almost any type of healthcare goods or services. More data are available on utilization than on the other components primarily because utilization data are routinely collected for administrative and billing purposes whenever a service is provided or a good is sold. Utilization rates indicate the actual level of activity as opposed to theoretical demand.

Because of the perceived relationship between demand and utilization, analysts sometimes work backward, using utilization levels as a basis for determining demand. However, utilization does not equal demand; depending on the circumstances, the level of demand may exceed utilization or, conversely, utilization levels may exceed reasonable demand for services. For example, there may be less utilization than expected because of limited access to services. On the other hand, some services may be overutilized for reasons (e.g., insurance coverage, physician practice patterns) unrelated to the level of demand.

Likewise, identifiable demand may not directly translate into utilization. Because marketers are concerned with what consumers actually do, situations in which the level of demand exceeds actual utilization may represent marketing opportunities. (See Pol and Thomas [2013] for a detailed review of the relationship between demographic characteristics and health status and health behavior.) Health services researchers commonly compare the assumed level of need with the observed level of utilization.

Proxy Data

Because propensity (to use health services) data about the residents of a particular geographic area are unlikely to exist, inferences based on knowledge gained from the analyses of other population segments may have to be made. For example, if the likelihood of the presence of HIV among Latinos is a function of Puerto Rican ancestry, a specified level of education and income, and residency in a highly mobile urban area, then developing a propensity score for the presence of HIV in various Latino populations should be possible. Thus, the propensity score for Latinos in parts of New York City might be 250, while in Miami this score might be only 45. In another example, the propensity for undergoing laser eye surgery might be related to certain psychographic or lifestyle segments. Thus, five lifestyle segments might be found to have a propensity score for laser eye surgery of 300 or more (or three times the average), in contrast to ten other lifestyle segments who almost never undergo laser eye surgery. Determining the potential market becomes possible by using such an approach to the extent that the distribution of lifestyles can be specified for a target area.

Factors Influencing Demand

Many factors influence the level of health services demand, and their interactions are complex. Although biological characteristics may predispose a person to certain health problems, other factors may ultimately determine the type and amount of services used. Biological factors are comparable to the healthcare needs described earlier and may or may not translate into utilization. Nonmedical factors, on the other hand, may be more of an influence on wants than on needs.

Knowledge of a population's characteristics (e.g., cultural background, lifestyle patterns) and existing structural factors (e.g., technology, health insurance, financing arrangements, healthcare providers) may allow a more accurate prediction of the type and level of services demanded than would knowledge of the actual level of morbidity. This section describes some of the factors that influence the level of demand.

Population Characteristics

The population characteristics that influence the demand for health services can be categorized in terms of their effect on health status and health behavior. These categories include psychological factors, demographic factors, lifestyle and psychographic factors, and other (mostly structural) factors.

Psychological Factors

The psychological factors correlating with demand include emotional responses, personality types, and attitudes evoked by health problems. The relationship between these factors and health behavior can be exceedingly complex—as in the case of a hypochondriac or in cases where fear of dying, for example, pushes one person to seek treatment but prevents another from consulting a physician. Fear, pride, vanity, and myriad other emotion-based responses play a large role in the demand for many elective procedures (e.g., breast augmentation, liposuction).

In industries where marketers pay more attention to psychological motivations, personality traits are often thought to drive consumer behavior. In healthcare, however, the individualized nature of personality makes directly correlating those personal traits to utilization difficult, and data on the relationship between psychological characteristics and health behavior are limited.

Attitude, as discussed in earlier chapters, is a relatively consistent, acquired predisposition to behave or respond in a certain way. In healthcare, customer attitudes toward the healthcare system, physicians, facilities, treatments, and so forth influence the decision to obtain healthcare goods and services. The preference, choice, or willingness to use an urgent care center rather than an emergency department, a health maintenance organization rather than a traditional health plan, or a chiropractor over an orthopedic surgeon may be a function of a person's attitude.

Attitudes are not restricted to patients or clients; they also apply to other customers such as physicians and other health professionals. The attitudes of physicians, for example, have been shown to affect what types of services they provide to which types of communities and which types of individuals. The wide variation in medical procedure rates from community to community and the absence of some services in certain communities may be partly attributed to provider attitudes.

Demographic Factors

Demographic characteristics exert a powerful influence on utilization. Of the various demographic attributes, age is one of the best predictors of health services use. Certain conditions are associated with specific age cohorts, and age influences the types of services used and the frequency of their consumption.

In the United States, utilization increases with age, reflecting the onset of chronic conditions and more frequent hospital care. The rate of hospitalization for persons younger than age 45 is low, and the lowest admission rate to US hospitals is recorded for the age-6-to-17 cohort. After age 45, however, admission rates increase dramatically; the rate for the 45-to-64 age cohort is more than double the 15-to-44 age group. In terms of emergency department utilization (for true emergencies), teens and persons in their early 20s (particularly men) account for a disproportionate share as a result of injuries and accidents. The elderly also account for a large share of emergency department utilization (NCHS 2012).

The sex or gender of the consumer is another influential factor. In the United States, women are more involved than men in the healthcare system and are heavier users of health services in general. Women tend to visit physicians more often, take more prescription drugs, and use most other facilities and personnel at a higher rate. They also are more aware of available health services and are quicker to turn to health professionals when symptoms arise. Perhaps more important from a marketing perspective is the fact that women influence others' use of health services. They often are in charge of making healthcare decisions for their spouse and/or children, accounting for more than 80 percent of healthcare decisions (HCPro 2007).

Racial and ethnic backgrounds influence demand in the United States. Clear-cut differences have been identified between African Americans and non-Hispanic whites in terms of their use of health services. Certain Asian populations and many ethnic groups display distinctive utilization patterns. In general, whites tend to use physicians at a higher rate than do the rest of the population, but African Americans are significantly more likely to use emergency department services. Additionally, some minority groups are more likely to use alternative types of care (e.g., folk medicine and acupuncture). The differences in utilization may be traced to the types of health problems experienced by minority populations and may reflect variations in their lifestyle patterns and cultural preferences. Perceptions and expectations of the healthcare system also likely differ between races and ethnicities (NCHS 2012).

Marital status is related not only to the level of demand but also to the type of services used and the circumstances under which they are consumed. Married people in the United States tend to have fewer health problems than the unmarried, widowed, or divorced, but, ironically, they use health services at a higher rate. The lifestyles associated with an unmarried status are believed to prompt more health problems, while the social support provided by a marital relationship is thought to contribute to more diligent use of health services (NCHS 2012).

A population's income level is probably one of the best predictors of utilization. A correlation exists between income level and the amount of health services used as well as between the types of services used and the circumstances under which they are received. Despite the health penalty that accompanies low income, the unhealthy poor tend to use fewer services than do the healthy affluent. This is true whether the indicator is for inpatient care, outpatient care, tests and procedures performed, or virtually any other measure of utilization (NCHS 2012). In the past, lack of health insurance or coverage under the Medicaid program was typically a reflection of poverty-level income, but this is no longer necessarily true in the era of the Affordable Care Act (ACA), which aims to expand coverage to the previously uninsured or underinsured poor.

The relationship between educational level and utilization is similar to that for income. The distribution of health problems in a population is associated with educational status, making it one of the better predictors of demand. The rate of hospitalization for the least educated segments of the US population is low, despite the higher prevalence of health problems in this group. More educated segments, although less affected by health problems, have higher rates of health services utilization. This higher rate is thought to be a function of the greater appreciation (by the better educated segments) of the benefits of healthcare and greater access to insurance coverage (NCHS 2012).

The relationship between religious affiliation/degree of religiosity and health behavior is probably the most idiosyncratic of any of the demographic associations. Research on this relationship is limited, so clear patterns are hard to discern. Further, in the United States, religious affiliation and participation are associated with so many variables that isolating the influence of religious involvement on utilization is difficult. Nevertheless, evidence indicates that health status (and the subsequent use of services) is correlated with measures of religiosity. This factor may be an important consideration for marketers in some communities where faith-based healthcare organizations are common (Benjamins 2003).

Psychographic or Lifestyle Factors

Psychographic or lifestyle factors exert significant influence on a population's healthcare wants, needs, and behaviors. In fact, health behavior and the propensity to use health services may be more highly correlated with lifestyle characteristics than with other variables. If the lifestyle classification of members of a population can be determined, the types of health problems that group will experience, as well as likely utilization patterns, can be estimated. To a certain extent, lifestyles override, or at least refine, differences in health services utilization based on demographic traits. See Exhibit 7.3 for a discussion of lifestyle segmentation systems.

Structural Factors

Other influential factors—mostly "structural"—often operate independently from the characteristics of the population. Advances in technology usually lead to higher levels of utilization of the services supported by the new technology. Some operations, like laser eye surgery, could never be performed without technological advances. Technological advances also have contributed to the shift from inpatient care to outpatient care and facilitated the emergence of home health care as a major aspect of healthcare delivery. The impact of technology has been particularly notable in the area of diagnostic testing. The variety of tests that can be performed has increased dramatically; the expanded use of home testing is just one example.

EXHIBIT 7.3
Lifestyle
Segmentation
Systems

Lifestyle segmentation systems have been used for decades in other industries but have never received wide acceptance in healthcare. For the most part, provider organizations depended on physicians or health plans to channel patients to them. For this reason, they did not need to know much about the characteristics of their patients.

Today's healthcare environment demands increased attention to customer **segmentation**. The market has become consumer driven, and individuals are taking a more active role in healthcare decision making. The pharmaceutical industry has led the way with a heavy investment in research on market segmentation. Healthcare providers who perform elective procedures—such as plastic surgeons, orthopedic surgeons, and eye surgeons—also need such information. As the health insurance landscape changes (owing much to the ACA), growing numbers of health plans, providers, and other organizations are expressing an interest in customer segmentation and target marketing.

Segmentation
The process of dividing a population into meaningful segments for purposes of market analysis and strategic planning

The first lifestyle segmentation systems—also referred to as psychographic segmentation systems (see Chapter 5)—were developed in the 1970s. This approach to segmenting the population was developed in response to some of the perceived deficiencies in demographic profiling. Marketers realized that people in the same demographic category could be grouped differently on the basis of lifestyle. For example, all senior citizens used to be grouped into the over age 65 category. Lifestyle research discovered that within this demographic category were at least two major subgroups: (1) active, financially secure seniors and (2) frail elderly with limited resources.

The concept behind all segmentation systems is the use of geodemographic data in conjunction with data on consumer behaviors, attitudes, and preferences. This information is used to generate distinct lifestyle clusters that cover the entire population. A specific set of attributes can then be assigned to each cluster. Marketers and researchers can then attach health characteristics to each cluster on the basis of these unique attributes.

The MOSAIC lifestyle system, for example, includes 71 lifestyle clusters grouped into 12 major categories. This system has been used by Experian to assign psychographic clusters to more than 135 million households. Such systems can be used to perform lifestyle analyses and, depending on the database, provide a wide range of demographic, socioeconomic, and consumer data linked to each psychographic cluster. Vendors of psychographic segmentation systems continue to expand the range of data, and the healthcare industry is slowly beginning to embrace a psychographic segmentation approach to market research.

Another factor unrelated to health conditions is the type and extent of health insurance coverage available to individuals and families. The availability of insurance has been identified as one of the best predictors of the demand for services. When insurers introduce copayments and/or higher deductibles into their insurance plans, the use of health services often declines in response. When insurance reimbursement for a service increases, use of that service tends to rise as well. During the years before the enactment of the ACA, the growing number of uninsured led to decreased demand for basic health services, an unfortunate consequence at a time when health problems and chronic conditions were increasing.

Reimbursement arrangements also influence practice patterns. To limit claims payments, health plans imposed restrictions on the services hospitals could provide. Similarly, changing reimbursement and regulatory pressures forced physicians to change their practice patterns, which in turn led to changes in utilization levels for certain procedures. ACA provisions, however, are changing this dynamic, making high-quality, coordinated care (not financial considerations) the driver of greater utilization and reimbursement. Increased Medicaid payments to primary care doctors took effect in 2013, and insurers are now required to spend "at least 85% of all premium dollars collected . . . on health care services and health care quality improvement" (HHS 2014).

The availability of health services in the form of facilities and personnel has an understandable impact on the level of health services utilization. In some situations, the demand for services is not being met because of a lack of facilities or personnel. In other cases, an oversupply of facilities or personnel may result in overutilization of health services. When new facilities or equipment are acquired, there is financial pressure to generate as much utilization as possible to recoup the cost of newly acquired resources.

One final factor to consider is the practice patterns that characterize different health service providers. Far from being an exact science, medicine involves frequent value judgments on the part of physicians and other practitioners. The volume and types of services provided by physicians in the same market area vary greatly, and even more striking differences can be observed from market to market (Fisher 2008). Local practice patterns may account for significant variations in utilization between groups of patients who have similar health problems.

The recorded level of utilization reflects a combination of a population's needs, wants, and recommended standards as well as the impact of the structural factors. Each category of demand poses a different challenge for healthcare marketers, but the real challenge is determining the correct combination of factors relevant for a particular situation. Identifying demand is clearly a multifaceted process that involves a number of different dimensions.

Using only one dimension of needs, wants, recommended standards, or utilization as a proxy may be appropriate in a particular situation, but ultimately a blended concept must be developed to more precisely determine the level of demand. Exhibit 7.4 discusses the elasticity of the demand for health services.

Healthcare marketers must be cognizant that demand is variable and is affected by a wide range of factors. The marketer not only should know that levels of demand vary from one population segment to the next and within the segment itself but also should anticipate (and respond to) the trends in either the population segment in particular or the healthcare system in general that would inevitably affect demand.

Historically, economists considered medical care to be the one service for which demand was inelastic. The assumption was if an individual was sick, she would consume health services, and if an individual received health services, she must be sick. Today, this assumption is understood to apply only to rare, life-threatening situations for which treatment is almost invariably given, regardless of other characteristics of the patient or the healthcare system. For every episode requiring life-saving efforts, there are thousands of situations in which healthcare is consumed—many involving individuals who are not technically sick. As a result of this realization, the demand for most health services is now considered to be relatively elastic.

A substantial body of evidence indicates that differences in demand exist among people with similar health conditions; indeed, one of the major factors that drove (and continue to power) the passage of the ACA was the disparity in utilization of health services. In reality, demand rises and falls in response to a variety of factors. In areas where few health services are available, for example, demand appears to be low. Conversely, in areas with an abundance of healthcare resources, demand appears to be high. A change in physician practice standards is likely to affect the demand for health services. At one point, for example, it may have been "fashionable" among OB/GYNs to perform cesarean sections on a larger proportion of their pregnant patients; as more scientific evidence accumulated, a trend away from C-sections emerged.

Perhaps the best example of the elasticity of demand is when the demand rises and falls commensurate with the availability of health insurance. Indeed, because insurance coverage is one of the best predictors of demand, those who are adequately insured demand more health services than do those who are poorly insured.

EXHIBIT 7.4
The Elasticity of
Health Services
Demand

Measuring Utilization

Health services researchers have developed a number of indicators for measuring utilization. Commonly used indicators are discussed in this section.

Facilities Indicators

The hospital admission rate is one of the most frequently used indicators of utilization because the hospital is the focal point for treatment in the healthcare system. The terms *admissions* and *discharges* refer to episodes of inpatient utilization. The hospital admissions rate is a proxy for other indicators, as admissions correlate with tests conducted, surgeries performed, and the allocation of other resources. Hospital care is both labor and capital intensive, so one admission represents significant healthcare expenditures. Admissions may be measured for an entire community or for one facility, or they may be broken down into components of utilization (e.g., clinical specialty, demographic attribute, geographic origin, payer category).

The term *patient days* refers to the number of hospital days a particular population spends in a facility and is calculated by the number of patient days accrued per 1,000 residents. This measure refines hospital admissions as an indicator by reflecting the total utilization of resources on the basis of patient days to adjust for variations in length of stay. Like admission rates, patient days may be calculated by diagnosis, type of hospital, patient origin, and payer category. Changes in reimbursement procedures have made patient days a more effective indicator of resource utilization.

The term *average length of stay* is a measure of the average number of days patients remain in the facility during a specified period. This indicator is also a good measure of resource utilization. Medicare and many other health plans reimburse hospitals on a per diem rate, making a facility's average length of stay an important financial consideration.

Several other facility indicators, each important in its own way, might also be used. Utilization rates may be calculated for nursing homes, hospital emergency departments, hospital outpatient departments, freestanding emergency centers, minor medical centers, surgery centers, and freestanding diagnostic centers, among others.

Personnel Indicators

One of the most useful indicators of utilization is the volume of physician encounters. This volume is typically measured in terms of *physician office visits*, although telephone or e-mail contact and physician visits to hospitalized patients are sometimes considered. The physician is the gatekeeper for most types of health services, and physician visits are a more direct measure of utilization levels than are hospital admissions, as most people avail themselves of a physician's services at some time but may never be admitted to a hospital. Physician utilization rates are often broken down by specialty because utilization among specialties varies dramatically.

Utilization rates also might be calculated for other types of personnel—typically independent practitioners who, like physicians and dentists, are not supervised by other medical personnel. Examples include optometrists, podiatrists, chiropractors, and mental health counselors and therapists. Other healthcare personnel—who generally cannot operate independently, but for whom utilization rates might be calculated—include home health nurses, physician assistants, nurse practitioners, and technical professionals. Physical therapists and speech therapists are other personnel for whom utilization rates might be developed if, for example, the analyst is involved in marketing rehabilitation services.

Other Indicators

As home health care has become more important, so has *home health care visits* as a utilization indicator. The scope of home care has expanded and now encompasses a broad range of services. Home health care utilization is typically measured in terms of visits by various types of personnel. Thus, a population's utilization might be considered in terms of the number of home health nurse visits or home health physical therapist visits recorded. Alternatively, the number of residences (i.e., the rate per 1,000) receiving home care visits might be calculated.

Drug utilization is yet another indicator of health services utilization. Although patient care providers typically have limited use for drug utilization data, analysts representing entities such as pharmaceutical companies find the information valuable because prescription drugs (rather than over-the-counter medicine) are thought to more accurately reflect utilization of the healthcare system. Although the level of prescription drug utilization can be determined from physician and pharmacist records, the rate of nonprescription drugs utilization must be determined in more indirect ways. Important recent research has demonstrated that patterns of drug prescribing can serve as a proxy for chronic disease prevalence (Cossman et al. 2010).

Exhibit 7.5 presents some of the health services utilization rates discussed here along with sample calculations for obtaining these rates.

An obvious goal of healthcare marketers is to increase utilization of the services provided by their respective healthcare organization. This endeavor, like much else in healthcare, is not always straightforward. As a general rule, increased volume results in increased revenue—and, presumably, increased profit for the organization providing the services. However, organizations are often required by regulation, community standards, or consumer demand to provide services that may not generate enough revenue to cover costs.

EXHIBIT 7.5
Commonly Used
Health Services
Utilization Rates

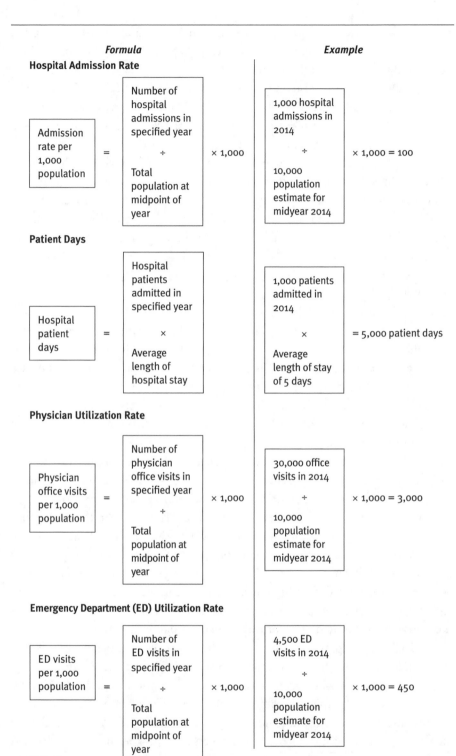

Further, ACA provisions require not-for-profit hospitals to demonstrate that they are meeting community needs regardless of the costs involved. In addition, because the fee schedules adopted by insurance companies and health plans limit the reimbursement amounts that organizations receive for many services, they may provide services for which the reimbursement is less than the cost of providing them. To further complicate the picture, a service that is profitable under normal circumstances may cause an organization to lose money if it attracts patients with no or poor ability to pay.

This situation has numerous implications for healthcare marketers. They must be familiar with the variety of services offered, the mechanisms for reimbursement, and the most desirable types of patients. In some situations, the sickest patients may be considered desirable, and in others, the target market may consist of healthy individuals. In some circumstances, a service might be provided at a loss to establish a customer relationship, and in other circumstances, services may be offered at a loss because volume in this service area has implications for down-the-road profit in a related service. Clearly, marketers in healthcare must be more intimately aware of the inner workings of their organizations than marketers in any other industry.

Predicting Demand

The current level of demand, however measured, is important information for marketers. Even more important is the anticipated future level of demand characterizing the population under study. Three of the techniques for projecting future demand are described in this section.

Traditional Model

The simplest and most straightforward prediction approach involves straight-line projections based on historical trends. For example, in the past it was common to review several years' experience with hospital admissions and then extrapolate the observed trend into the future. This approach was intuitive in that, if the trend had been upward, the assumption was that it would continue to rise. On the other hand, if the trend had been downward, the assumption was that the decline would persist into the future.

Few market analysts use this approach in today's healthcare environment. Developments external to the healthcare arena have such an effect on the demand for services and subsequent patterns of utilization that extrapolating from the past to the future is not practical. This situation forced the development of more sophisticated approaches to the **projection** of utilization.

Projection
The use of a statistical technique to calculate a future estimate

Population-Based Model

The most significant factor in predicting demand is the size of the population. The sheer number of people an organization serves has the greatest effect. Because of the importance of population size and because population projections are likely to be readily available and fairly reliable, the approaches that make up the population-based model have become the most common techniques for forecasting demand.

The simplest approach involves multiplying the projected population by known utilization rates. Thus, all population-based approaches depend on two components: (1) appropriate population estimates and projections and (2) accurate utilization rates. Various federal agencies provide population estimates and projections as well as information on utilization rates. Commercial data vendors also provide population estimates and projections.

Although some benefit can be derived from basing the demand estimates on the total population, the analysis typically examines utilization across various demographic factors. Changes in age distribution, for example, can have a major effect on utilization. Utilization patterns for males and females vary significantly and must be taken into consideration. To the extent that data are available, the population may be examined in terms of the influence of race and income on demand. In some cases, profiling the population by health insurance status may also be possible.

Projected utilization rates may be expressed, for example, in terms of hospital admissions or physician visits per 1,000 residents per year, patient days per 1,000 residents per year, live births per 1,000 women aged 15 to 44 per year, and so forth. These rates can be adjusted to account for regional differences when appropriate. The utilization rates of interest can be applied to different age and sex categories and adjusted for other attributes to the extent that the information is available.

Although the population-based model—in all of its permutations—is an intuitive, appealing approach, some caveats apply. The mobility of the population in contemporary America introduces an element of uncertainty into the projection process. The cohort effect (e.g., the changing characteristics of an age group as it grows older) also plays a role in determining differential utilization patterns. It is no longer safe to assume, for example, that the utilization patterns of 65-year-olds today will be the same as the patterns of 65-year-olds 20 years ago. Thus, applying an age-specific rate based on past experience to today's elderly may be risky.

Utilization rates themselves are subject to change for a number of reasons. Many of these factors have already been discussed, including availability of services, financing arrangements, and level of managed care penetration. Who could have predicted, for example, the decline in hospital admissions that resulted from the introduction of the Medicare prospective payment system and the emergence of managed care in the 1980s? Likewise, the ACA presents a new paradigm. Further, the frequency with which paradigm-changing developments occur makes predicting levels of utilization even more challenging.

Econometric Model

The econometric model comprises a variety of techniques for projecting future phenomena in complex situations. In its simplest form, the model is a type of time series analysis, attempting to statistically improve on the afore-mentioned projection that extrapolates past trends into the future.

Econometric approaches use equations that project utilization as a function of the interplay of independent variables. With a complex phenom-enon like the utilization of health services, **forecasts** based on multiple fac-tors make more sense than forecasts based on a single factor. Theoretically, the more factors used in predicting future utilization, the more accurate the prediction will be. Econometric prediction addresses these factors in a series of mathematical expressions. The equation ultimately used is the one that best "fits the curve" of historic demand. However, for this complex form of econometrics to work, projections are needed for numerous independent variables in the equation. Many analysts have attempted to apply the econo-metric model to predicting demand. Today, however, the model has limited use because of the unpredictability and instability of the healthcare environ-ment. See Case Study 7.1 for an example of the use of lifestyle analysis to predict the use of behavioral health services.

Forecast
A form of projection that incorporates likely future developments into the calculations

CASE STUDY 7.1
Using Lifestyle Analysis to Predict the Use of Behavioral Health Services

During the last quarter of the twentieth century, behavioral health ser-vices emerged as an important sector in the US healthcare system. This umbrella term covered many conditions, including psychiatric problems, emotional disturbances, substance abuse, hyperactivity in children, and other conditions considered treatable by mental health professionals. Behavioral health services were considered to be in a different category from the treatment of physical illness, and a separate industry devel-oped for the management of behavioral health problems. Many health plans carved out behavioral health services, and, eventually, national managed care plans specializing in such services emerged.

(continued)

By the late 1990s, the primary purchasers of behavioral health services—that is, major employers—were facing growing financial pressure because of increasing healthcare costs. Behavioral health services were particularly problematic because of the open-ended nature of many behavioral health conditions. At the same time, however, regulations that mandated parity between physical health coverage and behavioral health coverage were enacted. Employers who wanted to offer behavioral health coverage to their employees were faced with a major cost-containment challenge.

ABC Health Services was a major player in the behavioral health arena, reporting an enrollment of more than 3 million members in its managed care plans. ABC was faced with the same issue other behavioral health plans had to address: customers who could not distinguish between plans and were shopping for the lowest price. As a result, ABC was losing clients to other, sometimes less capable plans that quoted lower prices.

In response to this situation, ABC developed an innovative approach to the market using lifestyle segmentation analysis. On the basis of records maintained on enrollees who participated in its behavioral health plans, ABC believed the likelihood of using behavioral health services could be linked to different lifestyle categories among employees. ABC also thought that the type and intensity of services used could be correlated with lifestyle cluster.

ABC subsequently profiled existing clients in terms of its MOSAIC lifestyle clusters (see Exhibit 7.3). They found that approximately a dozen lifestyle clusters (of the 60 MOSAIC clusters at that time) were associated with a high propensity to use behavioral health services. Another ten lifestyle clusters were almost never associated with the use of these services. The remaining clusters did not appear to correlate with use or nonuse.

The cluster populated by middle-class suburban families tended to be characterized by high utilization levels, whereas the cluster populated by low-income rural families was characterized by low utilization levels. Furthermore, the older affluent suburban household cluster had a high propensity for using alcohol abuse services but not drug abuse services. On the other hand, the single, affluent, urban, high-rise cluster had a high propensity to use drug abuse services but not alcohol treatment services. Some clusters were characterized by episodic use of services (e.g., in response to some stressful event), and members of other clusters were characterized by recurrent use of services, indicating deeper problems.

ABC was able to use this information in marketing its behavioral health plan to existing customers and prospective clients. ABC representatives offered to profile the employees of existing customers, for example, to determine the extent to which the package of services offered by ABC was meeting their employees' needs. Profiling not only allowed ABC to more efficiently serve the existing client population but also helped the organization to predict future use of behavioral health services. The service mix could be subsequently adjusted to serve existing enrollees more efficiently and more cost-effectively.

To attract prospective clients, ABC distinguished itself from other behavioral health plans by determining a configuration of needs for the target group of employees. By serving in a consultative role, ABC demonstrated greater expertise than its competitors did in managing behavioral health clients. Further, ABC could offer a package of services tailored to the needs of its clients, rather than the one-size-fits-all plan offered by other firms. By developing an in-depth knowledge of the target population using lifestyle segmentation analysis, ABC was able to provide more effective services at competitive prices while raising the satisfaction level of employers and employees.

Case Study Discussion Questions

1. What is the conventional wisdom regarding the distribution of mental health problems in the population? Is it surprising to find that mental health problems are concentrated in different segments of the population?

2. What are the implications of this irregular distribution for marketing?

3. Which sensitivities surrounding the marketing of mental health services should the marketer be aware of?

4. Does the fact that hospitals often lose money on mental health patients mean that they should not market to the affected population?

5. Is this health problem one for which healthcare organizations might find social marketing useful?

Summary

Determining demand in healthcare is a complex task that requires marketers to develop an understanding of the many factors that influence the ultimate utilization of health services. From a marketing perspective, demand can be conceptualized as the ultimate result of the combined effect of (1) healthcare needs, (2) healthcare wants, (3) recommended standards of care, and (4) utilization patterns.

The demand for health services is surprisingly elastic. A number of factors influence the level of demand, including population characteristics (such as demographics, psychographics, and social group affiliation) and structural factors (such as availability of and access to health personnel and health facilities; financial arrangements, especially the availability of insurance; technological resources; and physician practice patterns). Some of the factors that contribute to demand are expected to be affected by provisions of the ACA.

A variety of indicators can be used to measure utilization rates. For hospitals, these indicators include use rates for admissions, patient days, and length of stay. Other indicators include use rates for physician office visits, procedures performed, and drugs prescribed. The utilization indicators chosen depend on the type of organization and the product being marketed. In healthcare, increased volume is not always a desirable phenomenon, and marketers must have enough knowledge about the organization's operations to know which services to promote and which to avoid.

Information on the demand for a service is typically unavailable, so marketers must develop ways to determine potential demand. Similarly, data on utilization rates for various types of services may not be readily available. Marketers must also be able to generate estimates and projections of the demand for services and likely utilization rates to develop an effective marketing plan. A number of methodologies are available for this purpose, including population-based and econometric models.

Key Points

- The demand for health services reflects the combined effect of healthcare needs, wants, recommended standards, and utilization patterns.
- Because demand is hard to quantify, the level of utilization is often used as a proxy for demand.
- The amount of sickness in a population influences demand but may be less important in determining demand than other factors.

- Because of the various factors influencing utilization, demand in the United States is relatively elastic.
- Frequently, a mismatch exists between service demand and actual service utilization; some needs go unmet, while some services are overutilized.
- Besides biological factors, demand is influenced by psychological, demographic, sociocultural, and economic factors.
- Psychographic (or lifestyle) attributes may exert significant influence on demand by affecting health status and health behavior.
- In healthcare, demand can be created where it did not previously exist by introducing new procedures or drugs, modifying diagnostic criteria, or identifying new health problems.
- Extrinsic factors—such as availability of services, technological developments, physician practice patterns, and insurance reimbursement rates—also influence the demand for health services.
- A variety of indicators can be used to measure utilization, including use rates for hospitals, physicians, other practitioners, and pharmaceuticals.
- Health services researchers have developed a variety of techniques for predicting utilization, including population-based and econometric models.

Discussion Questions

1. Why is demand in healthcare a complicated issue, and what are some components that might contribute to the level of demand?
2. What is the difference between healthcare needs and healthcare wants, and to what extent do the two overlap?
3. Why is the correlation between demand and utilization imperfect?
4. What are some demographic factors that influence demand?
5. What role do psychographic or lifestyle factors play in influencing demand?
6. Why may the mere presence of health services increase demand?
7. Can demand for health services be created?
8. What is the role of health insurance in determining demand?
9. Why do patterns of utilization vary widely from community to community when the communities generally share the same characteristics?

Additional Resources

American Association of Family Practitioners. 2010. "Health Care Reform Law Will Increase Demand for Preventive Services, Say Experts." www.aafp.org/news /government-medicine/20100728hcreformprevent.html.

Dixon-Fyle, S., and T. Kowallik. 2010. *Engaging Consumers to Manage Health Care Demand*. New York: McKinsey & Company. www.mckinsey.com/insights/health _systems_and_services/engaging_consumers_to_manage_health_care_demand.

Mulley, A. G. 2009. "Inconvenient Truths About Supplier Induced Demand and Unwarranted Variation in Medical Practice." *British Medical Journal* 339: doi.org/10.1136/bmj.b4073.

Sekhri, N., R. Chisholm, A. Longhi, P. Evans, M. Rilling, E. Wilson, and Y. Madrid. 2006. "Principles of Forecasting Demand for Global Health Products." www .cgdev.org/doc/ghprn/Demand_Forecasting_Principles,Sept-06.pdf.

HEALTHCARE MARKETING TECHNIQUES

Because marketing in healthcare encompasses a wider range of activities than marketing in most other industries, the topic is covered in the broadest possible sense in this book. The chapters in Part III review the marketing techniques used in healthcare, consider the advantages and disadvantages of their use, and assess their relative effectiveness. The extent to which these techniques can be transferred to healthcare from other industries is also considered.

MARKETING STRATEGIES

Healthcare organizations are often tempted to rush a marketing campaign into the field, but few can be successful without first designing a well-thought-out business strategy to guide the organization's marketing initiatives. This chapter describes healthcare marketing strategies and highlights the relevance of the traditional four Ps of marketing—product, price, place, and promotion. Factors influencing strategy development are reviewed, and the steps involved in developing a marketing strategy are outlined.

What Is Strategy?

Although used in a variety of ways by different students of marketing, the term **strategy** (for the purposes of this book) refers to the generalized approach taken to meet market challenges. A strategy establishes the tone for any marketing activity (tactic) and sets the parameters within which the marketer must operate. The strategy influences the marketing plan that is ultimately developed and guides subsequent marketing initiatives.

Strategy
A general approach to be taken to meet market challenges

Marketers often think of strategy in terms of the level to which it relates. For example, they might create a *corporate strategy* that deals with the overall development of an organization's business activities, a *business strategy* that indicates how to approach a particular product and/or market, or a *marketing strategy* that focuses on one or more aspects of the marketing mix. Marketing strategy is most relevant to this discussion and might be thought of as the marketing logic by which an organization hopes to achieve its objectives. The marketing strategy is reflected in the initiatives the organization applies to target markets, the marketing mix it selects, and the marketing expenditures for which it budgets.

Ideally, strategies are carefully thought out and deliberately formulated through enterprisewide strategic planning. The absence of an articulated strategy, however, does not mean that no strategy exists. Acts of commission or omission ultimately create a strategy, and even the absence of a strategy could be considered a strategic approach in a technical sense. As a result, many healthcare organizations end up with de facto strategies that are not deliberately formulated. This situation may result from lack of a formal strategic plan, failure to link marketing to an existing strategic plan, or failure to articulate marketing strategies clearly. In most cases, this situation results when the organization neglects to engage in formal market strategy development.

Unplanned strategies are referred to as *emergent strategies* and are derived from a pattern of behavior not consciously imposed by senior management. They are the outcome of activities and behaviors that occur unconsciously but nevertheless fall into a consistent pattern. Although many healthcare administrators would concede that they do not have a strategy in place, some form of strategy, albeit unstated, usually exists. See Exhibit 8.1 for a schematic on the role of strategy in an organization.

Why Is Strategy Development Important?

To a certain extent, strategies are developed for the same reasons any type of planning activity is carried out. All strategies should accomplish the following functions:

- *Provide direction for the organization or program.* The strategy should constitute the "which way" aspect of organizational development.
- *Focus effort on one of many possible options.* Because there will always be numerous strategic options from which to choose, focusing on a particular strategy prevents confusion of purpose and diffusion of efforts.
- *Unify the organization's actions.* The strategy should give the organization a purpose and unify the actions of its members.
- *Differentiate the organization.* The strategy should reinforce the organization's identity and distinguish it from competitors.
- *Channel the organization's promotional materials.* The strategy should guide the development of promotional documents, and all materials should present a distinct, consistent **image**.
- *Marshal the organization's resources.* The strategy should guide the allocation of resources to focus them on one approach rather than many.
- *Support decision making in the organization.* The strategy should implicitly establish criteria for framing issues that require a decision.
- *Provide the organization with a competitive edge.* Ultimately, strategy development is about positioning the organization in relation to the market, capitalizing on the organization's strategic assets, and creating a strategic advantage.

Image
The perception an organization wants to project about itself, its products, and its services

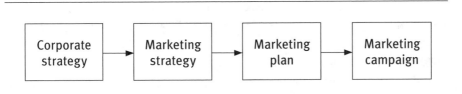

EXHIBIT 8.1
The Role of
Strategy in an
Organization

What Is the Strategy Development Context?

Strategic planning is a well-established activity in most industries and is often synonymous with corporate planning. The **strategic plan** is the primary mechanism through which an organization adapts to an ever-changing healthcare arena. The emphasis it places on market **positioning** underscores its central role in organizational development. A strategically oriented organization is one whose actions are aligned with the realities of its environment. The organization's strategic mind-set should ultimately spawn a marketing mind-set among its members or stakeholders (e.g., board, leaders, employees, physicians and other clinicians).

The strategic plan should guide the allocation of marketing resources, particularly when scarce resources are being dispensed. The plan should also serve as a basis for relationship development in an environment that has become increasingly driven by provider networks, integrated delivery systems, and referral relationships. The strategic planning process should address the appropriateness of existing links and identify potential new relationships.

Most important, the strategic plan should be a **call to action**. Many healthcare organizations have spun their wheels for years, waiting for a clear direction to present itself. The strategic plan should not only embody the organization's strategy but also convey the organization's vision and lay out the scenario for the kind of organization it wants to become. This vision should help marketers picture the marketing activities they must engage in to support the organization's strategic initiatives.

Healthcare administrators tend to rush headlong into marketing campaigns without regard for the strategic implications. Because marketing challenges often provoke heated, high-pressure situations, the tendency is to address immediate marketing needs without concern for the broader implications of these actions. This all-too-common scenario underscores the need for a strategic orientation at all levels of the organization.

Strategic plan
A comprehensive guide to action developed by an organization for carrying out a specific strategy

Positioning
The placement of an idea, an organization, or a product in the minds of the market population, relative to its competition

Call to action
A statement, usually at the end of a marketing piece, that encourages the audience to take initiative regarding the good or service being promoted

The Strategic Planning Process

The steps in the strategic planning process are summarized in this section. Although different perspectives exist on the steps and the sequencing of the process, the approach outlined here is a common one. The strategic marketing planning process is presented in Chapter 15 (see also Thomas [2003a]).

Step One: Plan for Planning

A good starting point for the strategic planning process is reviewing the organization's **mission** and **goals**. Because the organization likely spent considerable effort in defining its mission and establishing its goals, the process should confirm the validity of these concepts or provide a rationale for their modification.

Mission
The overarching purpose of an organization; the reason an organization exists

Goal
The ideal state or position the organization strives to achieve

Much of the activity at this stage is organizational in nature and focuses on identifying the key stakeholders, decision makers, and internal resources that should be involved in the planning process. A planning team should be established that includes representatives from all constituent groups, including stakeholders, key decision makers, and opinion leaders as well as representatives from key departments in the organization.

A general overview of the organization, its mission, and its current operations must be developed in step 4. However, step 1 clarifies the nature of the organization and the business it is in. For example, toward the end of the twentieth century, hospitals that continued to think they were in the hospital business rather than the healthcare business found themselves at a competitive disadvantage to hospitals that realized they had a broader mission. The redefinition of the mission of healthcare organizations that occurred in this period was a major contributor to the emergence of marketing as an essential healthcare function.

Step Two: State Assumptions

Assumptions might be made about the players involved in the local healthcare arena, the nature of the market area (and its population), the political climate, the position of other providers, and any other factors that might affect the strategic development process. Many of these assumptions are likely to have a marketing dimension; they may relate to the organization's position in the market, the nature of the competition, the distribution of the organization's facilities, and so forth. Although the planning team will undoubtedly refine its assumptions during the planning process, it should begin with some general ones—for example, "Managed care will continue to exert a major influence on the local market" or "We're number four in market share, and there is no way we will ever be number one."

Step Three: Gather Initial Information

The planning team begins the data collection process by gathering general background information on the organization, drawing from available organizational materials such as the following:

- Annual reports, press releases, and marketing pieces
- Resumés of management and key clinical and technical personnel
- Reports filed with regulatory agencies
- Business plans presented to funding sources
- Grant applications and certificate-of-need applications
- Executive committee minutes, planning retreat summaries, and evaluation studies

In addition, the team should conduct an inventory and assessment of existing marketing activities. Marketing initiatives that are already under way need to be cataloged, and existing marketing themes should be identified. Healthcare organizations that are new to formal marketing efforts may have a lot more marketing initiatives under way than they realize, although they may not recognize them for what they are. For example, an organization may offer perks to admitting physicians or conduct community health fairs without considering these initiatives as marketing activities.

Initial information should be gathered through interviews with knowledgeable persons (in the organization) representing various functional areas, vested interests, and perspectives. In large organizations, these interviews may be restricted to key administrators and medical staff and perhaps one or more individuals having a perspective on institutional history. In a small organization, such as a physician's practice, interviews with people further down the organizational structure may be necessary.

This step in the process should also identify the key constituents of the organization. To whom does it report? Who does it have to satisfy? If it is tightly held and private, a few entities that matter may exist outside the organization. On the other hand, a private, not-for-profit organization is likely to be accountable to its board members, regulators, major donors, and other interested parties. In a publicly held company, the board and the shareholders are important constituents. Other constituents to consider are patient groups, referring physicians, employee benefits managers, insurance plan representatives, and political officials. The list should include the full range of constituents that would conceivably be addressed by any type of marketing initiative, such as consumers (who need to be made aware of the organization's services), existing customers (whose loyalty needs to be strengthened), the medical staff (whose continued support must be ensured), and the media (who must be kept up to date on the organization's activities).

The information gathered should generate a description of the organization's **corporate culture**. This culture defines the organization's character, sets the tone for employee interaction, influences the organization's operations, and determines the extent to which the organization is amenable to the

Corporate culture
The values, beliefs, and attitudes that characterize an organization and guide its practices

planning process. It also typically determines the ease with which a marketing mind-set can be established within the organization.

The planning team is not likely to have all the answers to every question raised at this point, and typically more questions than answers are generated. Nevertheless, during this step, knowledge begins to accumulate and promising options and potential roadblocks begin to emerge.

Step Four: Profile the Organization

In step 4, the general description of the organization previously established is fleshed out in more detail. In profiling the organization, two important questions must be addressed:

1. *What is the organization's product or products?* This question may seem easy to answer, but few healthcare organizations can readily respond to this question. Organizations historically have not had to think in terms of discrete products. Furthermore, healthcare products are often complex and, unless their sole business is selling a healthcare widget, healthcare organizations offer products that may be difficult to classify. How does one conceptualize public health or occupational medicine, for example, as goods and services? Regardless of the complexity involved, specifying the organization's products is an important step in developing both general and marketing-specific strategies. (The nature of healthcare products is discussed in more detail in Chapter 6.)

2. *Who are the organization's customers?* In other words, who does the organization have to convince to purchase its services? The more multipurpose an organization is, the broader the range of customers it has. For a hospital, the list of customers includes patients, family members and other decision makers, staff physicians, referring physicians, major employers and business coalitions, insurance companies, and managed care plans. With the emergence of provider networks and integrated delivery systems, other care providers are also customers. The list does not stop there, particularly if the hospital is tax exempt (because of its not-for-profit status); its customers may include consumer advocacy groups, policymakers, legislators, regulators, and the press.

Step Five: Collect Baseline Data

Step 3 sets the stage for step 5, an intensive data collection agenda involving both internal and external data audits. Although the primary driver of strategy development is the external environment, a thorough organizational/internal self-analysis is equally critical.

The intent of the **internal audit** is to determine who does what in the organization, when and where they do it, how they do it, and even why and how well they do it. This self-analysis covers a wide variety of organizational features and can be incredibly detailed. The following lists the aspects of the organization that might be addressed in an internal audit:

Internal audit
The examination of internal data to assess organizational efficiency and effectiveness

- Policies and procedures
- Existing services and products
- Nature, number, and characteristics of customers
- Utilization patterns for services
- Sales volume
- Staffing levels and personnel characteristics
- Management processes
- Financial situation
- Fee/pricing structure
- Billing and collection practices
- Marketing arrangements
- Location of service outlets
- Referral relationships

The internal audit for a strategic plan typically involves some type of operational analysis. This analysis is likely to include, at a minimum, an evaluation of patient flow, paper flow, and information flow. The operational analysis may also examine staffing patterns, physical space considerations, and productivity. Although this information might not apply directly to most marketing initiatives, it is critical to any internal marketing effort.

The scope of the **external audit** (or environmental assessment) is determined by the nature of the organization and the issues under consideration. Macro-level trends are more important than micro-level trends for organizations involved in regional or national marketing initiatives. For most healthcare organizations, the external audit should focus on the local market because most marketing takes place there. An organization must consider the climate of the market area and determine what aspects of healthcare are relevant to the market area population.

External audit
The examination of the outside environment in which an organization operates; also known as *environmental assessment*

For marketers, the most important component of this step is market identification and description. The organization's market can be defined in a number of ways, and the definition used depends on the purpose of the analysis, the product or service being considered, the competitive environment, and even the type of organization involved in the marketing effort. Markets may be defined on the basis of geography, demographics, consumer demand, disease prevalence, and so forth. (Issues related to the identification of markets are discussed in Chapter 4.)

In a typical strategy development initiative, the first task is to profile the market area population. The type of information needed on the market area population varies with the nature of the project. Demographic data, including biosocial and sociocultural traits, are typically compiled first. At a minimum, the analyst would examine the population in terms of age, sex, race/ethnicity, marital status/family structure, income, and education; insurance coverage is also typically assessed. Furthermore, the migration process has taken on increasing importance in community analysis, and information on the volume and traits of migrants—particularly newcomers to the market area—may be useful.

The demographic analysis is often accompanied by an assessment of the psychographic or lifestyle characteristics of the market area population. Information on lifestyles can be used to determine the likely health priorities and behaviors of a target audience and any relevant subgroups. Often a reflection of lifestyles, the attitudes consumers display are likely to have considerable influence on the demand for almost all types of health services. Marketers must also consider the attitudes characterizing other constituents, such as referring physicians and policymakers.

A major component of the external audit is the competitive analysis. Organizations do not operate in a vacuum. Marketers must consider the healthcare environment and the other players in the arena. Any strategy must reflect the organization's position in the environment and in relation to its competitors. Competitors include providers within the same specialty or providers offering the same services as well as those outside the area that perform competitive services. For physicians, competitors include hospitals, freestanding clinics, and specialists who are "poaching" another specialty. Exhibit 8.2 lists examples of data collected during internal and external audits.

Step Six: Identify Health Status

The salient health characteristics of the target market are identified during the course of the external audit. Data on health characteristics offer insights into the health status of the population and, ultimately, into the types of health services the population requires.

Not all healthcare providers deal directly with reproductive health issues, but local fertility patterns exert a major influence on current and future patterns of demand, and a wide range of needs revolve around childbearing. Childbearing also triggers the need for such down-the-road services as pediatrics. Demands in this area may also encompass infertility treatments and treatments for conditions related to the male and female reproductive systems.

EXHIBIT 8.2
Data Collected
Through
Internal and
External Audits

Internal Audit	External Audit
Organizational structure	Market area
Corporate culture	Target market
Decision-making process	Consumer characteristics
Key influentials	Consumer perceptions
Staffing patterns	Utilization patterns
Sales volume	Competitors
Customer characteristics	Market positioning
Price structure	Market shares
Sources of revenue	Reimbursement trends
Profitability by service	
Referral sources	
Existing marketing initiatives	

Determining the level of morbidity in a population is also key. The incidence and prevalence rates for health conditions within a population provide a context for strategic development. To the extent possible, analysts must project incidence and prevalence rates into the future to anticipate service needs. Likewise, the level of disability in the population should be identified.

The levels of acute conditions, chronic conditions, reproductive health issues, mental health problems, and other health conditions are vital to understanding the healthcare needs of the market area population. The level of mortality and the leading causes of death within the market area population should also be studied. Market researchers are typically less interested in mortality than morbidity because the latter is more closely linked to service demand. Nevertheless, mortality data are almost always examined during this step because these data serve, to some extent, as a proxy for morbidity. Exhibit 8.3 describes the implications for healthcare marketing of the community health needs assessment provision of the Affordable Care Act.

Step Seven: Convert Health Status to Health Service Demand

Once the population's health status has been identified, marketers must then convert these characteristics into demand for goods and services. Demand can be conceptualized by service utilization (e.g., inpatient services, ambulatory care), diagnostic and therapeutic procedures, drug prescriptions, and other need indicators. Goods and services required by the population are a function of the needs identified in that population, such as care for acute conditions, chronic illnesses, reproductive health, and mental and behavioral problems. The amount of goods and services actually consumed, however, is determined by a variety of factors (see Chapter 7 for this discussion). For

EXHIBIT 8.3

Implications of the Affordable Care Act for Marketing

Community health needs assessment (CHNA)
An in-depth assessment of a community's population, health status, health-related issues, and unmet needs

The Affordable Care Act (ACA) of 2010 includes provisions that have significant implications for not-for-profit hospitals and, ultimately, for the marketing of those entities. Beginning in 2012, all not-for-profit hospitals are required by the Internal Revenue Service (IRS) to complete a **community health needs assessment (CHNA)** once every three years. In addition, not-for-profit hospitals are required to develop, adopt, and implement a public assistance plan to address community health needs within their service areas. The CHNA must include input from persons representing the broad interests of the community served by each hospital, such as those with knowledge of public health. The results of the CHNA must be made widely available to the general public.

For nearly 100 years, not-for-profit hospitals in the United States have enjoyed tax exemption by virtue of their charitable status. Exemption from federal, state, and local taxes was initially allowed when community hospitals operated primarily with uncompensated staff and charitable donations to provide free care to indigent populations. In 1956, the IRS began to require not-for-profit hospitals to promote the overall health of the community and to provide services for members of the community who are not able to pay.

Today's not-for-profit hospitals are much different from those in operation when the charitable provisions were first enacted. These hospitals provide secondary and tertiary care services that use advanced medical technology to perform complex diagnostic and therapeutic procedures. The role of hospitals in the treatment of chronic diseases, acute care, and trauma has expanded, and over time many have become wealthy institutions with power and presence in the community, in contrast to their almshouse roots. The apparent failure of some of these institutions to meet their community benefit expectations led to increased oversight by regulatory agencies.

Additional IRS revenue rulings in 1969 and 1983 established and clarified the *community benefit standard* requirements. These requirements were meant to ensure that adequate health services were available to members of the community who needed them. Bipartisan Congressional interest in the issue increased over time and resulted in the ACA provision titled "Additional Requirements for Charitable Hospitals." This provision imposed four new requirements for not-for-profit hospitals, including the CHNA requirements.

The ACA requires not-for-profit hospitals to systematically evaluate the health needs of community residents. They must identify medical and behavioral health needs, the health services currently available, important health service gaps, and unmet health needs. Consumer interviews, focus groups, and surveys must be conducted to ensure community participation and to incorporate the perspectives of residents into the availability of and access to health services. Projecting future health needs is an essential step in determining health service gaps, unmet health needs, and public assistance issues for the market area.

The ACA requirements go beyond any previous expectations in that the hospital must not only document the extent to which the organization is meeting the known healthcare needs of the community but also determine the unmet needs and then submit a plan for fulfilling these needs. If a CHNA reveals a gap in the services available to the community, the hospital must document that it has a plan to address this deficiency.

The CHNA presents three major implications for marketing:

1. To the extent that the hospital or health system is adequately providing a community benefit, the CHNA is a public relations boon—particularly if competitors are *not* meeting their obligations. Marketers can then present the hospital as a responsible community citizen that offers a wide range of benefits to the market area. The results of the CHNA should support the marketers' claim.

2. The hospital or those it engages to conduct the CHNA are given the opportunity to collect information from a wide variety of sources, including those who may not have had a voice in hospital decision making in the past. More important, the organization is given the opportunity to demonstrate that it is sincerely concerned about the overall needs of the community and is committed to meeting those needs.

3. The type of information generated by a CHNA should be compiled by marketers even in the absence of this requirement. This form of market research should reveal environmental opportunities and threats and should guide the development of the marketing strategy and targeted marketing initiatives. Marketers have every reason to be supportive of the CHNA and should encourage ongoing monitoring of market trends between CHNA assessments.

this reason, the actual health behavior of the target population needs to be considered.

Health behavior
Any action aimed at restoring, preserving, and enhancing an individual's health status

Health behavior (introduced in Chapter 7) refers to any action aimed at restoring, preserving, and/or enhancing an individual's health status. From a marketing perspective, information on health behavior provides insights into consumer behavior and the consumer decision-making process. Health behavior includes formal activities (such as physician visits, hospital admissions, and prescription drug consumption) and informal activities (such as wellness and fitness activities aimed at preventing disease or illness and maintaining, enhancing, or promoting well-being). Organizations employing social marketing, for example, are likely to require information on unhealthy lifestyles or risky behavior exhibited by the population. An understanding of the population's health behavior should supplement previously developed knowledge of the market area's health needs.

Utilization data are often the best source of information on health behavior, and healthcare organizations consider indicators of health behavior that are most relevant to their operations. To conduct step 7, hospitals are likely to examine the broad set of utilization indicators described throughout this book, while other organizations with limited operations are likely to focus on a narrow range of utilization indicators.

Step Eight: Conduct a Resource Inventory

A *resource inventory* identifies the facilities, personnel, and other resources of the organization that are available for or may be used to meet the healthcare needs of the target population. Sometimes the full range of available resources in the market area must be identified, but typically the focus of step 8 is on resources likely to be in competition with the organization doing the planning. Given the role of marketing in countering the competition, the resource inventory is a critical piece of the strategy development process. Here are some examples of resources commonly included in the inventory:

Accountable care organization
A structure involving a group of voluntary providers collectively held responsible for the overall cost and quality of care for a defined patient population

- Facilities
- Equipment
- Personnel
- Programs and services
- Funding sources
- Networks and relationships

The final category—networks and relationships—has been important throughout the era of managed care and negotiated contracts and is fundamental to this new environment of the **accountable care organization** (see

Exhibit 8.4). Such connections cannot be overestimated, and many organizations have come to view relationship building and **relationship management** as the responsibilities of the marketing department. The relationship building and management effort extends to organizations, medical personnel, and consumers.

In the future, patients are likely to use a provider because of their existing relationships (i.e., patients will form a relationship with their provider or health plan *before* they become sick rather than *after* they use the service or experience a medical episode). The existence of networks, integrated delivery systems, and strategic partners in the community should be fully addressed during strategic planning.

By step 8, the marketer has compiled a great deal of valuable data. On the basis of the information available, the marketer should be able to determine the following:

Relationship management
A focus on cultivating long-term relationships rather than short-term or onetime transactions

- Overall societal/healthcare/service trends
- Market area delineation
- Market area population profile
- Market area population health characteristics
- Level of demand for health services
- Current position of the organization/product
- Profile of current customers
- Resources available in the service area
- Gaps between needs and resources
- Future developments that will affect the organization

The state of the organization can now be frankly described and its position in the market assessed. Being thus informed, all parties can revisit the initial assumptions stated in step 2 and plan for strategy development.

Developing the Strategy

When should the strategy be developed? Different strategists may sequence the development of strategy at various points in the process. The development of strategy should occur when adequate baseline data have been acquired and analyzed. The sequencing of the strategy development process, as described in this section, depends on the nature and circumstances of the organization. The actual process of specifying a strategy is discussed later in the chapter.

EXHIBIT 8.4
Accountable
Care
Organizations:
The Future of
Healthcare?

According to the Centers for Medicare & Medicaid Services (2013), accountable care organizations (ACOs) are "groups of doctors, hospitals, and other healthcare providers, who come together voluntarily to give coordinated high quality care to their Medicare patients." ACOs are intended in part to make healthcare delivery more efficient, lower cost, better coordinated, and higher quality. This organizational structure is intended to address the long-standing problems in the US healthcare system of uneven quality, unsustainable costs, and fragmented care.

ACO implementation began in earnest in 2012 when Medicare began the Pioneer ACO program and the Medicare Shared Savings Program through contracts with fledgling ACOs. Today, many organizations have begun commercial payer ACO contracts, and several states have begun negotiating or implementing ACO contracts under Medicaid programs. At this early stage, it is too early to know whether ACOs will spur systemwide transformation of healthcare delivery. However, evidence from Medicare's Physician Group Practice Demonstration suggests that the ACO model holds promise. Still, many have raised doubts about the ability of the model to achieve its aims and concerns about the high cost and technical difficulty of establishing ACOs; the number of provider organizations that will sponsor or form ACOs is unclear at this point. Communities that have preexisting managed care or health maintenance organizations and/or pay-for-performance guidelines appear to be fertile ground for ACO development, but little else is known about the factors that contribute to ACO formation.

The implications of ACOs for healthcare marketing are yet unknown, but marketers may begin preparations in several areas in the event their organization launches or joins an ACO initiative:

1. *Marketing the ACO.* Few providers, consumers, and other customers will understand the concept initially, so marketers must make ACO information available to a wide range of existing and potential constituents. Marketers must adhere to the National Committee for Quality Assurance (NCQA) guidelines for promoting the ACO. According to NCQA guidelines, only accredited ACOs can advertise their accreditation status. Participating providers and other entities associated with the accredited ACO are not allowed to advertise the accreditation status or use the accreditation seal. However, the accredited ACO can list its participating providers and mention its accreditation status. Other guidelines—specific to

marketing and otherwise—will surely be added to ACO standards over time.

2. *Involving potential partners.* To convince potential partners to join an ACO, they must be given adequate data and information specific to the market area to convince them of the benefits of partnering. Marketers must be cognizant of the fact that, in some communities, competition for partners may already be ongoing between two or more ACOs. These partnerships may be "unholy alliances," but they can unite organizations that may have had a history of a lack of cooperation at best and competition at worst.

3. *Competing for customers.* Whether the marketers are attracting individual patients participating through a health insurance exchange, employees of a particular organization, or other groups of consumers, they must promote the benefits of ACO participation. If competition is tight, marketers must detail the merits of enrollment in their particular ACO plan. This situation makes an understanding of the market area population even more important.

4. *Internal marketing.* All personnel of an organization participating in an ACO must be made aware of this innovative organizational structure and what it means for customer service. Ongoing communication is necessary to ensure that all parties are fully informed and that misinformation does not rule the day.

As mentioned, while guidance on marketing ACOs is scant today, the future will see a proliferation of rules, recommendations, strategies, and warnings related to ACO marketing.

Set the Goal(s)

The goal(s) established during strategy development should reflect the information that has been compiled to date and should align with the organization's mission statement. As defined earlier, a goal depicts an ideal state and indicates where the organization would like to be at some point in the future. For example, the goal of a national medical products company may be to position itself as the low-cost provider of a certain product. For a local health services provider, the goal may be to establish itself as a niche player to take advantage of specified market opportunities. For the purveyor of a specific service, the goal may be to become the provider of choice for a particular segment of the market.

Set Objectives

Objective
A specific, concise, time-bound, formally designated target in support of a goal

Objectives should support the stated goal(s). To many, objectives are the tactics that support the strategic initiatives. For example, in support of its goal of expanding its orthopedic product lines, a hospital might set an objective that its orthopedic practice will recruit a sports medicine specialist within the next 12 months.

For every goal, a number of objectives are likely to be specified. Multiple objectives for a single goal are common because action will likely be required on a number of different fronts. As the planning team establishes objectives, any barriers to accomplishing the organization's stated objectives should be considered, identified, and assessed.

The possibility that pursuit of the objectives will bring about unanticipated consequences should also be considered. For example, a successful marketing campaign may overwhelm the service providers or otherwise strain resources. If the organization cannot deliver on the marketer's promises, negative consequences will likely result. A marketing campaign may alert competitors to the organization's strategic direction, or the campaign might alienate a party that had been a strong supporter of the organization. Although negative consequences cannot be totally eliminated, conceding their existence is the first step toward minimizing their impact.

Selecting a Strategy

In selecting a strategy, analysts must consider the organization's nature and mission, the market's characteristics (specifically, those of the customers), and the nature of existing competition. The chosen strategy will influence the public's perception of the organization and will carry long-term implications. Unfortunately, no standard list of strategies exists from which the organization can choose. Each situation is unique and will call for creative design.

SWOT Analysis

SWOT analysis
An assessment of an organization's strengths, weaknesses, opportunities, and threats

One technique that provides guidance in selecting an appropriate strategy is the SWOT analysis. The **SWOT analysis** examines the strengths, weaknesses, opportunities, and threats related to markets, organizations, or products (see Exhibit 8.5). It considers several dimensions of the situation simultaneously, thereby establishing a basis for subsequent strategy development.

The assessment of strengths reveals the attributes on which the strategist should capitalize. The weaknesses indicate aspects that should be minimized or ameliorated. The threats indicate aspects that should be neutralized

EXHIBIT 8.5
SWOT Analysis

The SWOT analysis has become a common technique for assessing the position of a healthcare organization within its market. A SWOT analysis involves an examination of the organization, its environment, and the manner in which the organization and environment interact. It is an important tool for strategists and marketers and has numerous applications in healthcare. It can be done for an entire organization or for specific subdivisions of the organization. Factors related to both the macroenvironment (societal) and the microenvironment (local) should be considered.

The four dimensions of the SWOT analysis are as follows:

1. *A strength is a distinctive skill, attribute, or competence that helps in achieving stated objectives.* Strengths can include marketing capabilities, management skills, image or reputation, and financial resources.
2. *A weakness is an attribute that indicates a vulnerability of the organization that hinders the achievement of its stated objectives.* Weaknesses might include inadequate working capital, poor management skills, lack of services, and personnel shortages.
3. *An opportunity is any feature of the external environment that has the potential to be a benefit during the pursuit of stated objectives.* Opportunities may take the form of gaps in the market, new sources of reimbursement, demographic shifts, weaknesses among competitors, and other potential areas for exploitation.
4. *A threat is an environmental condition or trend that may present problems with or prevent the achievement of stated objectives.* Threats may take the form of competitive activity, unfavorable demographic shifts, reimbursement changes, and other external developments.

The SWOT analysis should include data from both quantitative research and **personal interviews** with key personnel (e.g., stakeholders, key decision makers, opinion leaders). Because the identified strengths, weaknesses, opportunities, and threats guide further development of the plan, consensus needs to be reached on these attributes before proceeding with the planning process.

Personal interview
A data collection technique that involves face-to-face interaction and the administration of a survey by the interviewer to the respondent

or countered. Of the four dimensions, opportunities are perhaps the most salient for strategy development because an implicit goal of the chosen strategy should be to exploit opportunities that exist in the marketplace.

Strategic Approaches

Second-fiddle strategy
A marketing approach that concedes a subsidiary position in the market in favor of being an effective runner-up

Flanking strategy
A marketing approach that seeks to avoid confrontation with better-positioned competitors by bypassing their captive audiences and cultivating neglected target audiences

Market penetration strategy
A marketing approach that emphasizes extracting more product sales or greater service utilization from an existing customer base

New product strategy
A marketing approach that introduces differing quality levels or entirely new products into an existing market

Ideally, the marketing strategy supports the organization's mission and reflects the strategies embodied in the organization's strategic plan. Thus, if the strategic plan calls for positioning the organization as a caring organization, the marketing strategy should advance this plan. Sometimes, of course, a marketing strategy may call for a departure from this established approach. For example, a hospital that has adopted a "we're number two" approach against a powerful competitor may develop a world-class program and thus decide to take a much more aggressive marketing tactic to promote this new service. In light of this development, the hospital's **second-fiddle strategy** may be displaced by a **flanking strategy**.

Other approaches may involve a specific target market and a market-oriented strategy, while still others may revolve around a product or service line and a product-oriented strategy. One approach may address an aspect of the marketing mix, as in the case of a pricing strategy, while another may cut across the marketing mix and be broader in scope.

A **market penetration strategy** (existing market/existing product) focuses on efforts to extract more sales and greater usage out of existing markets by acquiring customers from competitors and converting nonusers into users. A *market development strategy* (new market/existing product) focuses on discovering new market sectors on the basis of different benefit profiles, establishing new distribution channels, developing new marketing approaches, and identifying underserved geographic areas. For example, a market niche strategy might be pursued by a healthcare organization that serves small segments of the healthcare market that competitors overlook or ignore.

A **new product strategy** or *service development strategy* (existing market/new product) focuses on modifying existing services by introducing differing quality levels and/or developing entirely new products. A *diversification strategy* (new market/new product) involves such actions as horizontal or vertical integration, concentric diversification, and conglomerate diversification—all of which involve extending the organization's operations to encompass additional services not previously offered.

The relationship between the product and the market can be depicted in five distinct configurations: (1) full service, (2) product/market specialization, (3) production specialization, (4) market specialization, and (5) selective specialization. This breakdown is illustrated in Exhibit 8.6. Examples of each of these relationships can be found in healthcare (although the term *service* should be substituted for *product* in most cases). The *full-service approach* was typical of most hospitals in the past, particularly during the production era following World War II. General hospitals attempted to be all things to all people, and their strategies reflected this orientation. This strategy promotes all products to all markets. A *product/market specialization approach* is typically adopted by an organization that supports a single service or service line for a defined market, such as in the case of a home infusion company that provides a discrete set of services to a narrowly defined market of home-bound pediatric patients.

Firms in the business of *product specialization* offer a distinct set of products that can be promoted to a number of markets in which consumers have one characteristic in common. For example, a firm specializing in assistive equipment (e.g., wheelchairs, walkers, home monitoring devices) promotes its products to consumers who have physical limitations and thus require assistive equipment. This firm's market would include the frail elderly, persons suffering from birth defects or childhood illness, injury victims, and those undergoing rehabilitation from surgery.

EXHIBIT 8.6
Product–Market Relationships

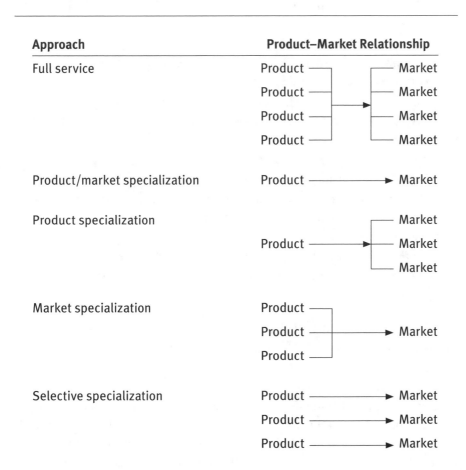

Approach	Product–Market Relationship
Full service	Product — Market Product — Market Product — Market Product — Market
Product/market specialization	Product ⟶ Market
Product specialization	Market Product ⟶ Market Market
Market specialization	Product Product ⟶ Market Product
Selective specialization	Product ⟶ Market Product ⟶ Market Product ⟶ Market

Organizations emphasizing *market specialization* typically develop a range of products geared to a certain market. Organizations that offer senior services or that specialize in women's healthcare goods and services are examples of enterprises pursuing market specialization. Pharmaceutical companies are probably the best-known example of firms engaged in *selective specialization*. Each drug constitutes a product line that is targeted to a specific market. For example, ABC Pharmaceutical's hypertension drug is marketed to the hypertensive market, its diabetes drug to the population affected by diabetes, its arthritis drug to the population of persons with rheumatoid arthritis, and so forth.

Another approach to strategy development examines the combination of market attractiveness and competitiveness found in the situation under study. For example, an area characterized by high market attractiveness and high competitiveness might call for a strategy involving investment and growth or, more likely, a strategy emphasizing selective growth in vulnerable areas. Different combinations of market attractiveness and competitiveness call for different strategies.

The following are examples of market-oriented strategies typically used in healthcare:

- *Dominance strategy.* The number one player in the market opts to focus on maintaining this position.
- *Second-fiddle strategy.* The runner-up in the market concedes its second-place status and acts accordingly (also called a *market-follower strategy*).
- *Frontal attack strategy.* The organization decides to confront the market leader or major competitors head-on.
- *Niche strategy.* The organization concedes that it cannot successfully compete for the mainstream market but instead concentrates on niche markets based on geography, population groups, or selected services.
- *Flanking strategy.* The organization outflanks the competition by entering new markets, cultivating new populations, or offering fringe products.

A sample strategy development process is presented in Case Study 8.1; the case applies the approaches just discussed.

The Four Ps

One approach to selecting a strategy considers the role of the marketing mix in establishing the strategic direction. The marketing mix is the set of controllable variables the firm uses to influence the target market. The mix includes the four Ps: product, price, place, and promotion (see also Chapter 2). As noted previously, the strategy could focus on any dimension of the four Ps or could cut across all four. Strategic approaches based on the four components of the marketing mix are addressed in this section.

Product Strategies

As the name implies, a *product strategy* focuses on one good (or product line) or service (or service line). The strategy is built around the qualities of the product, and the marketing approach attempts to capitalize on product attributes (e.g., quality, durability).

One example of a product strategy is a preemptive strategy. A preemptive strategy is used where only limited differences exist between the products in the same class. A preemptive strike attempts to convey something about a product that other competitors are reluctant to repeat because of the risk of being labeled blatant imitators. Another product-oriented approach focuses on the unique selling proposition, in which an organization establishes and communicates a product benefit that competitors cannot make or refuse to make. Marketers might also adopt a brand image strategy, which emphasizes psychological over physical differences between products. The aim in that case is to associate the product with symbols and characters that resonate with the target audience.

A positioning strategy attempts to define the comparisons between one product and another in the consumer's mind. The organization's task is to identify weaknesses in competing products and strengths in its own that can be reinforced to gain a competitive edge. Positioning indicates to customers how the company differs from current or potential competitors. A positioning strategy can be created through the following steps:

1. Identify competitors and competing products in the defined product category.
2. Determine consumers' perceptions of competing products.
3. Determine the relative position of competing products using a perceptional positioning map that graphically depicts the market.
4. Identify the gap within the market by assessing customer needs in relation to existing product offerings.
5. Select desired positioning.
6. Implement a promotional strategy.
7. Monitor and control the positioning process.

Pricing Strategies

Healthcare providers have seldom used pricing strategies, end users have not known the prices of health services before receiving them, and physicians

CASE STUDY 8.1
Hospital Strategy Development

A hospital management company recently acquired a 150-bed general hospital in a medium-sized city in the southeastern United States. Although the company had little knowledge of the local market when it acquired the facility, its first thought was to continue to run the facility as a general hospital. However, given that the hospital had not been profitable in offering general care and that it faced competition from three large facilities that had access to almost unlimited resources, the new managers chose to perform a situational analysis to determine the most appropriate strategy.

The managers commissioned a study of the immediate market area—the five-mile radius surrounding the hospital. This market area was examined in the context of overall trends for the metropolitan area. The analysts reviewed demographic trends to determine the future size and composition of the population as well as trends in service utilization. This information was used to develop projections of the future demand for health services in the urban area and the immediate market area. Particular attention was paid to the competitive situation to determine the services offered by other facilities, the existing market shares for those services, and the nature of existing managed care contracts and other negotiated relationships.

The analysis determined that the immediate service area was not likely to support a general hospital. The payer mix was not favorable, and other facilities controlled significant portions of the local market. Further, most area employers were tied to the provider networks of the two dominant systems in the community. The hospital did not have a large or strong medical staff. Given the existing provider networks involving competing hospitals, attracting additional physicians to the facility would have been difficult.

Having conceded that it could not operate effectively as a general community hospital and that confronting large, established competitors head-on was not practical, the managers considered other strategies. After analyzing the data, the managers decided that, under the circumstances, a niche strategy was appropriate for the hospital. It would identify niche services, and the corporate focus would be on exploiting those niches.

The hospital had previously developed an occupational health program that catered to the numerous employers in the area. Facilities were available, a basic program was in place, and adequate personnel were available to expand the program. Because no other entity was offering this service in the community, expansion of this program seemed like a logical next step. In addition, the hospital had a long-standing behavioral health program that had experienced some success in attracting patients, and some of the area's leading substance abuse experts were affiliated with the hospital. Thus, because a fledgling program was already in place, key personnel were available, and the market was underserved, the hospital also identified behavioral health (including substance abuse treatment) as a promising niche. Finally, in view of the large Medicare population in the general area and the lack of geropsychiatric services in the community, the hospital decided to add psychiatric services for seniors to the behavioral health component. This niche strategy focused on services that were not being adequately provided to the community.

One other niche was considered but eventually rejected. Market research indicated that minority group members—primarily African Americans—made up a large proportion of the community. The Hispanic population in the area was also growing rapidly. Further, mainstream providers historically had neglected these populations. A niche strategy focusing on these target populations was considered that would convert the hospital into a facility specializing in minority care. Because of the many unknowns surrounding this concept and the potential controversy such a strategy might generate, this idea was rejected.

After carefully assessing the situation, the managers conceded that the facility could not successfully operate as a general hospital and therefore chose to pursue a niche strategy. The approach has—in the short run at least—been relatively successful. The hospital has maintained a significant share of the occupational health and behavioral health markets in the city and has earned a reputation as a facility that does not offer a lot of services but that does a good job with the services it provides.

Case Study Discussion Questions

1. What factors raised concerns among the hospital's managers about the viability of the facility as a general community hospital, and how did the market analysis validate those concerns?
2. What steps were taken to determine the most appropriate focus for the hospital's services?
3. How would one classify the strategic approach the managers chose, and to what types of services did it direct them?

(the primary decision makers on healthcare purchasing) have seldom taken pricing into consideration. Further, the amount of reimbursement from third-party payers has often been established irrespective of the price set by the provider. For these reasons, healthcare has had few opportunities to compete on the basis of price. On the other hand, more **retail healthcare** businesses—such as personal health product manufacturers—are likely to use pricing strategies in much the same manner as do producers of other consumer health goods.

Retail healthcare
Healthcare products designed to attract discretionary consumption

Insurance providers are another sector of the industry for which price may be a factor. Although insurance premiums have been established according to the perceived risk to the insurer, the emergence of managed care plans prompted unprecedented competition. As managed care plans became more standardized during the 1990s, they were forced to compete on price. Because their products were essentially the same, price became a rational basis for competition. Interestingly, the health insurance exchanges introduced by the ACA have shed new light on the pricing practices of insurance companies.

A major drawback to the use of pricing strategies in healthcare is that organizations and practitioners have not been able to determine the cost of providing a service. The development of an intelligent pricing strategy requires some objective basis. Further, restrictions related to price fixing have prevented healthcare providers from using the fee schedules of other organizations as models.

Despite these barriers, a growing number of providers—particularly those performing elective procedures—are competing on price for services that are discretionary and typically paid for out of pocket. Most cosmetic surgery would be included in this category, and as competition has increased among ophthalmic surgeons, ophthalmologists performing laser eye surgery have also begun to compete on the basis of price.

Place Strategies

Place focuses on the manner in which a good or service is distributed. In healthcare, place refers to the location where services are rendered. An important aspect of place is the **channel** of distribution—the path a good or service takes as it travels from the producer to the consumer. Although this concept has traditionally applied to consumer goods, it can also be applied to health services.

Channel
The mechanism used to distribute a promotional message, good, or service

A variety of distribution channels are used to deliver health services. Primary care centers are typically located near potential patients (e.g., neighborhoods, heavily populated residential areas), whereas tertiary services are concentrated in medical centers, regardless of the proximity to population centers. Emergency services are delivered through a combination of distribution methods; ambulances travel to the patient and then take the patient to the hospital for treatment.

During the production era in healthcare, little emphasis was placed on the location of service outlets. Most intensive care was provided by hospitals, and patients were expected to travel to where the hospital was located. Physicians (particularly specialists) had the same attitude. Although primary care providers may have sought locations in the community that were close to patient populations, the overriding attitude was "if you build it, they will come."

The actions of some hospitals in the 1990s are an example of **channel management**. In the early 1990s, hospitals attempted to control the distribution of their primary care providers by purchasing and "controlling" physician practices. However, hospital administrators failed to consider that the product—physician practice patterns—could not be so easily controlled. As a result, such attempts largely failed. Although hospitals controlled the distribution of the practices, they were unable to control the products or prices these practices offered, thereby failing to benefit from their control of the distribution outlets.

Channel management
A formal program for reaching and servicing customers through a particular marketing channel

As the focus of healthcare shifted from the inpatient setting to the outpatient setting, healthcare providers were forced to pay attention to the location of services. Hospitals were largely immobile, but outpatient services could be established almost anywhere. Those who sought to compete with hospitals took advantage of their relative immobility and established facilities in proximity to target markets. Today, hospitals and health systems are engaging in another round of physician practice acquisition to manage channels.

The emergence of place strategies was driven by a new generation of healthcare consumers (baby boomers) with different expectations of healthcare providers. These patients brought a consumer orientation that demanded convenience of location and easy access to services. They placed a high value on their time and expected the same of service providers. The healthcare industry responded to this emerging consumerism by offering urgent care centers and freestanding diagnostic and surgery centers as convenient alternatives to traditional sources of care. The emphasis on place has also been encouraged by the employers and business coalitions that are paying a large share of the healthcare bill. Employers want their employees to have convenient access to services, not only to ensure patient satisfaction but to limit the time they are away from work using these services. In addition, one of the bases for competition among managed care plans is the convenience they provide to enrollees. To succeed, health plans found they had to establish networks of providers that were distributed in a manner that would meet the needs of their enrollee populations.

The combined influence of these developments has encouraged providers to take healthcare to the community. Expecting patients to come to the source of care is no longer a viable approach. The contemporary consumer demands convenient locations, and, in cases where locations cannot be changed, healthcare providers are working to improve the value of an existing location through more efficient patient-processing methods or redesign to create more appealing facilities.

Promotional Strategies

The most visible type of strategy used by healthcare organizations is promotion of the organization or its services. As healthcare marketing was coming into its own in the 1980s and 1990s, it focused on advertising, direct mail, and other traditional promotional strategies. The limitations of competition based on product, price, and place have encouraged healthcare providers to differentiate themselves through promotional strategies.

Promotional strategies should reflect the organization's overriding strategic orientation. If, for example, a hospital adopts a niche strategy, its promotional efforts should be focused on a narrow range of services and/or a targeted population. On the other hand, a hospital pursuing a full-service strategy should develop an approach that promotes the organization as a desirable choice for almost any service.

Similarly, a promotional strategy should reflect the organization's chosen approach to the market. If the organization has adopted an aggressive, hard-sell approach, the promotional strategy should reflect it. Conversely, if the organization has adopted a soft-sell approach, it would be reflected in initiatives to educate the market.

A promotions-oriented strategy can take a variety of forms. A *resonance strategy* strikes a chord with the consumer. The intention is to portray a lifestyle orientation that is synonymous with the target group and easily recognizable. For example, this approach might be used to promote a hospital-based fitness center. An *emotional strategy* plays on (and to) consumers' feelings—as in the case of children's health services.

In the contemporary healthcare arena, promotional strategies involve far more than advertising. Increasingly, healthcare providers have turned to personal selling and sales promotions to compete more effectively. To develop an effective promotional strategy, marketers must understand the various media (including social media) available to them and be able to craft a message with appropriate content and tone. (Promotional strategies are addressed frequently throughout the remainder of the book.)

The marketing mix concept discussed earlier has been adopted from other industries and applied to healthcare. Critics suggest, however, that the four Ps of marketing have never fit comfortably in healthcare. As healthcare providers become more service oriented, they too are criticizing this concept. Some have suggested the need to revise the four Ps and replace them with some other set of attributes that are more appropriate for contemporary healthcare. These conflicting views on the importance of the four Ps are a source of ongoing debate among health professionals.

Branding as a Strategy

Branding as a strategy is a relatively recent phenomenon in healthcare. A **brand** is a name, term, symbol, or design (or combination thereof) that signifies the goods or services of one seller or group of sellers. *Brand identity* refers to the visual features that create awareness in the mind of the consumer; these features include the brand's name, image, typography, color, package design, and slogans. The intent of the brand image is to distinguish in the eye of the user a company's product from competing products (Mangini 2002). The brand image indicates what business the company is in, what benefit the company provides, and why the company is better than its competition. Thus, brand identity is the visual, emotional, rational, and cultural image that a consumer associates with a company or product.

> **Branding**
> The creation of a brand for a company, service, or product
>
> **Brand**
> A name, term, symbol, or design (or combination thereof) that signifies the goods or services of one seller or group of sellers

Corporate branding is often confused with corporate identity or corporate image, but these three terms have different meanings:

1. *Corporate identity* refers to a company's name, logo, or tagline.
2. *Corporate image* is the public's perception of a company—whether that perception is intended or not.
3. *Corporate branding* is a business process that is planned, strategically focused, and integrated throughout the organization. It establishes direction, leadership, clarity of purpose, and energy for a company's corporate brand. *Brand associations* are attributes of a product or company that come to consumers' minds when they hear or see a brand name. An effective brand name evokes positive associations with the company. Therefore, the logic behind branding is simple: If consumers are familiar with a company's brand and perceive it positively, they are more likely to purchase the company's products.

A company's brand also has significant internal value. A strong corporate brand generates and sustains internal momentum. Employees have proven to be more committed to the brand's promise if it is understood and supported by every key player (Lake 2009). To maximize the effectiveness of its brand, a company must ensure that it is understood by all relevant audiences: customers, prospective consumers, business partners, the media, and employees. Corporate communication should reinforce the branding effort.

Branding is most effective for products that command a mass market, can benefit from advertising, and can be effectively evaluated by consumers. Few healthcare services have these characteristics. Because most healthcare is provided locally, few healthcare organizations need to develop national brand recognition. Furthermore, many organizations have been around for a long time, and efforts to rebrand them are often met with resistance. The national hospital chain HCA, for example, went through a period of renaming all of its hospitals with the HCA brand, only to have to revert to the hospitals' old names in some cases because of local resistance. The Mayo Clinic and the Cleveland Clinic are examples of healthcare organizations that successfully established national brands, but few organizations are in their league.

The lag in adopting branding strategies in healthcare has had both negative and positive consequences for healthcare marketing. The negative consequences include a lack of expertise and success in today's healthcare branding efforts. The positive consequence is that the healthcare industry can learn lessons from other industries. The emergence of the new healthcare consumer has prompted increased interest in branding among healthcare providers. This revitalized consumerism is being driven by well-informed consumers who are demanding choices.

For established retailers of healthcare products (e.g., pharmaceutical and personal health products companies), branding has been an inherent part of their strategy. In these cases, consumers are more likely to be familiar with the brand (e.g., Claritin, Band-Aids) than they are with the corporation that created it. The development of branding strategies in this segment of the industry reflects the relative ease of branding consumer products. According to Mangini (2002), several steps must be followed to establish a brand identity:

1. *Decide what to brand.* The organization must carefully consider the services it offers, the people who provide those services, the competition for those services, and the population the organization serves. Branding can focus on the entire health system, outpatient services, a prominent department, or a particular medical group. In addition, an institution may choose to focus on goods and services that are in high demand but difficult to emulate. No matter what the focus, effective brands are almost always linked to a target audience, such as women or senior citizens.

2. *Define the brand message.* The organization must decide what information to communicate about the service it wants to brand. For example, the focus may be on quality of care, convenience, or technology capabilities. Each of these approaches can be effective if the brand message relates to the target audience and the service being branded.

3. *Communicate the brand both internally and externally.* Internal communication is important to encourage and gain the staff acceptance and enthusiasm necessary for brand success. Staff members can be brought on board by giving them ownership of the branding initiative and rewarding them for their involvement in the campaign. External communication can take place through such channels as promotional materials and advertising. Most important, however, is that the message—both internal and external—is clear, consistent, and continuous.

The true test of a brand is the institution's performance. An organization must be confident that it can fulfill the promise of its brand. Every customer interaction must reinforce the brand identity, and that identity must be used to establish a relationship with consumers. If consumers have a positive interaction with the organization and are satisfied, they are potential sources of new business. Thus, information is key in determining how the institution is implementing its brand. It must develop a systemwide data collection, analysis, and reporting network so that it can continually assess the success of its brand and make necessary adjustments.

Once a brand is built, it must be constantly updated and revitalized. Brand revitalization does not simply mean creating a new logo or repackaging a product but also examining the company's point of differentiation. A successful branding process provides a framework that links the branding strategy to the business strategy. This linkage is essential because the commitment and involvement of executive management are key components of a successful branding strategy. Finally, once all key players understand the institution's brand identity and framework, documentation of the branding system can begin.

A number of important lessons about the healthcare branding process must be mentioned here:

1. A branding strategy must build consensus and ensure concurrence with the business strategy.
2. An organization's marketing department must be cautious about making changes to long-standing brand franchises. A strong brand, once tarnished, is difficult to reinstate.

3. An organization must follow a set of guidelines when developing its branding strategy, but it should also be flexible and allow carefully chosen exceptions to those rules.

4. An organization must consider its competitors' current and future brands.

5. To prevent inconsistency, an enterprise must secure commitment from every organizational level and all key players must reach consensus.

6. An organization must align its values with the values of its branding strategy.

Case Study 8.2 is an example of a successful branding initiative.

CASE STUDY 8.2
Establishing a Brand

One example of a successful branding initiative is the one developed by the Cleveland Clinic Foundation in Cleveland, Ohio. The outcome of its efforts demonstrates what branding can do for a healthcare organization and how a small outpatient practice can be transformed into a national brand.

The Cleveland Clinic was founded in 1921 by four veterans of World War I medical units and is now a leading American healthcare organization. From its start, the clinic was highly regarded for the quality of its specialty care, basic science research, and medical innovations. The clinic's initial marketing approach—typical of healthcare organizations in the premarketing era—targeted the physician audience in an effort to increase patient referrals. Promotional activities consisted of developing and distributing fund-raising brochures and disseminating press releases to the media.

In the 1990s, the clinic realized that healthcare consumers were looking for a trusted brand name and thus expanded its market research. This research indicated that local consumers highly respected the name *Cleveland Clinic*, so the organization focused on maintaining and protecting its brand through an integrated marketing effort. The 1990s also marked a period of hospital mergers and acquisitions in the healthcare industry, and the clinic played a significant role in this development. Over a two-year period, it merged with ten local community hospitals and formed the Cleveland Clinic Health System. The formation of this system presented a challenge in that the clinic had to decide how much it could share its brand identity without diluting it.

To address this challenge, the clinic established a four-tiered marketing approach that applied to all organizations using the Cleveland Clinic brand. Tier 1 members represent the core organizations—the conservators of the brand and directors of all marketing efforts. Tier 2 members include entities owned by the clinic but that have their own brand equity; in their advertisements, they are allowed to use only the words "Cleveland Clinic Health System" in half size under their own hospital name. Tier 3 includes clinic departments housed in hospitals the clinic does not own. They are not part of the clinic or the system, and the appropriate relationships are outlined in their advertising; they are prohibited from using the Cleveland Clinic name, logo, or tagline. Finally, Tier 4 includes organizations to which the clinic belongs. In these relationships, the clinic's logo may be used only in visual arrangement with the logos of other participating hospitals.

As this case shows, the Cleveland Clinic has been successful in supporting the integrity of its brand while extending the brand's positive image to other entities without diluting existing brand equity. Although not all healthcare organizations can be expected to have the same success as the clinic, this case illustrates how, with sound market intelligence and thoughtful planning, a successful branding initiative can be undertaken.

Case Study Discussion Questions

1. What changes in the marketplace led the Cleveland Clinic to reassess its marketing strategy?
2. What were potential negative consequences of expanding the brand "umbrella" too widely?
3. How did the clinic adapt its marketing strategy to the new organizational structure?
4. How is the clinic able to preserve its commitment to its mission while at the same time marketing a complex organization?

Summary

A well-thought-out marketing strategy is essential for any healthcare organization that hopes to compete in today's environment. Strategies set the tone for marketing activities and establish the parameters within which the marketer must operate. The strategy chosen influences the marketing plan that is ultimately developed and guides subsequent marketing initiatives. De facto strategies emerge in the absence of a formal corporate strategy. Strategies may be developed at different levels, from an overall corporate strategy to a specific marketing strategy.

The marketing strategy should be developed during the strategic planning process, thereby reflecting the overall corporate strategy. Strategy development follows a series of steps, from initial data collection through data analysis through the identification of strategic options. All key stakeholders should participate in the strategy development process.

Strategies are usually keyed to one of the four Ps of the marketing mix—product, price, place, or promotion. Customer relationship building and relationship management have become increasingly important in shaping strategy. A SWOT analysis may be used to inform strategy development.

A number of different strategic approaches are available to healthcare organizations; the type of organization and environmental circumstances determine the best approach to use. The chosen strategy should reflect the organization's positioning in the market. Most strategies consider the product–market relationship; options range from matching a specific product to a narrowly defined market to dispersing a range of products to a broad market. Branding as a strategy has become increasingly important in healthcare, although many healthcare organizations still face challenges in applying this approach.

Key Points

- Every healthcare organization should choose a strategy to guide its marketing activities.
- The marketing strategy should support the overall corporate strategy and guide the development of the organization's marketing plan.
- The chosen strategy performs a number of different functions, most important of which is to focus the entire organization on a common goal.
- If the healthcare organization does not proactively develop a strategy, a default strategy is likely to emerge that may not be in the best interest of the organization.
- Strategies can exist at various levels of the organization, from an enterprisewide strategy to specific strategies for individual departments or products.
- As with any strategy, the development of a marketing strategy should follow fairly rigid steps.

- Both internal and external data must be collected to develop an informed marketing strategy.
- Marketing strategies may reflect the organization's desired position in the marketplace, emphasize one or more of the four Ps of the product mix, and/or focus on the relationship between the organization's products and the market.
- Branding as a strategic approach has become more common among healthcare organizations, although certain attributes of the healthcare industry militate against a branding strategy.
- Although the ACA focuses primarily on health insurance reform, it does have certain implications for the marketing of health services.
- The ACA also has numerous implications for the marketing and pricing of health insurance products.

Discussion Questions

1. What are some of the different functions that a strategy performs for an organization?
2. What is meant by "the absence of an articulated strategy does not mean that no strategy exists"?
3. What is meant by "acts of commission or omission ultimately create a strategy, and even the absence of a strategy could be considered a strategic approach in a technical sense"?
4. What are the steps involved in the strategic planning process?
5. How should an organization's marketing strategy link to its strategic plan?
6. What types of strategies might an organization use, and what determines the best type of strategy to use for a particular situation?
7. What are some ways in which the product and market interface during strategy development?
8. What is the relationship between strategy development and the four Ps of the marketing mix?
9. What determines which of the four Ps is most relevant to strategy in a particular case?
10. Why is a branding strategy not universally employed by healthcare organizations?
11. Under what circumstances does a branding strategy appear to work best?

Additional Resources

Bashe, G. 2000. *Branding Health Services: Defining Yourself in the Marketplace.* Sudbury, MA: Jones and Bartlett.

Hillstead, S. G., and E. N. Berkowitz. 2012. *Health Care Market Strategy,* 4th ed. Sudbury, MA: Jones and Bartlett Learning.

Zuckerman, A. M. 2005. *Healthcare Strategic Planning,* 2nd ed. Chicago: Health Administration Press.

TRADITIONAL MARKETING TECHNIQUES

This chapter provides an overview of traditional marketing techniques as they are applied to healthcare. The promotional mix and media options are discussed, along with social marketing and integrated marketing. The pros and cons of each technique are discussed in turn.

The Promotional Mix

The promotional component of the marketing strategy could be considered the action component through which the marketing plan is implemented. *Promotions* refer to the techniques used to communicate with customers and potential customers for purposes of promoting an idea, an organization, or a product. Traditional promotional activities include public relations, advertising, personal sales, and sales promotion; for purposes of this discussion, direct marketing is also included. Each of these techniques is carried out through different means. The term *promotional mix* refers to the combination of techniques used for a given marketing campaign. The following sections discuss these techniques and their respective applications to healthcare.

Public Relations

Public relations (PR) is a form of communication management that uses publicity and other forms of promotion to influence consumers' feelings, opinions, or beliefs about an organization and its offerings. PR typically involves "unpaid" promotional activities, with marketing, communications, or other personnel carrying out PR activities as part of their job responsibility. The organization does not incur additional expenses or increases in overhead costs. PR activities include writing and distributing press releases (see Exhibit 9.1 for a sample), scheduling and holding press conferences, writing feature stories and producing public service announcements.

Publicity
Any promotion that generally draws attention to an organization but does not target a particular audience

Forms of Publicity

Publicity refers to any type of promotion that draws general attention to an organization without targeting a specific audience. This traditional form of

EXHIBIT 9.1
Sample Press
Release

U.S. Department of Health & Human Services   HRSA NEWS ROOM

Health Resources and Services Administration   http://newsroom.hrsa.gov

FOR IMMEDIATE RELEASE   CONTACT: HRSA PRESS OFFICE

Tuesday, October 29, 2013   301-443-3376

HHS awards $1.9 billion in grants for HIV/AIDS care and medications

More than $1.9 billion in grants have been awarded to cities, states and local community-based organizations the U.S. Department of Health and Human Services (HHS) announced today. This funding will ensure that people living with HIV/AIDS continue to have access to critical health care services and medications. The fiscal year 2013 awards were funded through the Ryan White HIV/AIDS Program.

"The Ryan White HIV/AIDS Program plays an important role in the fight against HIV/AIDS," said Secretary Kathleen Sebelius. "These grants will help make a real difference in the lives of Americans coping with HIV/AIDS, especially those in underserved urban and rural communities."

The Health Resources and Services Administration (HRSA), an agency within HHS, oversees the Ryan White HIV/AIDS Program, which provides funding for health services for people who lack sufficient health care coverage or financial resources to pay for treatment.

"The Ryan White HIV/AIDS Program helps more than half a million individuals each year obtain clinical care, treatment and support services," said HRSA Administrator Mary K. Wakefield, Ph.D., R.N. "The key to its success is the cities, states and community groups who know their populations and decide how best to allocate the funding they receive."

A total of $594 million was awarded to 53 cities to provide core medical and support services for individuals living with HIV/AIDS under Part A of the Ryan White HIV/AIDS Program. These grants are awarded to eligible metropolitan areas with the highest number of people living with HIV/AIDS and to areas experiencing increases in HIV/AIDS cases and emerging care needs. See a list of the Part A awards.

Approximately $1.16 billion was awarded in FY 2013 to 59 states and territories under Part B of the Ryan White HIV/AIDS Program. Part B grants include grants that can be used for home and community-based services, AIDS Drug Assistance Program (ADAP) assistance, and other direct services. In FY 2013, $309 million was awarded in Part B base

---

funding and $782 million was awarded for ADAP. In addition, 16 states received Emerging Community grants based on the number of AIDS cases over the most recent five-year period. Thirty-six states and territories were also awarded $10.1 million in Part B Minority AIDS Initiative grants. See a list of the Part B awards.

In FY 2013, approximately $178 million was awarded across the country to 357 local community-based organizations to provide core medical and support services to individuals living with HIV/AIDS under Part C of the Ryan White HIV/AIDS Program. Currently 351 Part C grantees are providing ongoing services. Part C grant recipients provide comprehensive primary health care in outpatient settings to people living with HIV disease. See a list of the FY 2013 Part C awarded grants.

These funds also will support states and communities in their ongoing efforts to pursue the goals of the National HIV/AIDS Strategy, particularly efforts to increase access to HIV care and reduce HIV-related health disparities.

To learn more about the Ryan White HIV/AIDS Program, visit hab.hrsa. gov. For more information about HIV/AIDS prevention, testing, treatment, and research, visit AIDS.gov.

The Ryan White HIV/AIDS Program is administered by the U.S. Department of Health and Human Services (HHS), Health Resources and Services Administration (HRSA), HIV/AIDS Bureau (HAB). Federal funds are awarded to agencies located around the country, which in turn deliver care to eligible individuals under funding categories called Parts. First authorized in 1990, the Ryan White HIV/AIDS Program is currently funded at more than $2 billion.

Source: Reprinted from HHS (2013).

---

promotion predates advertising and other marketing techniques. Following are some forms of publicity:

- *Collateral materials.* These are materials developed for the organization, program, or product being promoted. They include brochures, letterhead, business cards, social media content, and websites. A potential customer's first exposure to the organization, program, or product may be through such materials. In addition, collateral materials serve as a foundation for material developed for future or subsequent marketing efforts; are an inexpensive means of generating and maintaining **visibility** of the organization's activities; and convey basic information, such as location and directions, pertinent phone numbers, and e-mail addresses.

Visibility
A marketing campaign goal that raises the public's awareness of the organization, program, or product to increase consumers' top-of-mind recall

- *Public service announcements.* A no-cost advertisement that supports a public service campaign, a **public service announcement (PSA)** may be aired on radio or television, printed in a newspaper or magazine, featured on a billboard, or posted on the Internet. Although the no-cost aspect is appealing, the downside is that the advertising organization often has no control over the placement or timing of a PSA.

Public service announcement (PSA)
A no-cost advertisement that supports a community program or public initiative

- *Internal and external publications.* Staff of the communications department (or an overlapping function like marketing or community outreach) develop internal employee newsletters, annual reports, patient education pamphlets, and other publications geared to relevant groups within the organization (internal marketing) and outside of it (external marketing).

Sponsorship
Organizational support—typically financial—of a community project or event

- *Sponsorships.* **Sponsorship** involves support by the organization for a community project or event. This may include direct financial support through contributions or sponsorship of concessions (e.g., refreshment booth) or in-kind contributions such as volunteer time, food and beverages, and gift items (e.g., water bottles, T-shirts). The sponsor typically does not run an advertisement but may be mentioned in a "brought to you by" message. Although sponsorships may be done for altruistic reasons, they typically bestow goodwill and favorable attention on the generous organization. Additionally, sponsors receive substantial media coverage and improve their employees' morale. Unlike most forms of PR, sponsoring or underwriting a project or an event requires financial output.

Spokesperson
An individual—usually a celebrity—paid to deliver the organization's message or to speak publicly on its behalf

- *Spokespersons.* A **spokesperson** could be a national or local celebrity—such as an athlete, an actor, a community leader, or some other influential personality; a well-known mascot could also be a spokesperson. By associating the organization with a recognizable person or character, the organization hopes to be perceived in a positive way.

- *Community outreach programs.* Community outreach presents the organization's programs to the community and seeks to establish relationships with other community organizations. They may take the form of episodic activities, such as health fairs or educational programs, or ongoing initiatives such as "parish nurses" (fielded by churches to provide home visits and staff health fairs). This type of publicity emphasizes the organization's commitment to the community and its support of local interests. Although the benefits of community outreach activities are not as easily measured as the benefits of direct marketing activities, the organization often gains customers as a result of its health screenings, educational seminars, and referrals. Many consumers are not aware of the healthcare services offered in their own communities, and the organization's outreach efforts are a good way to raise **awareness**.

Awareness
Recognition of or familiarity with an organization or its product; the ultimate goal of a public relations effort

As noted in earlier chapters, healthcare organizations are typically regulated by state and federal government agencies. Decisions related to reimbursement rates and adding, eliminating, or changing a service may be controlled by government agencies. Organizations often must cultivate and maintain relationships with politicians and other policymakers and various government agencies—as well as initiate lobbying activities. In a large organization, the PR function is typically assigned responsibility for these activities or shares it with the government relations office.

Advertising

Advertising refers to any paid form of nonpersonal presentation and promotion of ideas, goods, or services by an identifiable sponsor, typically using mass media as the communication vehicle. The objectives of advertising are as follows:

- Promote products, services, organizations, and causes
- Increase product usage
- Remind consumers of the organization or product
- Build customer loyalty
- Introduce new products
- Offset competitors' advertising
- Support sales personnel in the field
- Alleviate sales fluctuations
- Educate consumers
- Maintain visibility

Not all of these objectives are relevant for every healthcare organization, and they are likely to be pursued selectively according to the type of marketing being undertaken.

Institutional advertising
Promotion of an organization rather than its products

Product advertising
Promotion of an organization's goods and services rather than the organization itself

Advertising is typically classified as institutional (or corporate) advertising or product advertising, depending on what is being promoted. **Institutional advertising** promotes the organization—its image, people, ideas, political issues, and any other traits or features but not its products. It may introduce or announce a new facility, present comparative information, or explain a public policy stance. **Product advertising**, on the other hand, promotes specific goods or services, not the institution itself. Historically, this type was less attractive to healthcare organizations, which tended, at least initially, to promote awareness of the institution rather than its products. At some point, large healthcare organizations realized that they could not be all things to all people and began to focus their advertising on specific services or service lines. Providers offering elective services shifted their advertising to tout the availability of laser surgery, facelifts, or pain management rather than the attributes of the organization.

Advertising is much more flexible than other traditional promotional techniques. An advertising campaign could be as simple as print ads in a local shoppers' newsletter or as complicated as a series of commercials that air on national television. This wide range of options comes with a wide range of costs, offers varying degrees of exposure to consumers, and requires varying degrees of effort from the organization. Ultimately, the scope of the advertising campaign is determined by the objectives of the effort, the types of product being promoted, and the nature of the target audience.

Personal Sales

Another tool in the promotional mix is personal sales—the conversation between a marketer or salesperson and one or more prospective purchasers for the purpose of generating sales. The primary difference between personal sales and advertising is that the former involves two-way rather than one-way communication. The primary objectives of personal sales are to (1) find prospects, (2) convince prospects to buy a product, and (3) keep existing customers engaged. These objectives involve researching prospects, providing after-sales service, forecasting future sales, and maintaining relationships with customers. Thus, the role of the salesperson requires not only selling but also developing a relationship with customers and serving as the organization's eyes and ears in the marketplace.

One advantage of personal sales is that the salesperson can get direct feedback from existing and prospective customers. If the customer expresses any misunderstandings or difficulties interpreting the information, the salesperson can correct the situation on the spot. Another advantage of personal sales is that the healthcare organization has more direct control over who receives the message. Hospitals that incorporate personal sales into their promotional mix report several benefits, including increased facility occupancy, improved medical staff relations, higher profitability, and increased market share (Powers and Bowers 1992).

Well-established personal-selling activities in healthcare include solicitation of physicians by pharmaceutical and medical supplier representatives, solicitation of consumers by insurance salespeople, and solicitation of hospitals by biomedical equipment representatives. Healthcare providers have become active in personal sales, and hospital representatives may solicit referring physicians, employers, and other organizations to promote the hospital's emergency department, sports medicine program, or particular service line. These activities have become increasingly important as interactions between individual physicians and individual patients have been displaced by interactions between groups of providers and groups of purchasers.

As with any promotional tool, however, personal sales has several limitations. First, it is costly. In addition to salary and benefits, the costs include travel expenses for sales staff, promotional materials, and technical support. Second, the number of customer visits a salesperson can make in one day is limited, as each visit can be time consuming. Third, the strength of the interpersonal connections made vary from one salesperson to the next. The sales message's "punch" (effect on the consumer) depends on the salesperson's training, disposition, and salesmanship as well as on customer attributes.

The more technologically sophisticated the service, the greater the need for personal sales. For example, a salesperson might be needed to explain the intricacies of a diagnostic technique or program, or a health system might use a sales representative to introduce new diagnostic technology to potential referring physicians. Personal sales are also important when a variety of decision makers (especially with differing perspectives) are involved or when an element of risk exists in the decision (e.g., committing to a managed care contract).

Personal sales can involve a combination of sales presentations, sales meetings, incentive programs, sample distributions, and participation in fairs and trade shows. Regardless of the personal sales mix, the selling process involves specific steps (see Exhibit 9.2).

Fund-raising is an aspect of personal sales that characterizes many not-for-profit healthcare organizations. Such organizations often rely on donations to support their programs or fund capital improvements, so organizations typically market themselves to potential donors to secure contributions. Although much of this effort may involve direct mail or telemarketing, major contributors typically must be contacted in person—that is, by a high-level representation of the organization acting as a "salesperson." Thus, many large not-for-profits maintain a "development staff" dedicated to soliciting funds directly from large donors.

EXHIBIT 9.2
Steps in the
Personal Sales
Process

Salespeople typically follow these steps when promoting an organization or a product.

Identification of the Prospective Customer

This first step involves identifying qualified potential customers. In
healthcare, for example, salespeople may identify potential referring
physicians, organ donors, or purchasers of biomedical equipment. In
some cases, the prospects are obvious—say, when contacting a hospital's purchasing office to promote routine products. In other cases—say,
when selling marketing research services to hospitals—the prospect
may be located in a variety of different departments (e.g., marketing,
research, business development) or at various levels within the organization, from research analyst up to vice president.

Pre-Approach

The second step requires the salesperson to learn as much as possible
about the prospects identified before the salesperson approaches
them. If the salesperson is offering supplies to a hospital, for example,
he or she should find out the hospital's level of supply use and its current suppliers. Likewise, a pharmaceutical sales representative must
first become familiar with a physician's prescribing practices and the
drugs he or she typically prescribes.

Approach

The third step occurs when the salesperson meets the prospective
buyer to establish a relationship. Healthcare sales are typically not
characterized by the wining and dining that often accompanies promotional activities in other industries. Because sales situations in healthcare vary, no standard approach to clients exists.

Presentation and Demonstration

This fourth step refers to the salesperson describing the attributes and
benefits of the healthcare product to the prospects. The two common
challenges here are that (1) many healthcare providers are not used
to receiving sales calls or visits and (2) salespeople may have difficulty meeting with the right person in a large healthcare organization.
Exhibiting at professional meetings is one way for a salesperson to
gain exposure to supplement presentations, demonstrations, and other
information channels.

Handling Objections

In this step, the salesperson seeks out, clarifies, and overcomes customer objections to buying. Because of the nature of healthcare, the sales representative is likely to take a consultative rather than hard-sell approach. Instead of trying to out-negotiate the customer, the salesperson is likely to address the customer's objections in a mutually beneficial manner.

Close

This step occurs when the salesperson asks the customer to order the product or otherwise consummates the sale. Establishing an agreement among the various parties initiates the fulfillment process. Closing a sale is often less straightforward in healthcare than it is in other industries, as many parties may have to participate in the purchase decision.

Follow-Up

After the sale, the salesperson follows up to ensure customer satisfaction and repeat business. In healthcare, relationship management is equally—if not more—important than in other industries, and ongoing contact with the customer is necessary.

Networking

While many sectors of the healthcare industry look askance at the wining-and-dining activities in other industries, a certain amount of networking is both inevitable and desirable for the purpose of the sale. Healthcare administrators (e.g., hospital administrators, physician practice managers) interact with those in similar positions to exchange information, flesh out ideas, and "do deals." Perhaps more so in healthcare than other industries, administrators are likely to know each other and run in the same social or professional circles. Likewise, physicians are notorious for hobnobbing with other physicians; this is certainly understandable given the importance of referral relationships in channeling patients to other physicians. Hospital and physician practice administrators also network with physicians as well.

Sales representatives of for-profit healthcare organizations are active networkers. They seek out prospects at professional meetings, in civic organizations, and at social events. Relationships developed at healthcare conferences or at the country club may be leveraged to a salesperson's advantage at some point in the future. The salesperson may offer to sponsor a meeting or a reception or may provide lunch to the employees of a networking partner or its practice. A representative will be present at such an event to answer questions and to get to know the people actually involved in decision making at the practice.

Sales Promotion

Sales promotion refers to any activity or material that directly induces resellers, salespersons, or consumers to buy a good or use a service. Enticements are offered to achieve a specific sales or marketing objective. The sales promotion mix includes health fairs and **trade shows**, exhibits, demonstrations, contests and games, premiums and gifts, rebates, attractive financing terms, and trade-in allowances.

Trade show
A convention at which vendors present their products to attendees

Although sales promotion methods have less application in healthcare than in most other industries, both "pull" and "push" incentives are frequently used. Pull incentives used to promote consumer goods also apply to personal healthcare products. They include discounts on the customer's next purchase, cash refunds, coupons, buy-one-get-one-free promotions, consumer contests, loyalty cards, free trials (or samples), free products, price reductions, and merchandising and point-of-sale displays. Manufacturers and service providers use push incentives to influence intermediaries to carry or deliver a product. For example, an optometrist might be offered incentives to carry (and presumably promote) a particular brand of contact lens solution.

Pharmaceutical companies use both pull and push strategies in promoting drugs to their target audiences. By using a pull strategy, they appeal directly to the consumer, recognizing that the consumer creates the demand for the product and pulls the product through the channel. In other words, the consumer requests that the physician write a prescription for the product, which ensures that at least one intermediary is distributing the product. When the consumer asks the pharmacy to fill the prescription, the consumer is again pulling the product through the supply chain because the pharmacy must order the pharmaceutical from the manufacturer to fill the prescription. At the same time, pharmaceutical companies offer samples and make sales calls to physicians to get them to push the product out to consumers.

For many provider organizations, holding or participating in health fairs is a form of sales promotion. Providers may offer diagnostic tests and distribute health education materials at these fairs, and the fairs give providers an opportunity to attain greater visibility and interact with patients who might not be familiar with them. Consumers who attend these health fairs, in turn, get the chance to enroll in local wellness programs, sign up for or obtain disease screening or tests on the spot, learn about medical risks and conditions, and (for those who test positive in screening tests) get a referral for diagnosis or treatment.

Exhibition at trade shows, professional meetings, and conferences is another form of sales promotion. These displays give organizations an opportunity to interact with hard-to-reach prospects, such as physicians and hospital administrators, who are often literally hidden behind their office doors. At exhibition halls, these consumers stroll straight up to the vendor's booth. The decision to exhibit and the type of display developed depend on the nature of the organization and its products as well as the characteristics of its target audience. In addition, an exhibit provides a unique avenue for conducting market research, as many of the best prospects are assembled in one location. Organizations that are not accustomed to or opt out of exhibiting may be missing out on this sales promotion format. Exhibit 9.3 lists ten tips for effective exhibit marketing.

Direct Marketing

Direct marketing involves an interactive system that uses one or more advertising media to effect a measurable response or transaction. Categories of direct marketing relevant to healthcare include direct mail, direct-response advertising, mail order, telemarketing, computerized marketing, and home shopping television.

Direct mail is a means of promotion whereby selected customers are sent advertising material addressed specifically to them. Direct mail traditionally has been distributed through the postal service, but more contemporary approaches may use e-mail transmission. Junk mail, e-mail spam, and unsolicited faxes are all products of direct-mail promotion.

Although many people find these types of solicitations annoying, they are considered effective marketing tools. Marketers like direct mail because it can target specific audiences and be personalized to the prospect's needs. Even if a campaign is able to achieve as little as a 2 percent response rate, marketers find direct mail to be reasonably cost-effective. Research has found that certain segments of the population are relatively responsive to mailed solicitations, and documents related to healthcare are less likely to be summarily discarded than others (Thomas 2008). Healthcare marketers find that direct mail works best when promoting an event, such as a patient education program or an open house. This approach probably does not work as well to stimulate action on an activity that does not have to be completed by a certain date (e.g., an elective procedure). Marketers of some elective procedures (e.g., laser eye surgery), however, have had reasonable success with direct mail. See Case Study 9.1 for an example of direct-to-consumer marketing.

EXHIBIT 9.3
Ten Tips for
Effective Exhibit
Marketing

Little guidance is available for healthcare organizations that want to be exhibitors at trade shows or professional meetings and conferences—perhaps because of the variations in marketing strategies and techniques used by different healthcare organizations. Nevertheless, general dos and don'ts are relevant to any organization that plans to exhibit. Here are ten of them.

1. Develop a Formal Exhibit Marketing Plan

Having both strategic exhibit marketing and tactical plans of action is a critical starting point. To make trade shows a powerful dimension of an organization's overall marketing operation, there must be alignment between the strategic marketing and the exhibit marketing plans. Trade shows should not be stand-alone ventures. Organizations should know and understand exactly what they wish to achieve at the show (e.g., shore up relationships with existing users, introduce new products/services to new markets).

2. Develop a Well-Defined Promotional Plan

An important component of exhibiting is promotion, including preshow, at-show, and post-show activities. Most exhibitors fail to develop a plan that encompasses all three areas. The organization's budget naturally plays a major role in deciding what and how much promotional activity is possible. Developing a meaningful theme or message that ties into the organization's strategic marketing plan helps guide promotional decisions. Exhibitors should know whom they want to target and develop different promotional programs customized for the different groups they want to attract. Target audiences can be reached through direct mail, advertising, public relations, sponsorships, social media, and the Internet.

3. Use Direct Mail Effectively

Direct mail is still one of the most popular promotional vehicles exhibitors use. From postcards to multipiece mailings, attendees are deluged with invitations to visit booths. Many of the mailings are based on lists of registrants, and as a result, everyone receives everything. To target the people they want to attract to their booth, exhibitors should use their own list of customers and prospects. Starting about four weeks before the show, exhibitors should mail materials to conference attendees at regular intervals. Distribution via first-class mail is recommended so that the mailing doesn't arrive after the show is over.

4. Give Prospects an Incentive to Visit the Booth

Regardless of the type of promotional vehicles used, exhibitors need to give visitors a reason to visit their booth. Limited by time constraints and distracted by a hall overflowing with fascinating products and services, people need an incentive to visit a particular booth. First and foremost, visitors are primarily interested in new offerings. They are eager to learn about the latest technologies, new applications, or anything that will help them save time or money. If an organization doesn't have a new product or service to introduce, it should put a new twist on one of its existing products or services.

5. Offer Giveaways That Work

Tied into giving visitors an incentive to visit the booth is an opportunity to offer a premium item that entices them. The giveaway item should be designed to make the exhibit more memorable and communicate, motivate, promote, or increase recognition of the company. Developing an effective giveaway takes thought and creativity. The company should consider items that (1) members of its target audience want, (2) help them do their jobs better, and (3) are not regularly available elsewhere. It should think about offering different gifts to different types of visitors. The company can use its website to tell visitors they can obtain important information, such as an executive report, if they visit the booth. Giveaways should be used as a reward or token of appreciation for visitors who participate in a demonstration, presentation, or contest or as a thank-you for providing information about their specific needs.

6. Use Press Relations Effectively

Public relations is one of the most cost-effective and successful methods for generating large volumes of direct inquiries and sales. Before the show, exhibitors should ask show management for a comprehensive media list to find out which publications are planning a special show edition. The company should send out newsworthy press releases focusing on what's new about its product or service or highlighting a new application or market venture. Press kits—including information about industry trends, statistics, new technology, or production—should be compiled for the press office. High-quality product photos and key company contacts should also be included in the kits.

(continued)

7. Differentiate Products or Services

Too many exhibitors are happy to use the "me too" marketing approach, and there is an underlying sameness about their marketing effort. In shows that attract hundreds of exhibitors, few stand out from the crowd. Because memorable exhibits are an integral part of a visitor's show experience, exhibitors should think about what makes their company different and why a prospect should buy its products or use its services. Every aspect of the exhibit marketing plan, including promotions, the booth, and the people working in the booth, should make an impact and generate curiosity.

8. Use the Booth as an Effective Marketing Tool

An organization's exhibit makes a strong statement about who it is, what it does, and how it does it. The purpose of an exhibit is to attract visitors so that the organization can achieve its marketing objectives. In addition to being an open, welcoming, friendly space, the exhibit needs to have a focal point and strongly communicate the benefit the exhibitor is offering to prospects. Displays that use large graphics are more effective than those that use reams of copy. Pictures paint a thousand words, and few attendees take the time to read lengthy copy. Presentations and demonstrations are critical parts of exhibit marketing. Exhibits should create an experience that gets visitors to use as many of their senses as possible.

9. Choose Exhibit Personnel Carefully

Exhibit personnel are a company's ambassadors, so they should be carefully selected. Before the show, they should be briefed on why the company is exhibiting, what it is exhibiting, and what it is expecting from them. Exhibit staff training is essential for a unified and professional image. The objectives of exhibit personnel should reflect the marketing plan, and staff should know how to close the interaction with a commitment to follow up. At the same time, the booth should not be crowded with company representatives, and specific tasks should be assigned to company personnel working the show.

10. Follow Up Promptly

The key to trade show success is effective lead management. The best time to plan for follow-up is before the show. Following up often takes second place to other management activities that occur after being out of the office for several days. The longer leads are left unattended, the colder and more mediocre they become. Exhibitors would be wise to develop an organized, systematic approach to follow-up. They should establish a lead-handling system, set timelines for follow-up, use a computerized database for lead tracking, make sales representatives accountable for leads assigned to them, and track the results of these efforts.

Source: Adapted from Friedmann (2009).

Direct-response advertising involves promotions via print or electronic media that provide an e-mail address or call-in number (typically a toll-free number) to potential customers. People who want to order a product or obtain more information are instructed to access the website or call the number. This approach has been used successfully in other industries and is now being used in healthcare. Physicians performing elective procedures, for example, may have an answering service to field such calls and provide information on laser eye surgery, hair transplants, weight-loss programs, or whatever service the practitioner is providing. Fitness equipment is also commonly promoted through television advertisements taking this approach.

Telemarketing is another form of direct marketing. Direct-response advertising is a form of telemarketing that involves inbound calls, but most people are more familiar with outbound telemarketing in which solicitors operating from a bank of telephone sets—often equipped with computer-assisted interviewing software—call people on a prospect list to offer a good or service. This technique, however, generated enough backlash among consumers that legislation was passed establishing a do-not-call list.

Telemarketing
Sales via telephone, through either outbound or inbound calls

Some telemarketing involves cold calls to individuals or households for which the demand for goods and services is unknown. More likely, the telephone numbers drawn from a sampling frame or randomly generated are keyed to certain characteristics of the target audience.

A more benign form of telemarketing in healthcare involves periodic contact with people who have expressed interest in a program or topic. Healthcare organizations assume that these people will be willing to receive calls describing such programs because of their implied previous interest and will not consider such calls an imposition. Hospital **call centers** frequently use this approach to follow up with existing customers or prospects.

Call center
A centralized communication hub established to capture incoming customer inquiries and generate outgoing marketing messages

Telemarketing is more expensive than direct-mail initiatives, but the costs are not unreasonable. Telemarketers' wages are relatively low, and the benefits gained by attracting a new patient are likely to be significant. Not all healthcare products lend themselves to this approach, but a surprising number do.

CASE STUDY 9.1

Using Direct-to-Consumer Advertising to Increase Drug Sales

After the Food and Drug Administration relaxed its rules on mass media advertising of prescription drugs, pharmaceutical companies began to engage in direct-to-consumer marketing. Rather than rely strictly on the prescription activities of physicians, the companies believed that direct appeals to consumers would increase overall pharmaceutical sales and at the same time convince consumers to request particular drugs.

To take advantage of this opportunity, GoodDrugs, Inc. shifted a portion of its advertising budget to direct-to-consumer marketing. This advertising was intended to supplement existing approaches—visits by sales representatives to physicians' offices, advertising in medical journals, and the presentation of educational seminars to physicians.

GoodDrugs planned and implemented a six-month television campaign to promote its best-selling (and most profitable) drug for indigestion. Because the drug was available only by prescription, the intent of the campaign was to raise awareness of the drug and get consumers to request their doctors to prescribe it.

At the end of the six-month campaign, GoodDrugs conducted a telephone survey of consumers in the media coverage area. The results were encouraging. Consumers had become aware of the drug: Half of the survey respondents remembered the advertisement associated with the drug, and a fourth of them recalled the drug's name. About 25 percent of those who had seen the advertisement said they had asked their doctor about using this drug for indigestion, and physicians wrote prescriptions for 71 percent of those who asked for one. Therefore, approximately 6 percent of the consumers who were exposed to the advertisement ended up with a prescription for the drug.

GoodDrugs marketers and sales executives were encouraged by the results of the television campaign. It had resulted in greater consumer awareness of their product, an increase in consumer preference for the drug, and an increase in desired physician prescribing behavior. As a result, GoodDrugs reworked its marketing budget, shifting resources away from personal sales and journal advertising and toward direct-to-consumer advertising.

Case Study Discussion Questions

1. What limitations were historically placed on pharmaceutical advertising, and what development encouraged drug companies to take more aggressive action?
2. What factors prompted pharmaceutical companies to shift some of their marketing efforts from physician-prescribers to consumers?
3. According to the GoodDrugs marketing team's evaluations, what were the results of the campaign?
4. What did the GoodDrugs marketers do as a result of this campaign?
5. How appropriate is it for pharmaceutical companies to market directly to consumers who may not be in a position to judge the merits of a particular drug?

Distribution of mail-order catalogs has been long used to reach consumers, but it has not been a traditional means of promoting healthcare goods and services. As the market for alternative therapies and do-it-yourself healthcare tests and treatments has grown, catalogs have become an important vehicle for promotion. In many parts of the country, if a consumer wants to purchase herbal supplements, natural remedies, or other unconventional treatments, mail order may be the only way to obtain some products. People are also turning to mail order catalogs and the Internet in search of better prices for prescription drugs. Although mail order catalogs are never going to become a mainstream promotional medium in healthcare, use of catalogs does have advantages. It puts product exposure directly in the hands of targeted consumers and can be relatively cost-effective because of economies of scale.

Venues for electronic marketing include the Internet and home shopping television channels. Home shopping channels capitalize on the fitness and wellness movement by selling elective goods such as fitness equipment, workout supplies, and skin treatments. Internet marketplaces, on the other hand, traffic in a variety of healthcare products, and aggressive e-mail and social media marketing carry messages about these products far and wide and quickly. Healthcare consumers frequently turn to the Internet as a first resort when locating and pricing consumer health goods. They also turn to the Internet for healthcare information, and the content posted online influences consumer decision making. Once considered a mechanism only for providing information about hospitals, health plans, pharmaceutical companies, and consumer products companies, the Internet has also become a medium for the aggressive marketing of a wide range of healthcare goods and services.

Exhibit 9.4 summarizes the role of various promotional techniques in healthcare marketing and the advantages and disadvantages to their use.

Media Options

Media plan
A document that outlines the objectives of a marketing campaign, its target audience, and the media intended to be used

Because advertisers and other promoters typically use various media as a means of communication, the media options available are an important consideration. For this discussion, the media are categorized into print media, electronic media, and display advertising. To capitalize on these media options, marketers should have a **media plan**.

Not only do marketers today have a wider variety of outlets for promotional activities, but they also have an abundance of publications (both print and virtual) in which they can advertise. In the 1950s, the advent of electronic media (TV and radio) introduced marketing efficiency by facilitating the information-dissemination process. In the 1980s, the emergence of cable television and satellite television allowed marketers access to almost unlimited transmission outlets. Now, the Internet links up billions of people worldwide, creating an enormous, 24/7 opportunity to interact with consumers. Marketers also have access to vast databases of information they can use to profile markets and target consumers.

Print Media

Print media
Any ink-on-paper medium used for promotional purposes

Print media is the most traditional vehicle for promoting organizations and products. Magazines, newspapers, journals, newsletters, and directories are common forms of print media. Although the "death" of print media has been widely reported, these reports are premature. Newspaper readership has indeed declined, but some demographic groups continue to be loyal print-media readers and magazine readership has remained steady.

Magazines—which are either popular aimed at the general public (e.g., *Self, Men's Health*) or trade aimed at professionals in a particular field (e.g., *Modern Healthcare, Healthcare Executive, Scrubs*)—offer many advantages to advertisers. First, they allow color production and ample space for images and words, and marketers can use the magazine's national readership data to target subscribers. Second, they have high potential readership, and readers expect them to include advertisements. Third, they have relatively long "shelf life" and can be read at the subscriber's leisure. Fourth, advertising in magazines can be cost-effective, depending on the audience. On the other hand, there are disadvantages to the use of magazines for promotion. Advertisements may appear in a magazine's "desert areas"—the spaces seldom noticed by readers or are lost in the surrounding clutter of a page. Monthly distribution is also problematic if marketers want to promote more

EXHIBIT 9.4
Matrix for
Promotional
Decision
Making

Promotional Technique	Uses	Audience	Time Frame	Relative Cost	Advantages	Disadvantages
Public relations	Awareness Visibility Service rollout	General public Stakeholders Decision makers Influentials	Short term within a longer-term strategic context	Primarily staff time with low out-of-pocket costs	Broad reach Low cost Short lead time	Not targeted Short shelf life
Communication	Awareness Visibility Education Relationship development/maintenance	General public Stakeholders Existing customers Employees	Ongoing with periodic flurry of activity	Primarily staff time with moderate out-of-pocket costs	Direct to target Low cost	Narrow focus Staffing costs
Community outreach	Awareness Visibility Education Relationship development/maintenance	General public Targeted consumer groups	Ongoing with periodic flurry of activity	Primarily staff time with moderate out-of-pocket costs	Ongoing presence Personalized Localized	High effort Long lead time
Networking	Awareness Business development Relationship development/maintenance Intelligence gathering	Key stakeholders Potential partners Potential referrers	Ongoing	Little additional cost	Ongoing Targeted	Time commitment
Direct marketing	Exposure Product introduction Call to action	Targeted consumer groups	Short term but with some lead time	Moderate costs	Focused Customized Multiple exposures	Low response rate High unit cost Short shelf life
Personal sales	Visibility Close contacts Relationship development	Influentials Potential customers	Regular periodic contact	Moderate to high costs	Face to face Ongoing Feedback on market	Sales force maintenance Cost
Advertising	Awareness Visibility Image enhancement	General public Targeted customer groups	Typically long term with long lead time	High costs	Many options Design options Easily targeted	Cost Negative connotation Short shelf life

Source: Thomas and Calhoun (2007).

frequently or have time-sensitive offerings. "Shoppers' magazines"—distributed to local consumers at no cost—are available in many communities and provide opportunities for promotions. Ad placement in these magazines is relatively inexpensive but may not be effective because these publications are considered "throwaways."

Newspapers come out either daily or weekly and have a national, regional, or local distribution. The advantages of newspaper advertising include extensive market coverage, timing flexibility, and the ability to use illustrations. On the other hand, newspaper advertising is a mass marketing approach that attempts to reach all audiences and does not differentiate among groups of readers; that makes it difficult for the advertising content to attract attention. In recent years, newspapers have suffered a declining readership, retaining the loyalty of few demographic groups. Depending on the market, newspaper advertising can be relatively expensive, so marketers need to ensure that the objectives of the marketing plan lend themselves to this medium. Alternative newspapers are usually weeklies that cover aspects of the news neglected by the mainstream press. In some communities, the readers make alternative newspapers appropriate vehicles for promoting healthcare products. These readers may support progressive causes or use alternative and innovative goods and services, such as holistic medicine or therapies. Special-interest newspapers devoted to health and wellness have also emerged, and some regular newspapers chronicle developments in the local healthcare arena and reserve sections for topics such as fitness and wellness and alternative medicine. These newspapers are advertising venues for many healthcare goods and services.

Journals are possibly more ubiquitous in healthcare than in any other industry. Every medical specialty and all allied health fields generate one or more journals, and most associations for health professionals publish at least one journal for their members (e.g., *Journal of Healthcare Management*, *Physician Executive Journal*). Some journals are highly specialized and do not carry advertisements, but others are mainstream—though still academic—and do feature ads (e.g., *Journal of the American Medical Association*, *New England Journal of Medicine*). Industry journals are effective vehicles for advertising because their audiences are targeted and effectively prescreened. Pharmaceutical companies are heavy advertisers in these publications, as are medical supply, equipment, and information technology vendors.

Change occurs rapidly in healthcare, and the lead time required to produce publications such as magazines and journals does not accommodate last-minute revisions or additions to advertising content. Newsletters, therefore, have become an alternative but equally valuable vehicle for publicizing new programs, services, or organizational changes. Although advertisements are rare in printed newsletters, e-newsletters (electronic or online) often accept product notices and promotional postings.

Directories have become an increasingly important means of gaining visibility. Some directories, such as state physician directories or hospital directories, are compiled for bureaucratic recordkeeping purposes. Such directories are generally not intended for commercial use, and an organization's inclusion may or may not be mandatory. Some directories are compiled for administrative purposes but subsequently shared with a larger audience (e.g., a health plan's provider directory). Another category of directories includes those commercially produced for distribution. One function of these directories is to make their listed organizations more visible, and organizations may have to pay a fee to be listed. These directories are typically sold to customers who need the information. There are directories of physicians, hospitals, information technology vendors, and so forth. A number of publishers compile and distribute directories as their primary business activity, and many such directories are posted on the Internet. Consumer-oriented print directories are being replaced with online directories. An online listing represents a form of advertising, but these web-based directories also post promotional content. For example, the website of a nursing home directory may feature ads by nursing facilities, home health agencies, pharmaceutical companies, and insurance plans.

Exhibit 9.5 compares the costs of various promotional vehicles, including print and electronic media.

Electronic Media

Electronic media include television, radio, the Internet, and cinema; each can be used for promotional purposes.

Television is the prototypical marketing medium. With television, a healthcare organization can build a high level of awareness of its offerings, reach large audiences, and demonstrate its products (using sound and visuals). In addition, television is accessible to almost everyone and 24-hour programming has become the norm, which have made advertisements highly visible. Promotion via television has its downsides, however. First, viewers may find commercial breaks irritating. Second, the medium is considered transient with a limited shelf life. Third, the ability to target specific audiences is limited. Fourth, television advertising is expensive, particularly given its unpredictable outcomes.

Historically, television advertising was concentrated on the national networks (ABC, NBC, CBS, and FOX). However, this has changed with the advent of cable television and satellite broadcasting. These channels and their programs developed their own following, which became conceptualized as market segments. Marketers learned the demographic traits of these segments on the basis of their viewing preferences. This development has enabled marketers to target television audiences much more precisely. For example, viewers of travel and food channels tend to be college educated (or higher), to have creative or academic careers or white-collar jobs, to have more disposable income, to live in cities, and so forth. Marketers seeking to target this segment would run a commercial on these travel and food channels. Advertising time is much less expensive on cable than on network television (see Exhibit 9.5).

Radio is often considered by listeners as a companion (as it is often turned on when one is driving or doing tasks around the house). The most important attribute of radio advertising is that it can precisely target an audience by playing at a specific time of day and on a specific station. Further, radio advertising time and production costs are relatively low, especially

EXHIBIT 9.5
Comparative
Promotional
Costs

Medium/Vehicle	Promotion Type	Cost
Billboard	Artwork	$3,000
	Installation	$5,000–$500,000, with a minimum 16-week contract
Cable TV	30-second commercial, prime time	$5,000–$8,000
Local network TV	30-second commercial, off–peak time	$100
	30-second commercial, prime time	$200,000
Direct mail	4" x 6" postcards, including postage	$1,000–$1,500
Internet ad	Pay per click	$0.60 cents; $1,200–$1,000 per month for an aggressive campaign
	Banner ad	$200–$1,200 per year
	Search engine optimization	$15,000+
Magazine	Ad	$1,200–$5,000 per month or per issue, depending on ad size and readership demographics
Newspaper	2" x 2" ad	$1,300 per week
Radio	60-second commercial on a rotator (with higher prices of time slots are selective)	$100–$1,000

Note: Costs vary from market to market. These figures should be used only for comparative purposes and should not be considered absolute rates.
Sources: Black Swamp Media Group (blackswampgraphics.com); Inland Empire Small Business Development Center (www.iesmallbusiness.com); Pole Positioning Web Marketing (www.polepositioning.com); Thomas (2008).

Infomercial
An in-depth advertisement that mimics the look and feel of a daytime talk show, news report, documentary, demonstration, or other presentation format

compared to TV commercials. However, radio has no visual attribute and is a transient medium. If the listener misses the commercial, he or she may not catch it again. In addition, the growth in number of radio stations has caused radio audiences to become fragmented and reduce in size.

One trend that electronic media had spawned is the **infomercial**, a portmanteau of information and commercial. Infomercials are advertisements that vary in length—from 30 seconds to one hour—and air on television or radio. They give a good or a service in-depth treatment, educating viewers on its features and benefits and presenting testimonies from fans, success stories, and corroborative data—all often in a casual, entertaining, upbeat, and easy-to-understand manner. Their format varies widely, ranging from daytime talk shows to news reports to documentaries and demonstrations. Whatever the format, infomercials focus on the product, not the advertiser (which is recognized but not directly discussed). Their intent is to soft-sell the good or service by implying that the advertiser (provider, supplier, or manufacturer) is the authority on the topic, thus attracting customers without having to overtly solicit them. "As seen on TV" infomercials are common examples, and a quick Google or YouTube search yields more examples (from both TV and radio) that feature consumer health products and provider organizations.

As mentioned in earlier chapters, most healthcare organizations—particularly those involved in direct patient care—were slow to warm up to Internet advertising, such as **banner ads** and popup ads. Consumer health products companies, on the other hand, were quick to take advantage of web-based or Internet marketing. Today, many healthcare marketers have a web presence, using not only banner and popup ads but also online directories, social media (see Chapter 11), mobile apps, and search engine optimization, among many other technology-enabled tactics.

Banner ad
A small, rectangular promotional graphic that appears in printed material or on a website

Goods and services are used in film sets or appear on screen as props or background scenery; this is why cinema has long been part of the electronic medium of advertising. Cinema advertising is not commonly used for healthcare products—at least not yet. However, as healthcare becomes even more consumer driven, as healthcare becomes a priority for the government and the public (as shown by the passage of the Affordable Care Act [ACA]), and as in-theater advertising spots become more common, healthcare marketers will most likely enter the cinema arena.

Display Advertising

Display advertising is a media form that includes outdoor advertising, transportation advertising, and posters. Outdoor advertising primarily involves billboards, although other types of signage (e.g., banners, portable signs) are also used. While billboard advertising has its critics, it is popular with hospitals, health plans, voluntary associations, and other healthcare organizations. Transportation (or transit) advertising consists of graphics, signs, or plaques placed on buses, taxis, and other commercial vehicles. Posters are bills displayed in public places to attract attention to an organization, a service, or an event.

Using display advertising, marketers can reach large numbers of people and build a high level of awareness of a product or an organization at a relatively low cost. Display advertising can be short or long term, can support local or national marketing campaigns, and can be strategically located. On the downside, display advertising is often subject to the effects of weather and criticized for despoiling natural settings.

Exhibit 9.6 compares the advantages and disadvantages of various print, electronic, and display media options.

Social Marketing

Social marketing can be defined as the application of commercial marketing techniques to the development and implementation of programs that influence the attitudes, knowledge, and behavior of target audiences for purposes of improving individual and community health status. It is used most often by not-for-profit healthcare organizations and government agencies seeking to change consumer behavior. It is considered social in the sense that the organizations involved typically do not engage in these efforts for their own benefit but for the benefit of the general public or some subgroup of the public.

A key difference between social marketing and direct marketing is the former's target audience and goals. Social marketing has a **population health** orientation and thus aims to affect the knowledge, attitudes, and behavior of large segments of the population rather than one consumer at a time. In contrast to the top-down approach of traditional marketing, social marketing uses a bottom-up approach, listening to the needs and desires of the target audience and building the marketing campaign on that basis. This focus on the consumer requires the use of **in-depth interviews** and constant reevaluation of the message. Social marketers research their target audience and then segment it into groups on the basis of common risk behaviors, motivations, and information channel preferences. The marketing mix is continually refined on the basis of consumer feedback. Instead of a sales pitch, the target audience might be exposed to an intervention (e.g., educational program, health screening initiative) aimed at changing attitudes or encouraging healthy behavior.

Social marketing takes advantage of various types of media to target audiences, tailor messages, and engage people for purposes of increasing knowledge, influencing attitudes, and changing behaviors. As population-based approaches have become more common (and now the focus of the ACA), the role of health communication has expanded. Community-centered prevention shifts attention from the individual to the group and emphasizes the empowerment of individuals and communities to effect change on multiple levels.

Population health
An approach to affecting the health status and health behavior of groups rather than individuals

In-depth interview
A data collection technique whereby the interviewer asks probing questions to elicit detailed information from the interviewee

EXHIBIT 9.6
Matrix for
Media Decision
Making

Medium	Uses	Audience	Resource Requirements	Relative Cost	Advantages	Disadvantages
Television	Exposure Service introduction Call to action		Production skills Creative skills	High	Consumer appeal Multiple exposures	Cost Negative connotation Short shelf life Competing ads
Network		General public			Broad reach	Diffuse impact
Cable		Targeted consumers			Targeted reach	Narrow impact
Radio	Exposure Service introduction Call to action	General public Targeted consumers	Production skills Creative skills	Moderate	Broad or narrow reach	Cost Short shelf life
Newspapers	Exposure Service introduction Call to action	General public		Moderate	Broad reach Low unit cost Frequent exposure	Cost Competing ads Short shelf life
Magazines	Exposure Service introduction Call to action	General public (but higher end)		Moderate	Moderate shelf life Design options	Cost Competing ads
Internet		General public Targeted consumers		Low	Appealing medium Interactive Ongoing	Incomplete coverage Spam annoyance
Display advertising	Public notice of products	General public	Limited production skills	Low to Moderate	Mass exposure	Untargeted/ downscale perception

The functions of social marketing in healthcare include the following:

- Increase knowledge and awareness of a health issue, problem, or solution
- Influence perceptions, beliefs, attitudes, and social norms
- Prompt a desired response
- Demonstrate or illustrate health-enhancing skills
- Show the benefits of behavior change
- Increase demand for health services
- Reinforce knowledge, attitudes, and behaviors
- Refute myths and misconceptions
- Coalesce organizational relationships
- Advocate for a health issue or a population group

Exhibit 9.7 describes the steps involved in developing a social marketing campaign. The steps in carrying out a social marketing program are illustrated in Case Study 9.2.

EXHIBIT 9.7
Ten Steps for
Developing
a Social
Marketing
Campaign

Most successful social marketing campaigns can be broken down into these 10 steps:

- *Step 1: Define Your Audience.* Be specific and learn as much as possible about the target audience. One way to define the target audience is to describe their demographics (i.e., heterosexual males between the ages of 14 and 18 who smoke). In addition, paint a vivid picture of the individuals *within* the group; understand their attitudes, feelings, beliefs, values, motivation, and culture—all the factors that might influence their behavior.

- *Step 2: Identify Evaluation Measures.* Evaluation is a big part of all prevention efforts: This is no exception. Evaluate whether the campaign was implemented as intended and if the specific goals were met. Start developing the evaluation strategy early in the planning process. Think carefully about the evaluation questions, the best ways to collect the necessary information, and the type of people to bring on board to help in the process.

  Establishing a direct correlation between the campaign and any observed outcomes may be difficult because a communications campaign does not exist in a vacuum. However, it's possible to evaluate broader, population-level changes in behavior and compare them to a baseline before the marketing campaign began. For example, Massachusetts is currently conducting a large-scale, multi-million dollar anti-smoking campaign, funded solely by a tax on tobacco products. To assess change, [the state] measures the difference in the number of cigarette packs sold before and since the campaign began.

- *Step 3: Identify Channels.* It's important to think about how to communicate the intended message. One option is to deliver the message *directly* to the target audience. Common marketing channels include television or radio commercials, interviews, and public service announcements. They include newspaper or magazine articles, editorials, and print ads; billboards; and banners across main streets. In addition, Websites; electronic mailing lists; bulk mailings; and special events, contests, and awards can also be used. In selecting appropriate dissemination channels, consider the costs involved. Think about where the target audience gets its information, and which channels they consider most credible. Also, keep in mind that the most effective campaigns combine mass media with other efforts, such as community events and small-group discussions.

Another option is to deliver the message *indirectly,* through intermediaries associated with the target audience. Intermediaries include people who work with these groups, such as coaches, teachers, and counselors; or other people who are respected, such as athletes, clergy, and community and political leaders. Intermediaries can also be credible organizations, such as citizens' advocacy groups and local agencies.

- *Step 4: Identify Benefits.* The exchange principle asserts that in order for people to voluntarily give something up or try something new, they must benefit in some way. Ask the following question: Why would the target audience want to adopt the behavior promoted in the campaign? Think about this question from the audience's perspective. For example, to convince people over 50 to start exercising, highlight benefits such as increased energy and protection against osteoporosis. But to convince young adults to exercise, "sell" the idea that going to the gym is a great way to get in shape and increase your sex appeal.

  It is also important to differentiate between long- and short-term benefits. People tend to gravitate toward short-term benefits: They're more immediate and enticing. Therefore, in the example above, increased energy—a short-term benefit—may be a far more compelling reason for people to exercise than developing stronger bones. However, only solid research will tell for sure.

- *Step 5: Identify Obstacles.* To achieve an exchange, it is also important to identify any *obstacles* that might prevent members of the target audience from adopting a given behavior. For example, when promoting treatment for alcohol and drug problems, find out whether treatment slots are, in fact available; whether members of the target audience have insurance coverage; and if the programs can be reached using public transportation. Another example is encouraging a group of adults to quit smoking. The sheer power of nicotine addiction, plus the strength of the habit of smoking, are both big obstacles that prevent many people from quitting. The prevention message must thus be compelling, and salient enough to overcome these barriers. In order for the "exchange" to work, the benefit of adopting (or giving up) a behavior must be greater than the cost.

- *Step 6: Determine the Message.* This is a critical step. When creating a message, be very clear about the behavior you want to

(continued)

elicit. Do you want the audience to make a telephone call? Send for information? Stop doing something—like smoking—or start doing something—like talking to their children about drugs? People who see or hear the message must be clear about what is expected of them.

Next, create a message that builds on what has been learned about the audience: their existing knowledge, concerns, and interests. Try to emphasize positive behavior change rather than negative consequences. For example, the message "Use a designated driver" offers people concrete information for how to get home safely, whereas "Don't Drink and Drive" simply tells people what not to do.

Finally, determine the tone and the style of the message. Tone is an elusive quality but is very important in a social marketing campaign. Determine if the message is intended to be informative? Emotional? Humorous? A combination of the above?

Remember: all the "pieces" of the message—headlines, illustrations, and copy—should work together to immediately establish what is being offered, what the benefits are, and who is advertising it. People should know at a glance what the message is about.

- *Step 7: Test and Refine.* It's very important to "pre-test" the message. The best way to do this is to test the message on focus groups that represent the target audience. Present them with several message samples and record their impressions and reactions. Then use their feedback to refine the message. Test the message for comprehension, attention and recall, strong and weak points, personal relevance to the target audience, and sensitivity to cultural and/or audience-specific characteristics.

- *Step 8: Collect Data.* Collect data to determine whether the message is having an impact. Data collection might involve conducting more focus groups, administering surveys, or doing telephone interviews. Data collection methods should be dictated not only by cost, but also by the questions you want answered and the kind of information you want to collect. Whenever possible, work with an evaluator to design and implement your data collection efforts.

- *Step 9: Modify Your Work, Based on the Data.* Even the best-researched campaign often needs some tweaking once it has been launched. Use the data collected to refine and adjust the message, communication channels, and promotion strategies. If something isn't working, a small alteration is often enough to improve it significantly. If unsure, go back to the target audience and ask them what they think.

- *Step 10: Write an Evaluation Report.* This is often required by the funder. Yet, even when it is not, creating a report is a helpful way to organize the information collected so that it can be shared with others and garner support for future efforts. In the report, present the intended, campaign accomplishments, broad lessons learned, and remaining tasks or recommendations for follow-up. Try to be concise, avoid jargon, and present a balanced set of findings.

When moving through each of these steps, always keep a clear picture of the target audience. The most valuable asset is knowledge of the audience. Don't ever underestimate just how critically important that knowledge is to the success of any social marketing campaign.

Source: Reprinted from Substance Abuse and Mental Health Services Administration (2013).

Integrated Marketing

Given the number of available marketing techniques and the fragmentation of media vehicles, determining the most appropriate tactic for a particular situation is a challenge. One approach that may help tie some of the parts together is integrated marketing. **Integrated marketing** (or integrated marketing communication) emphasizes a consistent overarching approach to the organization's promotional strategy. Its ultimate aim is to achieve synergy between the component parts of the strategy to make the entire effort more effective.

Marketers coordinate advertising campaigns across various media, supplementing television advertisements with marketing messages communicated via other media vehicles, such as print. For example, a print advertisement might capture a frame from a television commercial and include a tagline that summarizes the 15- or 30-second message, or a radio station may air an excerpt from the dialogue and the announcer's product claims from that same commercial. Integrated marketing involves the strategic choice of elements of marketing communication that effectively and economically influence transactions between an organization and its existing and potential customers or clients. This approach ensures that all elements are delivered synergistically.

Integrated marketing
A marketing approach that emphasizes consistency in the promotional strategy to achieve synergy between its component parts

CASE STUDY 9.2
The Texas WIC Program

In the mid-1990s, a social marketing program was implemented to increase enrollment and improve customer and employee satisfaction with the Special Supplemental Nutrition Program for Women, Infants, and Children (WIC) in Texas. (Although this case is 20 years old, the approach used here is relevant in today's environment.)

Participant observation, in-depth interviews, **telephone interviews**, focus groups, and surveys were used to identify the needs, preferences, and characteristics of four target audiences: (1) families eligible but not participating in the program, (2) program participants, (3) program employees, and (4) professionals who refer people to the program.

The results of this research were used to develop a comprehensive social marketing plan that included policy changes, service delivery improvements, staff and vendor training, internal promotion, public information and communications, client education, and community-based interventions. This plan was designed to change families' perceptions of WIC as a welfare program that provided free food to poor people by emphasizing nutrition education, health checkups, immunizations, and referrals. It included recommendations for lowering costs by repositioning the program as a temporary assistance nutrition and health program—"WIC—Helping Families Help Themselves"—in which families can maintain their pride and self-esteem as they earn their WIC benefits and learn about nutrition and other ways to help their families.

Because many women did not know they were eligible for the program and/or had trouble enrolling, the marketing plan also emphasized ways to help families understand eligibility guidelines, to streamline the certification process, and to make it easier for health and social service professionals to refer eligible women. Placement strategies recommended locating WIC clinics outside of government assistance venues, and professional training programs were developed to enhance employees' skills in dealing with customers and teach grocery store cashiers to process WIC purchases more efficiently and respectfully. Promotional efforts included a community outreach kit to reach referral sources as well as the use of mass media to reach eligible families.

The Texas WIC Program was launched in the fall of 1995. Program data were used to monitor the number of families who called the toll-free number for more information after the program was launched and, more importantly, the number of people participating in Texas WIC.

Telephone interview
A data collection technique whereby a survey instrument is administered by an interviewer to a respondent over the telephone

When results showed that increases in program enrollment were not sustained, mid-course revisions were made to improve program delivery. The program's caseload then grew from its baseline level of 582,819 in October 1993 to 778,558 in October 1998—an increase of almost 200,000 participants.

Source: Grier and Bryant (2005).

Case Study Discussion Questions

1. Why did the operators of the WIC program feel it was necessary to obtain information concerning consumers who used and did not use its services?
2. What methods were applied to develop a profile of users and non-users?
3. In what way did they position the program to make it more appealing to eligible beneficiaries?
4. How was the repackaged program promoted to the public?

Many factors have encouraged the use of integrated marketing. Tighter marketing budgets have squeezed available resources, and the fragmentation of the media has demanded some unifying force. The shift from mass marketing to target marketing and the rise of electronic media (especially the Internet and social media) have contributed to this development. Although integrated marketing appears to be an obvious step toward more effective marketing, it is inconsistent with traditional patterns of marketing behavior and is cumbersome to implement in some organizations.

If resistance can be overcome, however, an organization can derive major advantages from the marketing integration process. Its strategies will reinforce each other; its messages will be consistent and their delivery synergized; cost savings will ensue; and it will sustain a competitive advantage. See Case Study 9.3 for a description of an integrated marketing strategy.

Summary

A variety of established marketing techniques are available to the healthcare industry. All of these approaches are commonly used in other industries and have been adopted in varying degrees by healthcare organizations. Traditional approaches to reaching the organization's constituents include PR

CASE STUDY 9.3
Integrated Marketing Strategy

Many people who might benefit from hearing aids do not wear them. Further, those who might benefit from surgical treatment are even more unlikely to present for treatment. Among adults aged 18 years or older with impaired hearing, 78 percent do not own a hearing aid. As the US population ages, the need for hearing assistance will become nearly universal—but even today among the hearing impaired who are aged 65 years or older, 61 percent do not wear hearing aids. Research has found that although people would readily acquiesce to wearing eyeglasses to correct their vision, would have no problem taking pain relievers to alleviate aches, and would not mind having to walk with a cane, the prospect of having to wear a hearing aid would be difficult for them to accept.

The hearing and speech communications literature suggests that use of a hearing aid carries a stigma that implies the wearer is old, feeble, and incompetent. An article in the American Psychological Association's *Monitor on Psychology* described the denial and depression people associate with hearing loss. In addition, hearing loss, if not addressed with hearing aids, can lead to greater dependence on a spouse and withdrawal from social events. People do not want to admit their hearing loss to themselves because it connotes aging; nor do they want to admit it to others for fear of being viewed as incompetent.

Given all these considerations, when *Business Week* featured a hearing aid manufacturer in its Annual Design Awards, the product receiving acclaim was tiny and said to "nestle discreetly in the ear canal." Hearing aid sales surged when a prominent person publicly acknowledged that he had begun to wear one, likely because hearing aids were then perceived as more acceptable when associated with a popular and purportedly virile individual rather than one who was old and feeble.

A product with such a negative image as hearing aids clearly presents a challenge for marketers interested in stimulating sales. Research conducted to determine how to induce more favorable attitudes toward these personal, stigmatized products assessed the applicability and effectiveness of integrated marketing communication in the promotion of hearing aids. In addition, the research looked at whether a stigmatized product might best be approached through multimodality approaches, thereby reinforcing the advertising message.

A panel of respondents was established as a **test market**. The researchers contacted 4,344 participants at time 1, before being exposed to the aforementioned marketing communications. The attitudes of 3,351 participants were then measured at time 2, after being exposed to the combination of synchronized materials. Finally, the attitudes of 3,049 respondents were remeasured three months after being exposed to the marketing materials, at time 3.

Three advertising themes were tested in this study: warm and emotional, educational, and wedge of doubt. The warm and emotional print advertisement began with the question "Honey, can you pick up some nails?" A response of "Sure" was printed in the middle of the page, with a photograph of a can of escargot. The tagline printed at the bottom of the page inquired, "Is it any wonder hearing loss can frustrate those around you? Have your hearing checked. For you. For them."

The copy in the educational message stated, "Use your head once a year" and was placed above a photograph of headphones. The advertisement's closing copy read: "Annual hearing checkups help you spot changes in your hearing. Hear today. Hear tomorrow."

The wedge-of-doubt advertisement began with copy that warned: "If you think it's difficult admitting your hearing problem, imagine admitting all the mistakes you've made because of it." At the bottom, the advertisement read: "When you can't hear clearly, it's easy to misunderstand someone. And before you know it, people start thinking you've lost your mental edge."

Once these messages had been tested with various audiences, they were adapted for delivery via other media vehicles: mass media (including print and television ads) and private media customized to appeal to targeted individuals (including telemarketing phone calls and direct marketing mailings).

The analysis showed that consistent combinations of media (both mass or both private) were more effective than mixed media; the two private media (telemarketing combined with direct marketing) outperformed any two mixed media (telemarketing and print, telemarketing and television, direct marketing and print, or direct marketing and television). In addition, the private media combination outperformed the public media combination. Learning more about the product in a private setting appeared to increase acceptance.

Finally, the content of the message affected the impact of the particular class of media (mass or private). The integrated private media

(continued)

Test market
A group or population on which a marketing theme or concept is tested

(telemarketing and direct marketing) performed best, first with the wedge-of-doubt content and then with the warm and emotional content. The combination of two private exposures did not perform well in all cases—the combination with the educational advertising message was not effective. The wedge-of-doubt content, which worked best when delivered via the two private media, did not perform well in all cases, either; it performed the worst when delivered via a mass medium.

Marketing health services can be complicated. As this investigation demonstrates, rarely can a marketer choose a medium or an advertising message without considering the big picture. Media cannot be simply pasted together to achieve some seemingly critical threshold of ad weight; many mixed media can perform worse than fewer exposures of sensibly integrated media. Similarly, the choice of media outlets depends on both the product and the content of the ads. A well-thought-out combination of media and messages appears to have greater influence on consumers than a haphazard collection of media and messages.

Source: Adapted from Iacobucci and colleagues (2002).

Case Study Discussion Questions

1. What challenges are faced by those trying to promote hearing aids to the consumer market?
2. How do marketers test the effectiveness of a promotional message?
3. What type of message appeared to resonate most with consumers and why?
4. Did mass media or private media fare better in terms of promotional results?
5. What characteristics of integrated marketing contributed to the success of this campaign?

(e.g., publicity, communications, government relations), advertising, personal sales, and sales promotion. Direct marketing is a recent addition to the healthcare marketer's arsenal of techniques.

The technique of choice depends on the type of organization involved and the product being marketed, among other factors. Of special importance is the objective of the promotional initiative. Objectives vary with the situation; different aims (e.g., raise visibility, retain existing customers, change consumer attitudes, increase market share) call for different marketing techniques. A common theme among all promotional objectives, however, is effective communication.

Likewise, different circumstances call for different types of media. Marketers have the option of using print media (e.g., magazines, newspapers), electronic media (e.g., radio, television, Internet), and display media. There are advantages and disadvantages to the use of each type. Display media, such as billboards, are not as applicable to healthcare as most other promotional techniques but are nevertheless employed by various healthcare organizations.

Healthcare organizations are increasingly recognizing the importance of integrated marketing. This systematic approach to promoting an idea, an organization, or a product instills consistency in the marketing initiative and facilitates the coordination of a potentially broad range of promotional activities.

Key Points

- Healthcare marketers have access to a variety of promotional techniques that have been used historically in other industries, although some have to be modified for use in healthcare.
- Long before most healthcare organizations embarked on formal marketing initiatives, they relied on various forms of publicity for promotional purposes.
- Promotional activities that are not always recognized by health professionals as marketing include community outreach, networking, and government relations.
- Advertising has probably been the most visible form of marketing by healthcare organizations, although arguably not the most important.
- Although some health professionals have a negative view of advertising, it can serve a number of positive functions.
- As healthcare organizations became more involved in ancillary endeavors (e.g., fitness centers) and business-to-business marketing, personal sales became more important.
- Sales promotion is not typically associated with the marketing of healthcare services but is commonly used to promote consumer health products.
- As the consumer has become more important in healthcare, use of direct-to-consumer marketing has become more common.
- Direct mail and telemarketing are often employed to deliver the message directly to the consumer.

- Available print media include newspapers, magazines, journals, and other publications.
- Available electronic media include radio, television (network and cable), and the Internet.
- Available display advertising include posters, billboards, and other outdoor media.
- The promotional technique and medium a marketer chooses to use depend on the type of organization, type of product, and characteristics of the target audience.
- Integrated marketing involves the coordination of all promotional activities to communicate a consistent and uniform marketing message.

Discussion Questions

1. What role does the nature of the product play in determining the promotional vehicle to be used?
2. How important is the culture of the community when choosing a promotional technique?
3. Why is PR often a preferred form of promotion for healthcare organizations?
4. Can it be argued that a major function of promotional activities in healthcare is educating the healthcare consumer?
5. Why do many health professionals and even members of the general public resist the idea of using advertising to promote health services?
6. What steps are involved in the personal sales process, and under what circumstances is personal sales the most effective promotional technique?
7. What is the difference between a push and a pull approach in the context of sales promotion?
8. What developments in healthcare have encouraged the use of direct marketing?
9. What are the pros and cons to using different print media?
10. What are the advantages and disadvantages of using electronic media as opposed to print media?
11. What factors are encouraging the growing emphasis on integrated marketing among healthcare organizations?

Additional Resources

Advertising Age: http://adage.com

American Marketing Association: www.ama.org

HowStuffWorks.com. 2013. "How Do Television Ratings Work? How Do They Figure Out How Many People Are Watching a Show?" http://electronics.how stuffworks.com/question433.htm.

Kotler, P., and G. Armstrong. 2013. *Principles of Marketing,* 15th ed. Upper Saddle River, NJ: Prentice Hall.

Society for Healthcare Strategy & Market Development: www.shsmd.org

CONTEMPORARY MARKETING TECHNIQUES

The changes that the field of marketing experienced during its evolution eventually filtered down to healthcare. By the 1990s, healthcare marketing had adopted techniques from other industries and developed new healthcare-specific approaches. These program-based and technology-based techniques enable healthcare marketers to take advantage of contemporary technology. Despite their seemingly impersonal technical basis, these approaches focus on customer relationship development and management, not just the sale of goods and services.

The healthcare industry has not been a leader in the development of marketing techniques, and trends outside the field have ultimately influenced the form healthcare marketing has taken. Observers such as Scott (2009) contend that marketing has undergone a revolution so significant that marketers (inside and outside of healthcare) would do well to forget much of what they know about traditional marketing. The emergence of electronic modes of communication has led to a new paradigm, which makes traditional marketing techniques—at least as employed in the past—obsolete or, at best, woefully outdated. As Scott indicates in his book *The New Rules of Marketing and PR*, marketing is no longer about selling but about disseminating information; one-way "interruptive" marketing is no longer effective or even acceptable. Traditional media no longer control the playing field when almost anyone can become a new-media expert armed with what is essentially a free means of information distribution. In today's environment, content trumps style and information sharing replaces information hoarding.

The New Approaches

Since the 1990s, healthcare has experienced a number of trends related to marketing, including a shift in emphasis from image marketing to service marketing, from mass marketing to target marketing, from a one-size-fits-all philosophy to personalization and customization, and from a focus on a single healthcare episode to long-term relationships. These developments in healthcare, as in other industries, have benefited from the application of contemporary technology.

The marketing techniques that have gained momentum in healthcare can be divided into (1) techniques that involve programmatic changes that support marketing and (2) techniques that capitalize on information management. The former implies an innovative approach at a conceptual level and the latter a technology-based approach that may be applied to traditional or innovative marketing techniques.

One factor common to both types of techniques is the emphasis on *relationship management*. Relationship management is the process of getting closer to the customer by developing a long-term relationship through careful attention to service needs and high-quality care. It succeeds by keeping existing customers happy, ensuring repeat business, and recognizing the revenue potential of long-term relationships. The attributes of relationship management include the following:

- Focus on customer retention
- Orientation toward product benefits rather than product features
- Long-term view of customer relationships
- Development of ongoing relationships
- Multiple employee/customer contacts
- Emphasis on key account relationship management
- Emphasis on trust

All of the techniques discussed in this section incorporate at least some of these attributes.

Program-Based Techniques

Marketing techniques that are program-based require a rethinking of the programs offered by the organization in the context of the new marketing reality. These techniques include direct-to-consumer marketing, business-to-business marketing, internal marketing, and concierge services.

Direct-to-Consumer Marketing

As mentioned in Chapter 1, the customer—the ultimate end user of healthcare products—was initially written off as a marketing target. The physician made most of the medical decisions for the patient, and the health plan controlled its enrollee's choice of provider and the services obtained from that provider. Choice of drug typically depended on the physician's prescription, and the supply channels for medical goods and services generally focused on intermediaries rather than the end user. With the emergence of the healthcare "consumer," these practices have undergone dramatic change. Aided by access to state-of-the-art technology, customers are now expressing their preferences for everything—from physicians and hospitals to health plans and prescription drugs.

The direct-to-consumer movement was jump-started by the pharmaceutical industry. Pharmaceutical companies have spent more money and have been the most visible among healthcare organizations in attracting current and potential customers to their brands. (See Exhibit 10.1 for the pros and cons of direct-to-consumer marketing in the pharmaceutical sector.) Health insurers have followed this trend, albeit at a safe distance, by offering policies via the Internet and increasing the number of health plans aimed at individuals rather than groups. The implementation of the Affordable Care Act (ACA) has led to a surge in **Internet marketing** by insurance companies. The shift from **defined benefits** to **defined contributions** has made the ability to customize plan benefits to address the needs of individuals and groups essential if an insurer hopes to remain competitive.

The direct-to-consumer movement has not been lost on providers, with hospitals, physicians, and other practitioners launching technologically sophisticated websites to maintain contact with existing customers and to entice prospective customers. These sites are not only informational but also interactive—for example, patients can bid online for elective procedures (e.g., facelift by a plastic surgeon). Such features serve as direct negotiating and communication links between provider and consumer.

A number of factors have driven direct-to-consumer marketing:

- New regulations for drug companies
- Introduction of defined contributions, which increased health plan enrollees' latitude in choosing and customizing menus of services
- Providers' chase of discretionary patient dollars (e.g., elective procedures)
- Use of the Internet as a direct path to the hearts, minds, and pocketbooks of healthcare customers

Internet marketing
A marketing approach that uses the Internet to promote an idea, an organization, a good, or a service

Defined benefits
The set of covered services identified by the insurer and received by every plan member

Defined contributions
The set of covered services whose combination and value are identified by every plan member and not the insurer

Consumers, for their part, have eagerly accepted this onslaught of direct marketing attention, taking advantage of the available information to tailor offers to their needs. The Internet has become a favored vehicle for engaging individual customers, but print and electronic media have played a part, too. Direct mail appears to have made a comeback from its junk-mail reputation as well.

This aggressive and multilayered approach marks the end of one-size-fits-all marketing. For health plan marketers, this has meant promoting a variety of unbundled services to a variety of people with distinct needs and preferences, rather than offering a standard bundled program that applies to

EXHIBIT 10.1

The Pros and Cons of Direct-to-Consumer Pharmaceutical Advertising

Pros	Cons
Meets increasing demand for medical information	Interferes with the physician–patient relationship and pressures physicians to prescribe
Informs consumers about new treatments	Confuses the patient
Encourages people to seek medical attention for conditions or symptoms that might otherwise go untreated	Emphasizes pharmaceutical treatments when other treatment options may be preferred
Decreases the cost of healthcare	Increases the cost of drugs
Promotes patient compliance	Results in unnecessary drug use

Source: Adapted from Craig (1998).

all customers. Enrollees may now have a "cafeteria" option that allows them to select from a cafeteria-type "menu" the services they want covered. For example, in the past, insurers would have offered both an employer of a high school–educated, blue-collar workforce (Employer A) and an employer of a college-educated, professional workforce (Employer B) standard plans that covered identical benefits. In today's environment, however, insurers would sell Employer A a plan that reflects the specific needs and wants of its employees; this plan is inevitably different from the plan customized for Employer B —and other employee groups, for that matter.

Because of this consumer-driven market, healthcare marketers have had to rethink their approaches in more ways than one. As discussed in previous chapters, marketers today must be better in touch with end users to gain in-depth knowledge of their target audience's wants, needs, and preferences. To determine which groups or individuals want a particular good or service and to what extent they want standardization over customization, marketers must study consumer characteristics and behaviors at the household level, as they have historically done in other industries. They must understand the interrelationship between psychographics (lifestyle traits), consumer behavior, and demand for services.

Business-to-Business Marketing

Much of the discussion about healthcare marketing focuses on the patient and other end users, but a significant amount of healthcare marketing involves business-to-business transactions. The corporatization of the industry means that more and more relationships are forged between two or more corporate entities. Traditional doctor–patient relationships have been supplanted by contractual arrangements between groups of buyers and sellers of health services. Many hospital programs now target corporate customers rather than individual patients. Healthcare delivery also has been employing a business-like approach. All of these have contributed to the growth of **business-to-business marketing**.

Clearly, business-to-business marketing in healthcare is nothing new. Healthcare organizations are major purchasers of a wide variety of goods, and large organizations do business with hundreds of vendors. Business-to-business marketing involves building profitable, value-oriented relationships between two businesses and their respective staffs. Business marketers focus on a few customers, and the sales transactions are usually larger in scope, more complex, and more technically oriented.

Business-to-business marketing
The process of building profitable, value-oriented relationships among businesses

Business-to-business marketing has become integral to selling products or services to business, industrial, institutional, and government buyers. In past decades, innovative products, great engineering, or great salesmanship alone might have been enough to close a sale, but healthcare organizations no longer have the luxury of "build it and they will come" thinking. Statistical tools, data mining techniques, and marketing research techniques that work so well in the consumer product arena must be fine-tuned for business-to-business marketing in healthcare.

The factors involved in marketing to businesses are significantly different from those involved in marketing to individuals. Business customers and traditional customers do not buy in the same way; they are driven by different impulses and respond to different approaches. Business-to-business purchases are often considered group decisions, whereas business-to-consumer purchases are more personal.

Much of the business-to-business marketing in healthcare is fairly routine and resembles the process in other industries. Hospitals and other large healthcare institutions have purchasing departments with established procedures for dealing with vendors of goods and services. Those marketing nonroutine services to a hospital or health system face several challenges:

- *Finding the right contact.* A marketer trying to promote an innovative technology solution, an organizational engineering initiative, or a customer relationship marketing system may run into difficulty identifying the right person to talk to. Depending on the organization, the person handling this type of proposal may be in a marketing, an administration, an operations, or even a clinical department.
- *Arranging a meeting with or a presentation to the identified contact.* Hospital administrators are notorious for their crowded schedules, and waiting six weeks or more for an appointment—common in healthcare—would seem ludicrous in most other industries.

- *Waiting for a decision.* The initial contact person may not be the primary decision maker, so that individual may have to discuss the proposal with someone further up the chain of command. That could take many weeks or even months. The final decision then may not come until much later, especially if the proposal concerns a project that is not a priority.

Case study 10.1 presents an example of business-to-business marketing in healthcare.

Internal Marketing

Internal marketing refers to a provider's efforts to effectively train and motivate its customer service and support staffs to work as a team to generate customer satisfaction. It strives to get everybody in the organization working toward common objectives. It is based on the premise that the relationships among people who work together mirror the relationships between customers and suppliers. Its goal is to increase communication among staff members to maximize a marketing campaign's effectiveness.

Internal marketing is a combination of marketing, human resources, training, and behavioral science. It redefines employees as valued customers, with the rationale that anticipating, identifying, and satisfying employee needs lead to greater employee commitment. In turn, greater commitment improves the quality of services provided to external customers.

The marketing department is a logical focal point for internal marketing because of its knowledge of the organization's overall strategy and its appreciation of external customers' needs. It has the expertise to deploy these tools with regard to internal customers and the budgets and financial resources to do the job. Internal marketing begins with communication, and communication is the marketing staff's primary responsibility. For internal marketing to be successful, employees must be made fully aware of the organization's aims and activities. Amazingly, employees of large healthcare organizations are often unaware of the services or programs their own organization offers. Although such lack of awareness is evident to some degree in any organization, it appears to be an inherent characteristic of healthcare.

A deliberate effort is required to instill requisite knowledge about the organization and its services and to ensure that all employees are working toward the same goal. Employees must develop a basic understanding of the nature of their customers, especially as they are often isolated from the service-delivery aspects of healthcare operations. They may have little knowledge of the customer interaction process or, at best, only a partial understanding of service delivery.

CASE STUDY 10.1

Using Business-to-Business Marketing to Promote an Occupational Health Program

Meridian Medical Center (MMC) was a 100-bed hospital located in a suburb of a medium-sized city. In its 40 years of operations, it had undergone several changes in ownership and was currently an investor-owned for-profit facility. MMC offered a wide range of services, but its survival had depended largely on its ability to identify niches that were not being filled by larger, better-financed providers in the area. MMC had become the major local provider of inpatient psychiatric and substance abuse treatment as well as weight management services. Its business was driven by personal referrals, word of mouth, and the reputation of its clinicians.

For five years, MMC had operated a fledgling occupational health program, primarily in response to the needs of nearby industries. Hospital staff treated minor injuries and illnesses (mostly on an urgent care basis) and the occasional emergency case. They also administered drug tests, tuberculosis tests, and other tests required for certain classes of employees. MMC administrators recognized a growing market for employee health programs in the area and planned a promotional campaign to pursue additional occupational health business. Prior to initiating the campaign, MMC took advantage of some of its unused space to create an occupational medicine center with a dedicated entrance. The intent of the program was to provide high-quality care in a comfortable setting and efficiently return employees to their job.

A much different means of attracting businesses was required for the occupational health program because clients were not likely to be self-referred but sent to the facility by their employers. Thus, this initiative required business-to-business marketing. MMC hired a salesperson to call on area employers and familiarize them with the program and its services. The salesperson's ultimate goal was to establish relationships with local employers, which would guarantee they would use MMC for their occupational health needs.

The salesperson had a clinical background and thus could discuss occupational health services intelligently. The challenge was to use personal sales to convince employers that MMC was the best choice in the area. Fortunately, the occupational health field was not well organized in the city, so presenting MMC's program as a dedicated resource

(continued)

generated a favorable response. In addition, the salesperson had to convince employers that sending their sick or injured employees to the emergency department or a private physician was not cost-effective or practical. Once MMC gained a foothold in a couple of companies, others began to express an interest in signing on.

While personal sales became the primary means of promoting the program, other traditional promotional techniques were used as well. Prior to the first sales call, MMC held a grand-opening ceremony and invited human resources staff from the area's businesses. MMC was fortunate in getting an endorsement from the local chamber of commerce, which recognized the unmet need. The salesperson gave presentations to various business groups and service organizations to reiterate the benefits of the program. MMC sponsored local events put on by the chamber of commerce and other groups involved in community development. It offered discounts for seasonal services (e.g., flu shots, allergy shots) and lifestyle-related services (e.g., cholesterol testing, smoking cessation, weight management). (See Chapter 9 for the discussion of these promotional techniques.)

Through personal sales, public relations, sales promotion, and other marketing techniques, MMC established itself as the first choice for occupational health services in the area. Because of the program's growth, MMC added more clinical staff and two salespersons.

Case Study Discussion Questions

1. How did MMC attract clients for its traditionally offered services (e.g., substance abuse, weight management)?
2. Why did occupational health require a different means of promotion from MMC's traditional services?
3. Who were the actual customers for occupational health services?
4. What preparations were required of MMC prior to promoting its occupational health services?
5. Why was personal sales the method of choice for this business-to-business marketing initiative?
6. What other promotional techniques were used to supplement personal sales?
7. In what ways did MMC try to differentiate its services from those provided by other health facilities?

Unfortunately, investment in internal efforts has always been a paltry fraction of most marketing budgets and is probably even smaller in healthcare than in other industries. Internal marketing is typically overshadowed in the budgeting process. Organizations that are frantically trying to boost revenues and cut costs may not appreciate the need to spend money on marketing to their employees. They miss the point that employees are ultimately those who deliver on or carry out the promises they made. Lack of investment may also result from a conscious decision by executives who dismiss internal efforts as feel-good pseudoscience, even though research consistently demonstrates that poor service (which stems more from people problems than from product problems) is what pushes customers away and into the arms of competitors.

Furthermore, internal marketing is an important implementation tool. It facilitates communication and helps squelch resistance to change. It informs and involves all staff in new initiatives and strategies. Internal marketing initiatives are relatively simple to develop if the marketer is familiar with traditional principles of marketing. Internal marketing is based on the same rules that govern external marketing and is similarly structured; the main difference is that the customers are staff and other internal stakeholders. Simply, internal marketing is nothing mysterious; most of it is common sense. Among the most common features of internal marketing programs are workshops, special events, company anniversary celebrations, appreciation dinners, brown-bag lunches, off-site/satellite office visits, internal newsletters, bulletin boards, e-mail newsletters, intranets, and broadcast e-mails. Case study 10.2 describes an example of internal marketing.

Concierge Services

In the late 1990s, healthcare providers witnessed the emergence of **concierge services**; some providers have restructured their practices to adopt this model. Concierge services are customized, personal, and on-demand services provided to clients who pay extra for the privilege. Some healthcare organizations have simply introduced practices borrowed from the hospitality industry, while others have restructured their practices to meet a broad range of health-related needs for a small, select patient population.

Concierge services Customized health services offered to customers who pay a premium for the personalized attention

Some organizations have adopted concierge services as part of their customer service approach. Hospitals may offer valet parking or gourmet food options for hospitalized patients. Large physician practices may offer certain services at little or no additional cost, such as help with health insurance filing, referral scheduling, and transportation. Concierge practices—usually involving one or a small number of physicians—accept a limited number of patients who pay an annual fee in addition to the cost of care provided.

CASE STUDY 10.2

Internal Marketing at SouthCoast Rehabilitation Center

SouthCoast Hospital operated 240 licensed beds, 30 of which were devoted to inpatient rehabilitation. The rehab facility was located in a separate building and primarily provided services to patients discharged from critical care units of the hospital who had been admitted for stroke, heart attack, or trauma. The facility was the only one of its kind operating in the market area and thus had no competition.

As Medicare and other insurers attempted to reduce the cost of care, increasing restrictions were placed on the provision of rehabilitation services on an inpatient basis. As with many other health conditions, the emphasis (and the reimbursement) was being shifted to outpatient care. This development created a challenge for SouthCoast in that it had historically focused on inpatient care and left outpatient rehabilitation services to other providers in the community. Now, the organization was forced to expand the limited outpatient services it offered and compete with other providers; the good thing was that it was known as the premier provider of rehab services in the region and had an excellent facility. However, it had not yet developed its outpatient program, which would require a marketing effort. The marketing staff embarked on a research initiative to determine the perception of SouthCoast's rehab services both in the market area and inside the organization itself. It was anticipated that much of its outpatient business (like its inpatient business) would come from internal referrals.

The goals of internal marketing research were to discover whether the physicians and staff (i.e., administrators, staff physicians, other clinicians, social workers, and discharge planners) knew of SouthCoast's rehabilitation services (both inpatient and outpatient), to assess whether they were using the services or otherwise referring patients to the facility, and to determine what was needed to generate more patients from internal sources. Marketing personnel had never conducted internal research before and were somewhat stunned by their findings from **surveys**, interviews, and **focus groups**.

First, some administrators were unaware of the availability and nature of the organization's rehab services. While many specialists routinely referred their recovering patients to the facility, many did not. Other staff members also were not aware of these services; this group included discharge planners who influenced the disposition of patients once their inpatient care was completed. Second, among those who

Survey
A data collection technique that involves the use of a questionnaire administered in any number of ways

Focus group
A data collection technique that involves eliciting opinions and perspectives from a panel of individuals who interact under the direction of a leader

did know about the facility, few actually referred their patients to it. For example, the two major orthopedic surgery groups operating at the hospital seldom referred patients to the facility. Third, because of the limited outpatient rehab services in SouthCoast, many staff had established relationships with other rehab providers in the community.

Clearly, an internal marketing initiative was needed, so marketing developed a plan for increasing awareness and utilization of the outpatient rehab services. Among the activities that were planned for this purpose were as follows:

- Grand opening of the outpatient services, including tours of space, for all staff and physicians
- Informational sessions for those within the hospital who should be making referrals—including physician staff, patient advocates, social workers, and discharge planners—as well as admissions and financial services staff
- Monthly employee newsletter describing the activities of the rehab facility, spotlighting key staff, and featuring successful rehab stories
- Promotional materials (e.g., keychains, refrigerator magnets, post-it notes) bearing the outpatient rehab center's contact information

Every six months after the introduction of the internal marketing campaign, SouthCoast rehab staff conducted an assessment of the effectiveness of the initiative. At the first six-month mark, the outcome evaluation found that the level of awareness had risen substantially, the willingness to refer had increased, and the perception of the service had become positive. The real proof, however, was in the utilization level. Independent of any external marketing, the number of internal referrals had increased dramatically in a matter of months. Subsequent research revealed that all of these indicators continued to trend up, and SouthCoast was able to carve out a significant share of the outpatient rehabilitation market.

Case Study Discussion Questions

1. What development led to a need for SouthCoast to shift its emphasis from inpatient rehabilitation to outpatient rehabilitation?

(continued)

2. Why did SouthCoast now face a competitive situation that had not been an issue in the past?
3. Because the rehab facility was well established, marketing staff made certain assumptions about the internal awareness of the rehab services. What surprises awaited them when they conducted internal research?
4. What possible reasons could there be for the lack of awareness (and subsequent lack of referrals) of the rehab services?
5. What steps were taken as part of the internal marketing campaign?
6. What other activities might have contributed to the internal marketing effort?

The concept behind concierge services is simple, if somewhat controversial. Participating physicians agree to accept only a small number of patients (e.g., hundreds rather than thousands) in exchange for an annual fee (currently ranging from a few hundred dollars per year for limited services for an individual to several thousand dollars per year for expanded services for a family). These services may include 24/7 access to the physician or other staff member, immediate telephone response, same-day appointments, longer office consultations, and house calls. The physician may even accompany the client to visits with other healthcare providers to serve as an "interpreter." In most cases, existing insurance continues to pay for covered services.

The number of concierge practices is still small, but this approach appears to be gaining momentum—partly driven by customer dissatisfaction with health insurers. Most of these practices have been initiated by physicians, although hospitals are becoming increasingly involved in establishing concierge services. Since the first model was developed in Seattle in the 1990s, concierge practices have emerged mostly on the East and West Coasts. A handful of national chains of concierge practices have also appeared.

Concierge services are not without critics. Observers inside and outside medicine have condemned them as avaricious and likely to contribute to the already serious shortage or maldistribution of physicians. If large numbers of physicians reduce their patient loads from 5,000 to 300, many patients are left without access to physicians. Indeed, established patients converting to a concierge practice must be among the first to sign up or face the prospect of finding another doctor.

The concierge trend reflects broader changes that are affecting society in general and healthcare in particular. Many observers point to managed care as a factor that has induced dissatisfaction and disenchantment among physicians. Features of managed care such as the assembly-line approach, oversight imposed by nonclinical personnel, and limitations on utilization have led physicians to take some radical approaches. Some physician practices do not participate in managed care and may not accept insurance. Similarly, direct-pay practices accept only out-of-pocket payments—but at half of the managed care rate. (How the ACA will affect such practices is too early to tell.) Methods of reimbursement may not be the main factor in the rise of concierge medicine, but the baby boomers may be. Typically well-to-do, aging baby boomers have quickly become targets for concierge practices. Not all concierge members are upscale baby boomers, however; some Medicare managed care plans have added concierge services as well.

The public has not accepted the concierge concept to the extent anticipated. Not only is it a departure from the type of medical practice most healthcare customers are comfortable with, but also the extent to which patients are dissatisfied with their existing providers may have been overestimated. In addition, some physicians have found that the 24/7 demands of concierge medicine are an unanticipated burden. As a marketing paradigm, concierge services make a lot of sense, but whether it turns into a widespread form of medical practice remains to be seen—especially in the struggling economy that the United States has been experiencing in the past five years.

Technology-Based Techniques

Technology-based techniques take advantage of available state-of-the-art technology. Pioneered in other industries, these techniques are increasingly being adopted by healthcare marketers who recognize the contributions technology can bring to the marketing effort.

Database Marketing

Database marketing (closely linked to customer relationship management) is a well-established component of marketing in most industries—but not in healthcare. Although patient care does not easily lend itself to the retail-oriented applications of this marketing technique, health professionals are increasingly recognizing the ways in which healthcare can benefit from some aspects of database marketing.

Database marketing involves collecting, storing, analyzing, and using information about customers and their past purchase behaviors to guide future marketing decisions. Ultimately, database marketing involves two main activities: (1) building a comprehensive database of customer profiles and (2) launching direct marketing initiatives based on those profiles. The direct marketing that results is considered database marketing if it is response and outcomes oriented. The integrated data set created through this process can be analyzed to discern consumer-related patterns relevant to the marketing process. This knowledge can be used to create a communication vehicle that allows the healthcare organization to target relevant prospects and deliver the appropriate message.

A number of constraints are implicit in database marketing in healthcare. These constraints are legal or ethical and often relate to issues of privacy, confidentiality, and data security. The repercussions from disclosing the medical condition of a customer are much greater than those from disclosing grocery store purchases or even financial transactions. The enactment of the **Health Insurance Portability and Accountability Act (HIPAA)** in 1996 focused the spotlight on the issue of patient data confidentiality (see Chapter 16).

The application of database marketing to patient care is challenging in that the healthcare customer's decision-making process is much different from that of other consumers. For one thing, patients may not be well informed about the attributes of various healthcare goods and services. Further, products must generate adequate margins to be candidates for database marketing, and some health services do not qualify on this score. Even the establishment of a database marketing system may be hindered by the fact that healthcare is much more complex than most other enterprises and includes numerous data collection points. Adapting database marketing to healthcare requires a certain level of sophistication and a relatively expensive technology solution capable of handling these complexities. The ideal system for healthcare database marketing is difficult to conceptualize, however, because of the convoluted decision making and financing arrangements in healthcare. The variety of coding systems (see Chapter 6) alone presents challenges to the development of database marketing applications. Healthcare providers must invest a lot of effort in the process, which is a challenge when many healthcare executives are not attuned to direct consumer marketing. In the past, the limitation was the technology itself, but today the impediment is the complexity of healthcare.

Database marketing cannot be imported from another industry without extensive modification, as patients and clients cannot be treated the same way as fast-food customers or car buyers are treated. Nevertheless, the potential applications of such a database to healthcare are almost unlimited. While the complexities pose numerous challenges, they can also be viewed as an opportunity or a reason to develop a database structure. The data mining potential from a well-designed customer database is considerable. Any choice-driven program—whether an affinity program (e.g., senior program), a concierge service, or a fund-raising initiative—is a natural candidate for database marketing. Pharmaceutical companies already use a version of database marketing in their direct-to-consumer campaigns. Health plans also are using this approach to segment their enrollee populations, and hospitals

Health Insurance Portability and Accountability Act (HIPAA)
1996 legislation that limits access to and protects individuals' protected health information

may introduce new programs to a "captive audience" through their customer databases.

Customer concerns about privacy can be addressed by having an opt-in/opt-out feature and letting patients indicate their preferred means of contact. With these features in place, database marketing appears ideal for a number of healthcare areas. Two obvious—but different—examples include the operation of wellness programs and the promotion of retail goods and services.

In other industries, database marketing is used for **cross-selling**, **up-selling**, follow-up sales, and so on. Overt solicitation in healthcare may be a turnoff for an organization's customers, but if conducted in the right way it can be an effective means of increasing customer uptake. For example, if a patient registers for an educational program (and gives consent for subsequent contact), she may be offered follow-up resources. Likewise, many healthcare organizations promote ancillary goods and services (e.g., pediatric services to obstetrics patients), and patient data inform the bundling of services that benefit the patient. The degree to which healthcare customers will accept more aggressive database marketing depends on how the technique is implemented. Clearly, the call to action that pharmaceutical companies have issued through their direct-to-consumer marketing has been well received by patients (if not by physicians). If database marketing is employed to help the customer obtain more information, then it is likely to be perceived as a positive outreach. Still, the potential for backlash exists—whether it is mild and simple as a customer requesting to be removed from a solicitation list or as serious and complex as a customer feeling anxious about their sensitive medical information.

Cross-selling
A sales approach that encourages the purchase of additional products and services related to the initial purchase

Upselling
A sales approach that encourages the purchase of an upgraded (and more expensive) product over a lesser and cheaper option

Customer Relationship Management

Well-developed and well-executed *customer relationship management* (CRM) programs are generating substantial returns for many businesses, and new technologies only add to the possibilities. Healthcare organizations are beginning to recognize the benefits of CRM and are predicted to increase spending on CRM activities. At the same time, CRM is still largely misunderstood by many health professionals and provider organizations; they must significantly change their mind-sets to realize the true benefits of CRM. The most important benefit of CRM is its contribution to the ways in which the organization defines its customers, segments them into meaningful categories, determines their needs, and provides services to them. Organizations need to balance the value they provide to customers with the value CRM generates for the organization.

Marketers should identify which of the organization's goals can be addressed using CRM and, based on those goals, create subsequent internal plans and implementation activities. Some common goals and objectives of technology-driven CRM programs include the following:

- Improving customer service and satisfaction
- Reducing the number of negative customer experiences
- Allocating resources more efficiently
- Reducing expenses related to customer interaction
- Attracting prospects and retaining existing customers
- Anticipating customers' needs and building stronger relationships over time
- Improving clinical outcomes
- Increasing profitability

Because customer satisfaction is a key metric for defining the organization's success, a CRM strategy can contribute to that goal. Given that most hospitals already use patient satisfaction as a key performance indicator, it should not be a big leap for management to see the value in CRM strategies, which enhance customer satisfaction in all areas of the system. Marketers can then introduce the more aggressive objectives of improved patient volume, revenue, and profitability.

Existing businesses often have difficulty changing the institutional mind-set from one that is driven by sales or operations to one that is driven by customers. Healthcare organizations in particular seem to have difficulty making this shift. For this reason, healthcare marketers are often not able to integrate every aspect of their organization into a CRM program, and they probably should not try.

The success of CRM programs hinges *not* on how comprehensive or complex a program is but on how well coordinated and orchestrated it is. CRM strategies could be applied to the following areas:

- Disease management for a group of chronically ill patients
- Physician-to-physician marketing
- Community health screening or prevention
- Specific product lines, such as cardiology, oncology, women's health, maternity, or sports medicine
- Urgent care services
- Promotion of the organization's website or establishment of an online community
- Call center or customer service functions
- Identification and servicing of the organization's top-ten referring physicians

- Identification and servicing of the organization's top-ten leading accounts or clients
- Frequent customer program or other affinity club

Case Study 10.3 describes efforts to promote heart health using CRM.

Internet Marketing

Although healthcare providers were slow to jump on the Internet marketing bandwagon, some healthcare organizations came to lead the way with certain aspects of online marketing. Hospital websites, for example, have become important sources of health information, and increasing numbers of healthcare consumers search online. Patients and caregivers alike use the Internet as a resource both before and after a physician visit. Because Internet users are seeking information, an Internet-based promotion can be more customized than, say, a television advertisement.

Observers have noted a progression in healthcare organizations' Internet marketing initiatives over time. The first stage simply involved a brochure-type website that identified the organization and described its work. The next stage introduced more service line and health content and more interactive features and applications. Websites became increasingly integrated with their organization's marketing efforts or other information technology applications. A growing number of health systems began pushing customized health information and medical records out to consumers, allowing e-mail communication with physicians, and carrying out some level of disease management online. Some are now using their websites as tools for establishing and maintaining customer relationships. Today, many healthcare organizations' websites include unique, sophisticated features. The *Hospitals & Health Networks*'s Most Wired Survey (www.hhnmostwired.com) is a useful indicator of what health systems are doing with information technology. Some of the early pioneers in this arena were Columbia/HCA; Kaiser Permanente; United Healthcare; and academic medical centers such as the University of Alabama at Birmingham and the University of Iowa.

Most healthcare organizations devote part of their marketing budget to online brand promotion. To assess the value of providing information online, many are attempting to determine their return on investment (ROI) by measuring whether physician visits are increasing, more prescriptions are being written, more coupons are being redeemed, and more products are being sold. Answering the ROI question enhances the appeal of Internet marketing (over offline marketing) for those skeptical about this methodology.

According to Scott (2009), the best websites focus on content that pulls customers, markets, media, and products together in a common location. A website should be the point at which all of an organization's online

CASE STUDY 10.3

Promoting Heart Health Using Customer Relationship Management

The Customer Potential Management Marketing Group (CPM) was a pioneer in applying CRM to the cardiology market. This company developed a program for three hospitals, which were part of a national healthcare system comprising more than 100 acute care hospitals in 17 states. The three participating hospitals (Hospital A, Hospital B, and Hospital C) ranged in size from a small local hospital to a large regional medical center.

The overall objective of the CRM marketing campaign was to educate the hospitals' customers about the early warning signs of a heart attack and encourage them to take a proactive role by determining their heart health. It also was designed to build awareness of the national healthcare system's local cardiology services and to drive early intervention and service utilization. It used the Consumer Healthcare Utilization Index (CHUI), a predictive index developed by CPM to select the individuals in each market area most likely to benefit from the campaign information. Targeted people were referred for a heart health exam, for which they paid a fee. The campaign also included a matched control group that did not receive any promotional material or services.

The area's referring physicians and providers were briefed about the campaign and encouraged to participate in screening patients. This was in keeping with the campaign's aim to involve physicians while promoting the hospitals' cardiology services and extending information to more patients. The study was designed to do the following:

- Identify people at risk for a heart attack, and initiate an early intervention (i.e., low-cost heart health exam)
- Provide consumers with beneficial education (regarding heart attack signs and symptoms)
- Strengthen relationships with primary care physicians and cardiologists
- Increase total charges attributed to cardiac-related services

The CRM approach involved delivering segmented messages to male and female prospects drawn from the databases of the three facilities. Solicitations were limited to one per household and targeted to persons aged 35 or older living in households reporting at least $30,000 in annual income. The campaign material consisted of a 7.5 × 5–inch, 4-color informational piece with two versions—one for males and one for females. The primary offer was a heart health check, which included an electrocardiogram (EKG) screen with a free EKG wallet card; body mass index measurement; lipid screen; and cardiac education booklet. The secondary offer was a free take-home health risk assessment. The cost per package (including printing and postage of the material) differed for each hospital—according to how many pieces were printed and how many pieces were mailed—and ranged from $0.71 to $1.39. Package prices for Hospitals B and C were higher because they printed large quantities for future mailings.

CPM staff maintained a complete record of organization-initiated communications—outbound dialogues with customers and prospective customers through direct mail. These communication records were matched to individuals and households in the database to assess activities, behaviors, and service utilization regarding the product line being promoted. Respondents were tracked through their appointment activity, and a response was tallied when a member of the target audience scheduled a heart health exam.

A 5 percent sample of the system's CRM database was flagged as a control group for each hospital. The control group was selected using the same criteria for selecting the organization-initiated communications groups. Members of the control group did not receive the mailing, but their activity was tracked in the database to compare activities, behaviors, and service utilization with those of the people who did receive the mailing.

The list of individuals with high predictive index scores compiled by Hospitals A and B returned significant positive results. Although Hospital C also reported positive results, fewer data were available for this site (e.g., EKG results were not available). At Hospital A, nearly half of those who signed up for the heart health exam had abnormal EKG readings. When combined with those whose EKG showed minor abnormalities, the percentage of people with some sort of abnormal reading rose to 54 percent. At Hospital B, 61 percent of those who signed up for the heart health exam had abnormal EKG readings.

The real measurement of success is a simple value proposition that demonstrates dollar for dollar the revenue received for revenue spent. Furthermore, an accurate calculation of ROI must take into account utilization (among the control group) that might have occurred without the campaign. The use of CHUI methodology to target potential cardiology

(continued)

patients clearly benefited the participating hospitals. The combined results for the first six months of this campaign are as follows:

- Patient response rate: 5.36 percent; control group response rate: 1.61 percent
- Marketing response increase: 333 percent
- Net profit: $1,868,711
- Marketing lift after factoring out the control group: $1,684,643
- ROI: $44.78 for every $1 spent on marketing

The results for the first six months demonstrated that this health system was successful in identifying the most appropriate individuals for cardiology services and generating a high return on the marketing investment. These results demonstrated that ability of the CHUI to target at-risk people for intervention by offering appropriate education, health maintenance, and wellness programs.

Case Study Discussion Questions

1. What was the organization's objective in applying the CRM approach to its customer pool?
2. In what ways did the initiative intend to change the knowledge, attitudes, or practices of the hospital's customers?
3. What were the characteristics of the promotional package used for this initiative?
4. How receptive were the organization's patients to this initiative?
5. What tangible benefits did the organization derive from this initiative?
6. How was ROI measured, and what did the evaluation reveal?

initiatives intersect, including podcasts, blogs, news releases, and other online features (see Chapter 11 on social media). A content-rich website should mesh the organization's resources in a cohesive and interesting way that efficiently informs the audience.

The Internet is also a major channel in the direct-to-consumer movement. By providing free online information, education, advice, summaries of scientific studies, tools, and shared experiences, pharmaceutical companies are communicating better with consumers. Well-established sites include

Schering Plough's claritin.com and Medtronic's medtronicdiabetes.com. In another notable effort, the National Headache Foundation and Astra Zeneca teamed up to create a Migraine Mentors at Work program (migrainementors .com). Consumer-advocacy organizations have been particularly aggressive in establishing sites for the benefit of consumers, such as HIVTribe's hivtribe. com and the American Cancer Association's cancer.org. These sites—online extensions of a workplace-based education/disease management program— provide users with information on how to manage their illness.

Healthcare marketers are successfully using offline techniques to draw consumers to their sites to search for information or respond to specific offers. They invite consumers to their sites to find a physician, view photos of newborns, sign up for a health screening, or take advantage of other features. Once consumers are online, marketers can convert Internet surfers into prospects by capturing personal information in a customer database and encouraging them to sign up for interactive health news and medical reminders. This tactic enables hospitals to extend their marketing reach in a more personal way than just advertising on television or through the mail.

While healthcare organizations have typically not been on the cutting edge of online approaches, many are taking advantage of contemporary technology—such as one that powers secondlife.com. Second Life is a virtual community and gaming system that uses state-of-the-art technology to enable users to develop a cyber persona and an accompanying world, interact and socialize with other users, create group activities, trade virtual properties and services, and so forth. The application has a three-dimensional modeling tool for "sculpting" objects and introducing animation. Case Study 10.4 describes a hospital's employment of Second Life for marketing purposes.

Many developments in healthcare Internet marketing are expected to continue. Contemporary technology allows marketers to do the following:

- Better integrate online initiatives with more traditional marketing programs
- Leverage targeted marketing campaigns to generate new referrals and patient encounters for service lines like cardiology, oncology, and orthopedics
- Focus on online customer relationship management strategies
- Increase direct-to-consumer online marketing
- Increase multicultural marketing as the industry gains a better understanding of the healthcare needs of diverse populations
- Better integrate the entire media mix
- Position the Internet as the ultimate relationship management tool

CASE STUDY 10.4
Hospital Takes Its Grand Opening to Second Life

In partnership with Cisco Systems, Palomar Pomerado Health in San Diego was able to hold a grand opening three years before it started operations by creating a simulated version of the real-life Palomar West Medical Campus using Second Life. The health system claimed that the facility was the first US hospital to be unveiled in this manner.

By entering Second Life, virtual visitors could tour the facility and see some of the amenities of the $810 million, publicly financed hospital, which now serves California's largest public health district. Under the direction of Palomar Pomerado's chief innovation officer, the facility was designed from the ground up to be integrated with leading-edge technology, including medical technology. Its Second Life presence offered patients and the healthcare community a chance to explore these innovations in the virtual world years before the physical facility opened.

Virtual visitors also helped Palomar Pomerado test some of its ideas regarding the use of leading-edge technology at the new facility and the opportunities futuristic concepts present for the healthcare industry at large. The system even used Second Life to test some technology proposed for deployment in Palomar West, such as radio frequency identification (RFID). Virtual patients taking the tour could wear RFID-enabled bracelets that not only tracked them but also guided them to areas of the facility in which their services or treatments were scheduled to take place. Thus, a virtual patient slated for day surgery could automatically have the hospital elevator land on the correct floor, according to the information programmed into the RFID bracelet. The idea behind the testing was that if the technology worked in a virtual setting, it could be adopted in the real world. Some of the concepts tested were not yet considered feasible in today's environment, but they were explored in advance.

Looking ahead, Palomar Pomerado planned to use Second Life to host industry events and meetings with healthcare leaders, policymakers, and others to discuss a variety of topics, including clinical and operational issues as well as the design and architecture of technology that could apply to the physical Palomar West setting.

Source: Adapted from McGee (2008).

Case Study Discussion Questions

1. Why have hospitals and other healthcare organizations been slow to adopt contemporary technology for nonmedical purposes?
2. What are the advantages and disadvantages of opening up development plans to the public and encouraging their feedback?
3. By using Second Life technology for the hospital's virtual grand opening, was Palomar Pomerado in danger of creating unrealistic expectations among future customers?
4. How do you think Palomar Pomerado's cutting-edge approach is likely to be perceived by the traditional healthcare community?
5. How likely are other healthcare organizations to adopt this approach in presenting themselves to the public?

Consumer Engagement

Consumer engagement refers to the process of establishing a relationship with a customer or a prospective customer and involving the person in bringing about a desired behavioral change. The growing interest in consumer engagement stems primarily from the perception shift from "patient" to "consumer." For example, a physician or other clinician might engage a patient to encourage compliance with a proposed treatment, a health plan might engage an enrollee to encourage a healthier lifestyle that would reduce healthcare use, and a wellness practitioner might engage a client to encourage active participation in a fitness program. In each case, engagement is built on the provider's understanding of the background, needs, and motivations of the customer; the most effective means of communicating with the customer; and the type of relationship that facilitates the customer's movement through the phases of awareness, action, and maintenance. (See Prochaska, Norcross, and DiClemente's [1995] stages-of-change model later in this section.)

Consumer engagement
The process of identifying and profiling consumers and subsequently involving them in desired behaviors

   Patients' participation in their own care is clearly a key to reducing health risks, improving outcomes, and lowering costs; without this involvement, the efforts of the healthcare providers are likely to be wasted (Demchak 2007). Noncompliant patients are not only detrimental to their own health but also costly for the overall healthcare system. Managing to improve or eliminate pre-diabetes symptoms is much less expensive than the lifetime treatment of diabetes. Regular visits to a primary care office are more effective healthwise and costwise than any visit to an emergency department. A prevention check-up and screening are preferable to a hospital stay, and purchasing and taking prescription drugs as ordered by the physician is obviously better than going without.

Implementing effective consumer engagement efforts involves considerable rethinking by both healthcare customers and providers. Patients and clients were told for decades to turn their healthcare and decision making over to the physician or hospital. Physicians, on the other hand, were trained to look at patients as separate from their environments and to rely on laboratory and other tests rather than listen to a patient's story. Providers, in general, were not paid for preventive care but were rewarded for "downstream" clinical care. Health insurance companies discouraged the use of services rather than ensured that each plan member received the right care at the right place at the right time. Much of this thinking has evolved and continues to evolve (albeit gradually)—thanks to many direct and indirect factors, including federal and state regulations, influential studies and reports, quality improvement and safety initiatives, the patient and family involvement movement, public demands for provider tranparency and accountability, and the ACA, just to name a few.

Encouraging Engagement

Healthcare researchers and experts have found that customer participation is fundamental to truly transforming the healthcare system. Patients today are encouraged to engage in a number of ways, such as selecting their own providers and health plans, monitoring and managing their own symptoms and illnesses, adopting and maintaining healthy behaviors, and interacting more deeply with their providers. Healthcare organizations, practitioners, insurers, and employers are offering incentives to urge patients, enrollees, and staff to get involved in supporting consumer-directed health plans.

The most promising approaches to supporting consumer engagement are those that are participatory rather than didactic, involve family members, and have multiple dimensions. Interventions tailored to the individual's existing ability to initiate change yield good results. If members of the targeted populations are asked to take small, but realistic steps (e.g., reduce the number of cigarettes per day rather than quit smoking cold turkey), they have a greater chance of succeeding and moving on with confidence to the next step.

Segmenting customers into groups based on their capacity to change could prove beneficial, especially if the segmentation is based on clinical risk factors. Segmentation can enable marketers to customize their strategies to address the unique challenges associated with each stage of engagement in a particular group. If engagement strategies are implemented before risks increase or health worsens, patients could require less acute care as their self-management skills improve and they gain confidence. Other stake-holders, such as providers and employers, could use similar techniques. Together, insurers, providers, and employers can help increase engagement by addressing the specific challenges customers face as they begin to manage their health. Outreach at the community level could help provide the local momentum needed to activate a specific population. Reaching out to those who are more motivated to become role models and opinion leaders may help to hasten change in the community.

The capacity to change depends on the customer's state of knowledge, attitudes, access to support resources, and other factors. The potential to change status determines the approach an organization may take to engage that person. One such approach was developed by Prochaska, Norcross, and DiClemente (1995), who identified the five stages of change: pre-contemplation, contemplation, preparation, action, and maintenance. (These stages are similar to those of the consumer decision-making process discussed in Chapter 5.)

A consumer in the pre-contemplation stage is not ready to use a service and needs to be educated about it. A consumer in the contemplation stage may be aware of the service but needs to adjust his or her attitude toward it. A consumer in the preparation stage is ready to take action and needs to be exposed to the service options available. A consumer in the action stage has committed to address the issue but needs supportive services. A consumer in the maintenance stage needs reinforcement. Thus, the stage of change becomes a major determinant of the type of marketing activity pursued. (See Exhibit 10.2 for a depiction of Prochaska, Norcross, and DiClemente's stages-of-change model.)

What Must Marketers Know?

Effective consumer engagement requires meeting customers where they are and progressively moving from a generalized approach to an individualized approach. As long as marketers continue to use a one-size-fits-all approach, they are likely to see little response from target audiences. Marketers need to recognize that customers are unable to make these changes on their own and that the entire healthcare system needs to engage them. An essential task in this process is educating providers on the different levels of engagement and the ways to tailor messages accordingly. Marketers also need to understand

- what types of interventions have the greatest effect on outcomes,
- how various interventions affect customers at each level of engagement, and
- how populations with low literacy or without health insurance (who tend to have lower health status) can be engaged.

EXHIBIT 10.2
Stages-of-
Change Model

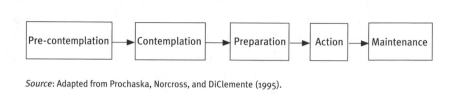

Source: Adapted from Prochaska, Norcross, and DiClemente (1995).

Financial incentives are commonly used to motivate consumer behaviors, although different consumer segments are likely to respond differently to such enticements. Even more important, marketers need to determine whether responsiveness to incentives leads to sustained behavior change and increased engagement.

Although much more research is required before the consumer engagement endeavor is thoroughly understood, some early conclusions can be drawn with regard to what makes an engagement approach effective. For a customer to benefit, he or she must

- possess adequate knowledge about health problems and preventive measures,
- be motivated,
- have the capacity to change,
- be offered meaningful incentives,
- be provided appropriate pathways for action, and
- receive reinforcement for positive behavior.

For those involved in fostering consumer engagement, the tools for change include an in-depth understanding of the target population, meaningful segmentation of this population, a proactive intervention package, targeted communications, ongoing support, and regular monitoring of consumer activity.

Limitations to Contemporary Marketing Techniques

Certain barriers exist to applying some of the more innovative and technology-based techniques discussed in this chapter.

First, adopting these techniques to healthcare may not be practical. Many healthcare organizations do not have the personnel or technical resources necessary to implement such techniques. They may lack the information technology infrastructure needed to support these approaches or may be unable to access the data on which these techniques depend. They are not likely to know how to implement database marketing or CRM without bringing in outside consultants.

Second, in healthcare, not only are the necessary data often lacking but concerns exist about the confidentiality of the patient data used in some of these contemporary marketing techniques. HIPAA restrictions have made many healthcare organizations reluctant to use—even legitimately—personal health data. Questions about the appropriateness of using patient data for marketing purposes reinforce these concerns. The conservative nature of health professionals poses a barrier to the use of data, while professionals in other industries would have no qualms about doing so.

Contemporary marketing techniques are being slowly but surely incorporated into healthcare—particularly into areas that have fewer reservations about the use of data (e.g., pharmaceutical distribution). The demands of a competitive and consumer-driven system need to be approached through new marketing techniques, and contemporary consumers are likely to insist on having more and more access to, and interaction with, healthcare providers. Ultimately, the challenge for healthcare is to use modern marketing techniques to establish and maintain customer relationships without violating or even giving the appearance of violating patient confidentiality.

Summary

Among the contemporary techniques that are programmatic are direct-to-consumer marketing, business-to-business marketing, internal marketing, and concierge services. Those that are technology-based include database marketing, customer relationship management, and Internet marketing. Techniques that involve information technology and intensive use of data have tremendous applications in healthcare but remain controversial. The enactment of HIPAA legislation, for one, has made many healthcare organizations reluctant to use personal health data for marketing purposes. The Internet has changed healthcare marketing, just as it has revolutionized marketing in other industries. That is expected to continue in the future.

Contemporary approaches to healthcare marketing emphasize customer relationships, and consumer engagement is its most recent incarnation. Experience has shown that promoting health services to consumers is becoming increasingly challenging. Customers and consumers are now at the stage where they understand the importance of availing themselves of a service. Although many are already engaged in their own healthcare and decision making, others must be convinced to proactively participate in managing their health and interacting with their providers. That task falls on healthcare marketers.

Key Points

- Healthcare has moved beyond traditional marketing techniques and adopted more sophisticated techniques that take advantage of information technology.
- Much of this shift has been driven by the need to develop and maintain relationships rather than simply sell products.
- Electronic forms of communication—mainly the Internet—have revolutionized the marketing of healthcare goods and services.
- To employ contemporary marketing techniques, marketers require in-depth knowledge of the target audience.
- Direct-to-consumer marketing recognizes the importance of the consumer as the end user and targets identifiable segments of the population.
- As healthcare becomes even more corporatized, organizations' transactions with other businesses have increased, necessitating business-to-business marketing approaches.
- Internal marketing focuses on internal customers to create a culture that fosters customer service and turns all employees into marketers.
- Aggressive healthcare organizations offer concierge services to cater to customers who desire special attention, and an increasing number of traditional health professionals are adopting concierge practices.
- Database marketing takes advantage of information technology to create a repository of customer data that can be used for relationship development and management and in follow-up sales efforts.
- Customer relationship management builds on database marketing to establish intensive relationships with customers.
- Internet marketing has become healthcare marketers' main medium of interface with target audiences.
- Consumer engagement is a way to positively influence customer behavior, and the task of promoting that engagement falls to healthcare marketers.
- The conservative nature of healthcare is a barrier to using contemporary marketing techniques, and the fear of violating HIPAA and patient confidentiality limits the use of personal health data for marketing purposes.

Discussion Questions

1. What marketing and/or healthcare factors are encouraging the adoption of contemporary marketing techniques?
2. In the pharmaceutical industry, why is direct-to-consumer marketing a radical departure from traditional approaches to marketing?
3. What developments in healthcare have encouraged the growth of business-to-business marketing?
4. In what ways can a healthcare organization use a customer database?
5. What factors have influenced the trend toward establishing long-term relationships, as opposed to trying to secure an immediate sale from the healthcare consumer?
6. Why is healthcare reluctant or cautious about using patient data or even applying technology-based marketing techniques?
7. As Internet marketing has matured, how have healthcare marketers taken advantage of it?
8. Why has consumer engagement become such a concern in healthcare, and what is the marketer's responsibility with regard to promoting it?

Additional Resources

Arrogant Healthcare Marketing Bastards: www.thinkinterval.com/arrogant-health care-marketing-bastards

Cellucci, L. W., C. Wiggins, and T. J. Farnsworth. 2014. *Healthcare Marketing: A Case Study Approach*. Chicago: Health Administration Press.

Second Life: secondlife.com

Shankland, S. 2003. "To DTC or Not to DTC? Direct to Consumer Advertising Can Seem Like a Prescription for Futility." *Marketing Health Services* 23 (4): 44.

11

SOCIAL MEDIA AND HEALTHCARE MARKETING

Within the past decade, a form of web-based communication called **social media** has emerged and spread rapidly. Although no concise definition of the term exists, it is an umbrella description for a variety of communication modes enabled and supported by Internet technology, such as social networking, blogging, file sharing, and podcasting (just to name a few). Social media are distinct from traditional media (TV, radio, print—also known as "industrial media") in that they connect people and allow direct interaction among a community of users, offering immediacy and flexibility. This chapter discusses the basics of social media and their application to healthcare marketing.

Social media
A variety of communication modes that use Internet technology to support innovative forms of interaction between people

The Basics of Social Media

Social media were developed for purposes of person-to-person interaction and have been primarily popularized by millennials—the generation of young, technology-savvy consumers. With roots in new-generation cell phone and Internet applications, social media technology allows individuals to maintain contact with friends, family, and other associates at any time from anywhere. Social media represents a revolution in communication, and its growth has been phenomenal.

Social networking numbers alone are remarkable. According to Pew Research Internet Project (2013), 73 percent of adults who regularly go on the Internet use social networking platforms—with Facebook being the leading site, followed by LinkedIn, Pinterest, Twitter, and Instagram. Similarly, eMarketer (2013) reported that social networking grew worldwide from 1.47 billion users in 2012 to 1.73 billion in 2013 (about 1 in 4 people). It also estimated that this audience would climb to 2.55 billion by 2017.

Social networking—perhaps the most common type of social media—is only one dimension of this communication mode. Social media users, with their desktops, tablets, or smartphones, can also create and post content—whether comments, pictures, videos, audios, or blog entries. Such **user-generated content** power sites that rely on visitor submissions and/or responses to those submissions—the YouTube and Wikipedia models, for example. In addition,

User-generated content
A website model that relies on user submissions and/or comments; the discussion thread is part of the content

social media host various types of peer-to-peer activities, from news updates to online collaboration to viral marketing to entertainment sharing. Social media have not eliminated the need for information gatekeepers in various industries, including healthcare, but they have helped shift the control of information from those gatekeepers to the consumers.

Each type of social media allows its users to create a "community," and this community is given a forum to contribute perspectives and knowledge on a wide range of topics, encompassing current events, politics, religion, pop culture, society, economics, commerce and consumerism, history, science, and healthcare, just to name a few. These are real-time (and often unfiltered) inputs or discussions that readers and other virtual community members can freely access in perpetuity with an Internet search or a visit to social media sites. Exhibit 11.1 describes the common types of social media.

EXHIBIT 11.1
Types of Social
Media

New types of social media (along with their specific platforms) are constantly emerging. Here are the most common types at the time of this writing.

- *Social networks.* These websites require every user to create a profile that showcases basic data (e.g., name, gender), interests, and other information the user wants to share; attaching pictures to a profile is highly encouraged. A profile then becomes the "face" of the user, allowing him or her to connect with the profiles of friends, family, colleagues, and even total strangers; to communicate with this network; and to share updates, media, content, and so on. Leading social networking platforms include Facebook, LinkedIn, Google+, and MySpace.

- *Blogs.* One of the oldest and most popular forms of social media, a blog (a contraction of web and log) is an online journal whose entries are organized by categories or by *tags* (codes that help search engines find entries easily and thus makes them a marketing tool). Blogs have evolved over time. They are no longer used exclusively for personal thoughts but are now a tool and medium for instructors/professors, marketers, and other professionals and businesses. They are no longer text-only but are multimedia. Many websites—from those posting news to those selling goods and services—have a dedicated blog. "Vlogs" (or video blogs) have emerged as well. Popular blogging platforms include WordPress, Blogger, and Tumblr.

- *Microblogs.* Microblogs feature short posts—usually restricted to a few lines of text, an image or photo, a short video, or a link. They are particularly suited for quick updates and distributing content via mobile devices. Notable microblogging platforms include Twitter (for text), Instagram (for photographs), and Vine (for video). Facebook, Google+, and LinkedIn all have their own microblogging features.
- *Content communities.* Content communities present the text, images, and videos submitted by their users or members. These users also comment on or discuss the content. YouTube, Flickr, and Scribd are examples of content communities.
- *Wikis.* Wiki websites are user-generated databases. One of the best-known wikis is Wikipedia, an online encyclopedia. Another site is WikiLeaks, a controversial wiki that posts information from whistleblowers.
- *Podcasts.* Podcasts comprise audio, video, PDF, or other content that can be downloaded or streamed either for free or through a paid subscription. The term itself is a portmanteau of "pod" (from iPod) and "broadcast" (as the content is "aired" or transmitted electronically).

Other types of social media include (but are certainly not limited to) ratings and reviews (e.g., Yelp, Angie's List); social bookmarking (e.g., Pinterest, Digg); forums and discussion boards (e.g., Reddit, Craigslist); 3D virtual worlds or gaming (e.g., Second Life, World of Warcraft); music and movie streaming (e.g., Pandora, Netflix); and media, science and technology, and pop culture aggregators (e.g., Mashable, BoingBoing, Buzzfeed).

A Healthcare Consumer's Tool

Not surprisingly, social media have become popular with people interested in healthcare issues (Sarasohn-Kahn 2008). It is hard to imagine a healthcare consumer today (even someone who is not technologically savvy, per se) who would not research his or her health condition or diagnosis on WebMD or watch a related video on YouTube, find more information about a physician or another clinician by using Google or Healthgrades or by asking friends on Facebook, or check out posts by those undergoing similar experiences on Twitter and WordPress. Online forums focused on specific diseases are burgeoning (e.g., Diabetes Daily), along with countless general healthcare and personal journey blogs (e.g., The Health Care Blog, Heart Sisters).

Healthcare and social media are natural partners. Social networks are user-friendly, and the posts are in real time, which helps when a patient and a doctor are trying to make a healthcare decision "on the fly." Blog entries (video, audio, and text), online articles, and forum discussions are stamped with a time and date, allowing healthcare consumers to disregard old and obsolete (and thus possibly dangerous) information. Because healthcare information is fluid or everchanging, it is disadvantageous to rely on only industrial media as sources; a printed brochure or an aired program cannot be changed once new information emerges. Social media, on the other hand, are not permanent and thus better suited for the dissemination of updates and other new material.

See Exhibit 11.2 and Case Study 11.1 for social media's application in a healthcare setting.

EXHIBIT 11.2
Social Media and the Healthcare Industry

The following statistics illustrate social media's role in healthcare:

1. More than 40% of consumers say that information found via social media affects the way they deal with their health.
2. 18- to 24-year-olds are more than twice as likely than 45-to 54-year-olds to use social media for health-related discussions.
3. 90% of respondents from 18 to 24 years of age say they would trust medical information shared by others on their social media networks.
4. 31% of healthcare organizations have specific social media guidelines in writing.
5. 19% of smartphone owners have at least one health "app" on their phone. Exercise, diet, and weight management apps are the most popular types.
6. From a recent study, 54% of patients are very comfortable with their providers seeking advice from online communities to better treat their conditions.
7. 31% of health professionals use social media for professional networking.
8. 41% of people say social media would affect their choice of a specific doctor, hospital, or medical facility.
9. 30% of adults are likely to share information about their health on social media sites with other patients, 47% with doctors, 43% with hospitals, 38% with a health insurance company and 32% with a drug company.
10. 26% of all hospitals in the U.S. participate in social media.

11. The most accessed online resources for health related information are: 56% searched WebMD, 31% [searched] on Wikipedia, 29% [searched] on health magazine websites, 17% used Facebook, 15% used YouTube, 13% used a blog or multiple blogs, 12% used patient communities, 6% used Twitter and 27% used none of the above.

12. Parents are more likely to seek medical answers online, 22% use Facebook and 20% use YouTube. Of non-parents, 14% use Facebook and 12% use YouTube to search for health care related topics.

13. 60% of doctors say social media improves the quality of care delivered to patients.

14. 2/3 of doctors use social media for professional purposes, often preferring an open forum as opposed to a physician-only online community.

15. YouTube traffic to hospital sites has increased 119% year-over-year.

16. International Telecommunications Union estimates that global penetration of mobile devices has reached 87% as of 2011.

17. 28% of health-related conversations on Facebook are supporting health-related causes, followed by 27% of people commenting about health experiences or updates.

18. 60% of social media users are the most likely to trust social media posts and activity by doctors over any other group.

19. 23% of drug companies have not addressed security and privacy in terms of social media.

20. The Mayo Clinic's podcast listeners rose by 76,000 after the clinic started using social media.

21. 60% of physicians' most popular activities on social media are following what colleagues are sharing and discussing.

22. 49% of those polled expect to hear from their doctor when requesting an appointment or [a] follow-up discussion via social media within a few hours.

23. 40% of people polled said information found on social media affects how someone coped with a chronic condition, their view of diet and exercise and their selection of a physician.

24. [To] more than 1,500 hospitals nationwide [that] have an online presence, Facebook is most popular.

Source: Reprinted with permission from referralMD (2013).

CASE STUDY 11.1
Virginia Blood Services' Facebook Events

When the legal age for donating blood in Virginia was lowered from 18 to 16, Virginia Blood Services (VBS) began to explore new methods of communicating with potential donors—particularly first-time donors—and attracting them to blood-collection events. VBS consulted with a marketing firm on how to use social media to reach those audiences.

It quickly became apparent that using social media was appropriate for reaching not only those as young as 16 but also college-aged students. Upcoming blood drives on college campuses signaled an opportunity to market the events in a way that would be applicable to both demographics. With a target population of high school and college students, the challenge of drawing interest and engagement was greater.

VBS developed a strategy of using Facebook Event to organize and promote a series of blood drives on campuses across the state. The events were linked to VBS's Facebook profile, which was already disseminating content and news. The success of this strategy was measured through the RSVP feature, which indicated who and how many would be attending, might be attending, or would not be attending a specific event. A related measure was the visibility of the feature. People without Facebook profiles could not see the event information unless it was made available to the public. People with profiles, in contrast, not only could see the event but also could become a "fan" and RSVP to the event; the Newsfeed feature would then publicize this intention to attend or participate. In a circle of friends, the more people planning to attend, the more people are influenced to attend or would know about the event. In the case of VBS, even if just 1 in 20 invited to the blood drive says "yes" or "maybe" to participating (which endorses the activity), then hundreds—if not thousands—of people who were not even invited would find out and could sign up themselves. In this way, the RSVP would likely take on a life of its own.

The immediate success of VBS's Facebook Event strategy was palpable: In just one week, several hundred people had viewed the promoted events and more than a third of them responded using the RSVP feature. For a blood drive at the University of Virginia, for example, VBS received 165 yeses, 64 maybes, 56 nos, and 247 no responses. More than 500 people viewed the event page in less than 7 days.

But the real results came after the blood drives, when the initiative was evaluated. Data were compiled on people who actually attended (as opposed to those who merely said yes), who were viable donors, who donated "double-reds" (i.e., a certain type of blood), and who were new donors. Because people generally use their real names on Facebook, VBS was able to develop a small programming script that matched donors in the database with the Facebook Event log of names. The final tally was a remarkable 28 percent increase in new donors, all solicited through Facebook. For some of the events, the double-red total increased more than 20 percent.

Case Study Discussion Questions

1. What demographic did VBS seek to penetrate, and why did it think an innovative method would be required to do so?
2. In addition to Facebook, what other forms of social media might VBS have employed?
3. What characteristics of Facebook and other social networks make them ideal for this type of campaign?
4. How effective was the VBS campaign, and how do the results compare with what might be expected using traditional marketing methods?

A Modern Marketer's Medium

The growth and popularity of social media have revolutionized marketing in all industries. The medium continually exhibits to marketers that target audiences (assuming they are "wired") not only are highly accessible anywhere and at any time but also are a conduit who can rapidly and widely spread a marketing campaign's message. Modern marketers realize that social media are part of contemporary communications' ecosystem that includes TV, radio, and print; thus, most marketers have integrated all these media to capture consumers with enjoyable and seamless promotions that are visible on the web, on mobile devices, on TV and the radio, and in print.

Social media marketing usually involves creating content and feeding it to appropriate online channels (e.g., social networks, blogs, news aggregators) to attract enough attention that it is willingly shared across platforms or it goes **viral** (i.e., an epidemic-like dissemination of content). When a brand's corporate message is posted and then passed on from user to user on a social network (by being reposted or retweeted, for example), it presumably resonates because it appears to come from a trusted third-party

Social media marketing
The promotion of an idea, a good, a service, or a brand using various types of social media

Viral
The rapid, epidemic-like dissemination of content on the Internet

source rather than generated by the brand or company itself. Obviously, this repetition increases the visibility of the message and its creator. The greater the number of people it reaches, the greater the likelihood it will bring more traffic or visitors to the company's website.

Because going viral tends to start on social networks, marketers tend to first post promotions on their organization's Facebook page and follow it up with a brief announcement on Twitter. Word of mouth becomes "word-of-mouth on steroids" (also known as electronic word of mouth or eWoM) when social networks are employed because of their capability to reach and attract even those who are not direct followers or fans. This is why social networks are referred to as earned media rather than paid media.

Earned media
The free exposures, publicity, or word of mouth that a brand, a product, an initiative, or content receives

Paid media
Ads and/or sponsorships purchased to promote a brand, a product, an initiative, or content

Owned media
Online channels that an organization develops, maintains, and cultivates for marketing and other purposes

Earned media refer to the free exposures, publicity, or word of mouth (likes, reposts, retweets, favorites, up votes, shares, recommendations, and other mentions) that a brand, a product, an initiative, or content receives. **Paid media**, on the other hand, refer to ads and/or sponsorships purchased to promote a brand, a product, an initiative, or content. A term related to these two is **owned media**, which are online channels (e.g., website, blog, Facebook page, Twitter feed) that the organization develops, maintains, and cultivates for marketing and other purposes. These terms are illustrated throughout this chapter.

Innovative healthcare marketers have long appreciated the advantages of social media for promoting healthcare organizations and their products. If the key functions of healthcare marketing are to inform and educate current and potential customers, then there is no better vehicle than social media to facilitate these activities. To this end, marketers have persuaded hospitals, health systems, and other healthcare organizations not only to launch their own websites, actively participate in social networking, and offer online courses but also to continue cultivating their web presence to disseminate information, encourage information sharing, support customer involvement and interaction, and welcome customer feedback. Furthermore, many have written blogs, hired or paid bloggers, sponsored content, published online advertorials and white papers, engaged in e-commerce, posted videos, created podcasts related to certain medical conditions or procedures, and so on—all to attract and retain healthcare consumers. Pharmaceutical companies have been at the forefront of these social media efforts, but even government agencies have done their part to support their missions and increase their online visibility.

Social media allow all users—whether individuals, groups, or organizations—to choose whom or what to follow. By choosing accordingly, marketers can narrow down a target audience. While this strategy may not be particularly helpful to providers of patient care, it could benefit individuals and groups practicing retail medicine or offering elective procedures as well as companies selling consumer health goods.

An equally important advantage of social media for healthcare is it gives organizations an opportunity to interact directly with their constituents or stakeholders. This personal interaction between the amorphous hospital and a flesh-and-bone patient, for example, can instill a feeling of loyalty from the patient and her family and friends. It communicates that the organization (regardless of who is running the account) cares that a particular patient is happy or sad, satisfied or angry, well or ill. A social network account (assuming it is run ethically and carefully) humanizes the business and makes it relatable, makes it seem as if it is listening to customer concerns.

Healthcare Consumers' Use of Social Media

Healthcare consumers who rely on social media—and the Internet as a whole—to address their healthcare issues currently outnumber the healthcare organizations that have a social media presence. This is understandable— not only because there are obviously more people than businesses but also because organizations (unlike private citizens) face legal and regulatory risks if they make false or careless moves online. For example, a hospital could get fined under HIPAA privacy rules for transmitting or sharing (online and offline) without the patient's consent—and for any other activities that it fails to safeguard—**protected health information**.

Consumers, on the other hand, are not daunted by social media. They use these channels to find answers to their health-related questions and commiserate about their conditions. They look up symptoms and treatments, specialists and practitioners in their community, and other patients' experiences. They are eager to share information with (as well as obtain information from) those they trust, and they are willing to give out their personal and medical data *if* doing so would benefit them. Their expectations of providers mirror the instant-gratification nature of social media: They want a response (or at least an acknowledgment) from individual practitioners and organizations within a short time. If they feel ignored, slighted, or unsatisfied, they are highly likely to broadcast this negative perception to their social media followers (and these people's followers and beyond), generating bad public relations for the provider in question.

Protected health information
A patient's identifiable healthcare data, including physical and mental health status, treatment record, and insurance and payment information

By the Numbers

Clearly, not all members of US society are users of social media, and different segments of the population adopt new technology at different rates. The same can be said of healthcare consumers.

As illustrated in Exhibit 11.3, the use of social media for various health-related activities varies depending on the demographic characteristics of customers. According to a study by PricewaterhouseCoopers Health Research

EXHIBIT 11.3
Social Media
Activities by
Healthcare
Consumers

| | Selected Characteristics | | | | | |
Activity	All	18–24	55–64	College Degree	‹$25,000	$25,000–$50,000
Post about health experiences	25	54	11	22	28	29
Comment on health experiences	26	53	14	27	27	29
Post review of meds, doctors, etc.	20	38	6	16	19	20
Share health-related videos, images	20	43	2	14	20	20
Share health symptoms/behavior	22	44	6	17	23	23
Join a health-related cause	23	44	8	20	24	28
Support a health-related cause	28	55	12	29	30	35

Source: Data from PricewaterhouseCoopers Health Research Institute (2012).

Institute (2012), the following traits describe survey respondents who said they avail themselves of social media or online resources:

- Male
- Age 18 to 34
- College educated
- Household income between $25,000 and $50,000
- Private insurance or Medicaid coverage

Interestingly, however, when all factors are taken into consideration, the group actually most active in engaging social media for healthcare purposes comprises females who are between 18 and 34, have no college degree, and earn between $25,000 and $50,000 annually.

Part of facilitating the use of social media by healthcare consumers is understanding who they trust online. According to Pricewaterhouse-Coopers Health Research Institute (2012), consumers are most willing to share health-related information online with providers (physicians, nurses, and organizations), patient advocacy groups, and patients they know. They are least likely to share health information with patients they do not know,

Party	Percent of Willing Consumers
Other patients you know	46
Other patients you don't know	25
Hospital	55
Doctor	60
Nurse	56
Health insurance company	42
Drug company	36
Retail pharmacy	48
Patient advocacy organization	54
Government organization	45
Gym or fitness center	34
Alternative healthcare setting	36

Source: Data from PricewaterhouseCoopers Health Research Institute (2012).

EXHIBIT 11.4
Healthcare Consumers' Willingness to Share Health Data Online

a gym or fitness center, a drug company, or an alternative care provider (see Exhibit 11.4).

Patient-Oriented Websites

Patient-oriented websites are online communities dedicated to health and wellness. They offer robust resources on myriad diseases and illnesses, symptoms and risk factors, treatments and cures, and medications and side effects—all usually written in easy-to-understand language, organized alphabetically, highly searchable, and laid out in a simple but attractive way. Collectively, these sites offer patient stories, health and industry news, expert medical insight, health apps and other tools, patient and provider blogs, educational literature (from newsletters to articles to research studies), links to other resources, support groups, discussion and chat forums, e-learning or webinars, advocacy opportunities, disease prevention and health monitoring guides, interactive social media platforms, and so much more. Most important, they empower patients as well as their family members or caregivers by equipping them with credible information, putting them in touch with those who have similar challenges and with health professionals, and giving them tools for self-management. (Similar digital communities are available for physicians and other health professionals, such as Sermo.com and Imedex.com; these communities may also be beneficial to patients and other healthcare customers.) Some of today's patient-oriented websites include the following:

- Alliancehealth.com
- Carepages.com
- Curetogether.com
- Dailystrength.org
- Everydayhealth.com
- Healthcommunities.com
- Inspire.com
- Organizedwisdom.com
- Patientslikeme.com
- WebMD.com

Many of these sites are accessible to casual Internet searchers, but others—because of confidentiality issues—require users to sign up for an account to take advantage of all the features. Exhibit 11.5 showcases one of these patient-oriented sites.

The Value of Social Media Engagement

In healthcare organizations, the social media realm is typically assigned to the marketing or communications department. Such a department appears to be the logical place from which to run social media initiatives, but relegating the effort this way suggests that top management has not bought into the value of social media.

Gleaning Benefits from Inbound Messages

Typically, "outbound" messages (those posts that originate from the organization and are transmitted to followers) get more attention than do "inbound" messages (those posts from followers directed either at the organization or to other followers), but both are equally important because they are critical sources of information.

One benefit of inbound messages is that they give an opportunity to hear honest opinions, identify concerns, and counter negative or incorrect perceptions. Consumers are out there talking honestly about products (goods and services) and people, so the organization must listen. For example, a plastic surgeon found out that some of his former patients were giving him poor reviews on Yelp and Healthgrades. It had never occurred to the surgeon to check review sites or that his service was being discussed in front

EXHIBIT 11.5
PatientsLikeMe

PatientsLikeMe was cofounded in 2004 by three MIT engineers after a family member of two of the founders was diagnosed with ALS (Lou Gehrig's disease) at an early age. Wanting to help patients like this to manage their condition, the trio conceptualized and built PatientsLikeMe, a health data–sharing platform designed to not only transform the way patients manage their own conditions and the way the healthcare industry conducts research but also improve patient care overall.

Today, members of PatientsLikeMe can share and learn from real-world, outcome-based health data. The organization's partnerships with trusted nonprofit, research, and industry leaders give members access to information that can improve products, services, and care. In addition, users can search the database, monitor their health, and connect with others who know firsthand what they are going through.

According to the company, "we are passionate about bringing people together for a greater purpose: speeding up the pace of research and fixing a broken healthcare system." Because much of healthcare data are private or proprietary, the development of breakthrough treatments takes decades and patients are unable to get the information they need to make important treatment decisions. To this end, PatientsLikeMe created a depository to which patients can add their specific symptoms, diagnoses, treatments, medications, stories, and so forth and from which other patients, caregivers, physicians, researchers, pharmaceutical and medical device companies, and anyone else can learn to ease and enrich the lives of those afflicted with a condition.

PatientsLikeMe has more than 200,000 members, who report their real-world experiences on more than 2,000 diseases—from the rare like ALS to the common like depression, fibromyalgia, multiple sclerosis, and psoriasis. Through health profiles, members can manage their health between doctor or hospital visits, document the severity of their symptoms, identify triggers, note their responses to new treatments, and track medication or treatment side effects. They also learn from the aggregated data of others in the same situation, getting and giving support in the process.

Source: Adapted from "About Us" and "Our Philosophy," www.patientslikeme.com.

of millions of people. After investigating these claims, he found out that the reviewers were not downgrading him but another physician with an identical name. Still, the surgeon was disheartened, but he learned a great lesson the hard way. Providers cannot ignore this type of feedback, and they should incorporate what they have learned into their marketing efforts.

Another benefit of inbound transmissions is that they contain additional details about patients. Despite the incredible amount of clinical data collected and stored by healthcare organizations, providers really do not know their customers. For whatever reason, patients are not reluctant to share many aspects of their lives on social media. Their social media posts give marketers (and providers) a glimpse into patients' life circumstances and other personal factors, providing insights that can be used to better serve customers.

Developing a Social Media Strategy

As noted by PricewaterhouseCoopers Health Research Institute (2012), business strategies that include social media can help healthcare organizations take a more active role in managing an individual's health. Thus, organizations need to coordinate internally to effectively use the information gleaned from the social media space and to connect with their customers in ways that build and increase trust. Trying to do this, however, is filled with pitfalls; to avoid them, organizations must provide the right leadership and invest adequate resources. Exhibit 11.6 lists the areas in which organizations may need to invest money and staff (Sargent 2011).

Marketers can transform customer comments and testimonials on social media (earned media) into relevant content that may be used for personal sales, advertising (paid media), and other promotional techniques. Additionally, marketers may tap into social media chatter to gauge public perceptions of the organization, its staff, and its services and to de-escalate any bad publicity.

See Case Study 11.2 for an example of one organization's social media strategy.

Monitoring Social Media

Social media monitoring entails tracking the content of various channels, especially those controlled by the organization (owned media). This is important for determining the volume and general sentiment of online chatter about a topic or the organization's brand, products, services, staff, or providers. Media monitoring has a long history in marketing, and it is now applied to social media.

Furthermore, social media can be mined to assess a brand's visibility, measure the impact of promotional campaigns, identify opportunities for engagement, discover competitor activity, and curb or anticipate impending crises. It can also alert marketers to emerging trends—what goods and services prospective customers might be interested in, what technologies they are using or prefer, what questions and concerns are they raising, and so on.

EXHIBIT 11.6

Social Media Areas That Require Resource Investment

Social media consultation may be helpful in the following areas:

- *Social Media Strategy*—What are your goals? Where will you invest your time on social media? What is your message? How can you monetize your social media efforts? Are you looking for a hard or soft return on investment (ROI)? A social media strategist can work with you to address these questions and formulate a plan that works for your business. The cost? Usually $500 and up.
- *Social Media Policies*—Once you have a plan in place, you need to establish social media policies. These are guidelines for your staff that cover appropriate use, showing employees where they are empowered in social channels, and where they need to exercise caution. Well written policies can be priceless, so it's worth investing $250 or more to have your own custom policy created.
- *Social Communications Calendar*—When do you post on your blog? What goes on Facebook? How often should you tweet? What do you say? A communications calendar can help you plan social media content that aligns with your strategy, enabling staff to express your messages in the right way at the right time. Monthly management of your social communications plan may run $500/ month or more.
- *Outsourced Engagement*—Hiring someone to tweet and post on your behalf may sound good, but this is one area I advise clients to be cautious about. There are many risks if you outsource the voice of your business, and the cost to your reputation can be high when things go wrong. With that in mind, if you choose to outsource your tweeting, posting and blogging, hire someone you can work closely with to collaborate on plans and create content. This will cost upwards of $50/hour or $500+ a month.

Source: Reprinted with permission from Claravon Consulting Group.

Understanding these buying signals can help marketers and sales people target relevant audiences and design the most appropriate campaigns.

Because of the the volume of activity and the conversations set to "private," monitoring social media has become a challenge and a full-time activity. However, marketers may use free or proprietary monitoring and analytics tools—such as Hootsuite, Klout, SDL, Argyle Social, and BackTweets, to name just a few—to help in this regard. The data and insights gleaned with the help of these tools can influence and shape future business decisions.

CASE STUDY 11.2
Hello Health

Hello Health, a Brooklyn-based primary care practice, is a paperless concierge service that eschews the limitations of insurance-based medicine. It is popular and successful, largely because it employs powerful social media tools and web-based technology. Its patients can go on their respective doctor's Facebook page to read about his or her personal interests. Patients who need a consult but cannot visit the office can send an instant message to their physician for quick and free advice. For complicated issues, patients are asked to come into the office. Appointments are booked online, and most communication is done electronically.

Many of the services of Hello Health require a nominal signup fee, which enables patients to participate in "cyber visits" with their personal physician. More than 300 patients enrolled in the year it launched, and the high demand forced the practice to open another office. Because it is a software company first and a healthcare entity second, it ensures that its participating practices are at the cutting edge of cyber medicine. The Canadian software company Myca, which established Hello Health and markets its products, provides practices with back-office support, such as billing for "remote care."

Hello Health has found that important by-products of using social media and web capabilities are patient-centered healthcare and patient happiness. For healthcare consumers who do not have adequate health insurance, the Hello Health model has particular appeal. For a fraction of the cost of an insurance premium, an enrollee can get easy access to a physician but pay only when care is rendered. How the Affordable Care Act might affect and thus alter this model remains to be seen.

Source: Adapted from Hawn (2009).

Summary

The emergence of social media as a communication mode has revolutionized marketing in healthcare and in other industries. Social media have become the primary means of interaction for many segments of society—in the United States and abroad. In addition, social media have proven to be a promising marketing tool. Social networking alone is expected to amass 2.5 billion users by 2017, so marketers cannot ignore social media's wide reach.

Perhaps the greatest benefit of social media marketing does not lie in the great number of people a marketing message could reach but in the great amount of consumer insights all those people could impart about a brand, a product, or an initiative.

The common types of social media are social networks, blogs, micro-blogs, content communities, wikis, and podcasts. Other types include but are not limited to ratings and reviews, social bookmarking, forums and discussion boards, virtual worlds or gaming, music and movie streaming, and information or data aggregators.

Healthcare consumers' use of social media has exploded. It ranges from exchanging information and sharing experiences on Facebook and disease-specific chatrooms to watching videos on YouTube to reading hospital/provider/patient blogs to participating in online support groups to researching symptoms and treatments on websites. Social media enable consumers to interact directly with other consumers, physicians and other clinicians, and other resources in real time and from any place. Although still a controversial use of social media, sharing personal health information online has become a practice for some social media users.

Pharmaceutical companies and consumer health product manufacturers have embraced this mode of communication, creating online communities around their products. Healthcare delivery organizations have started to do the same, going as far as posting professionally produced videos that show their top physicians and staff performing surgeries or explaining available treatments. At the very least, many providers rely on social media to promote their services and upcoming events and to encourage consumers to participate in their programs.

A brand, a product, an initiative, or content promoted on social media could "go viral" and garner exposure to millions of social media users all over the world. This is why social media channels are viewed as earned media, not paid media. Earned media are the mentions, likes, recommendations, and reposts gained by a campaign that cost nothing but could mean everything, while paid media are ads or sponsorships a campaign buys to attract attention or maintain visibility. Healthcare marketers who employ social media marketing could leverage their owned media (website, blog, Facebook page, Twitter feed, and other channels created, cultivated, and controlled by their respective organizations) with both earned and paid media.

Healthcare marketers should develop a social media strategy that integrates social media with other components of the marketing effort. This strategy should be well thought out and may require the involvement of a social media consultant. Part of this strategy is tracking and analyzing social media activities related to the campaign. Doing so would determine the impact of social media on the initiative's goals and objectives.

Key Points

- Social media revolutionized communications among consumers and between customers and businesses in all industries, including healthcare.
- Social media have the advantage of being free, accessible to all—and in real time and from anywhere, and flexible enough to support content in various format (e.g., text, images, video).
- On social media, users themselves can provide content, making reliance on the traditional gatekeepers of information unnecessary.
- The common types of social media are social networks, blogs, microblogs, content communities, wikis, and podcasts.
- Social media marketing has taken hold in healthcare and in other industries.
- Social media are widely used by not only healthcare consumers but also healthcare organizations, including providers, vendors of consumer health products, health insurance companies, and drug manufacturers.
- Different demographic groups use social media at different rates, thereby affecting the marketing strategy.
- Healthcare marketers benefit from being able to push information to social media users and to receive instantaneous feedback from members of online communities.
- Healthcare marketers should develop a social media strategy that integrates social media with other components of the marketing plan.

Discussion Questions

1. Define social media. How does social media marketing differ from traditional marketing techniques?
2. What are the attributes of social media that account for their widespread popularity?
3. What types of healthcare organizations have most rapidly incorporated social media into their marketing efforts?
4. What are some of the barriers to applying social media to healthcare issues and activities?
5. What are the common types of social media, and how do they differ from each other?
6. Why is the notion of user-generated content attractive to users of social media?

7. How have social media shifted the control of information away from traditional gatekeepers of information to the consumers of information?

8. Why is a social media strategy important, and what factors need to be considered in developing such a strategy?

Additional Resources

Healthcare Social Media Monitor: http://hcsmmonitor.com

PricewaterhouseCoopers Health Research Institute. 2012. *Social Media "Likes" Healthcare: From Marketing to Social Business.* New York: PricewaterhouseCoopers.

Thielst, C. B. 2013. *Social Media in Healthcare: Connect, Communicate, Collaborate,* 2nd ed. Chicago: Health Administration Press.

Timimi, F. K. 2013. "Healthcare: Don't Fear the 'What Ifs' in Social Media." http://blogs.einstein.yu.edu/healthcare-dont-fear-the-what-ifs-in-social-media/.

12

GLOBAL HEALTHCARE MARKETING

This chapter explores the reasons that healthcare has undergone globalization, the trends in medical tourism (also known as global medicine), and the four categories of medical tourists. The strategies and techniques that international healthcare marketers may employ to help their organizations develop a medical tourism program are discussed.

The past two decades ushered in the **globalization** of healthcare. This movement has meant, among others, the adaptation of the US healthcare system to the needs of immigrants and foreign nationals as well as the expansion of American healthcare interests overseas. Despite worldwide political, social, and economic unrest—which has caused many people to cut back on international travel, has made certain visas more difficult to obtain, and has put money transfers between countries under scrutiny—the medical tourism market is thriving and is expected to grow in the coming years (*International Medical Travel Journal* 2013).

Globalization
The worldwide expansion and interconnectedness of organizations and their associated economies and influence

Factors in US Healthcare Globalization

For years, advocates, policymakers, and other groups in the United States have called for modifying the country's healthcare system to accommodate its growing immigrant population. Furthermore, prestigious medical facilities have had a long history of providing clinical treatments and services to foreign notables. Various reports also detail the extent to which US hospitals and other healthcare organizations serve immigrants and foreigners (Derose, Escarce, and Lurie 2007), attract patients from other countries (Van Dusen 2008), and establish satellite facilities abroad (Are 2009). A growing number of Americans, in turn, have sought care overseas (OECD 2011). None of these developments is surprising for several reasons.

First, the Internet, computers (desk and mobile), and other technologies have shrunk the world, so to speak, and made it more accessible. Today, thanks to these advances, news and messages from even the most remote parts of the earth can spread almost instantaneously, people in different locations can open and close business deals or conduct commercial (and other) transactions without having to meet physically, massive amounts of data and information can be acquired in mere minutes, and human connections can be made at anytime and from anywhere. This revolution in international communication has exposed people to many other cultures, traditions, perspectives, and practices—along with their economic, political, social, and religious realities.

Second, multinational corporations have flourished, not only expanding trade between countries but also exerting resources and influence that rival those of nation-states. Their pan-national power has spurred more globalization. For-profit hospital chains, among others, recognize the potential for overseas expansion.

Third, immigration to the United States surged in the 1980s and has been growing since. For the US healthcare system, this has meant adopting strategies and practices that are sensitive to the needs of foreign-born patient populations, such as interpreter services; literature and signage in different languages; organization-wide cultural training for staff and clinicians; and recruitment of leaders, providers, and employees who reflect the diversity of healthcare customers.

Fourth, the forces of supply and demand have been at play. Population growth in the United States has been slow, and utilization of health services—particularly high-dollar inpatient services—has been on the decline (York, Kaufman, and Grube 2013). As a result, some sectors of the industry (such as hospitals and high-end elective surgery providers) have been left with unused capacity, leading some organizations to cast a wider net in hopes of attracting patients from distant shores. Further, the economies of many developing countries have been growing (e.g., China, Brazil), and the demand for modern health services in those nations has outstripped the supply. This mismatch has brought people seeking both elective and nonelective healthcare to the United States and to other countries with sophisticated medical technology.

In light of such tourism (and to leverage the reputation of those healthcare organizations that have already gained a foothold overseas), many US-based providers have stepped up their efforts to establish facilities in foreign markets with the greatest demand. At the same time, some countries have developed facilities whose services, medical staff (some of its members were educated and trained in the United States), equipment, and overall quality and outcomes are equal to or superior to those of US healthcare. As a result, they have attracted a worldwide following, including Americans. In many countries with a centralized, government-controlled healthcare system, private-sector healthcare has emerged and thrived because of the citizens' dissatisfaction with the system.

Fifth, the middle class—which currently stands at 2 billion and is expected to rise to 4.9 billion worldwide by 2030, owing mostly to the growth in Asia and other developing countries (Rohde 2012)—has increased demand for high-quality and accessible healthcare. This has put pressure on resource-constrained health ministries to improve services. Individuals with greater disposable income are more willing and able to pay for—or at least share the cost of—top-quality health services. For provider organizations seeking to expand their infrastructure and services (and hence increase revenues), the prospect of investing in burgeoning markets is inviting.

Trends in International Healthcare

Attracting Foreign Healthcare Consumers

In and around the 1950s, US medicine became the standard that other countries emulated. Despite the many problems inherent in the American healthcare system, droves of health professionals from other countries come to the United States every year to train and work, multiple foreign governments routinely study its models and approaches to medical care, and thousands of people from all over the world seek care in its facilities. These countries have borrowed American ideas regarding health insurance, information technology, and market competition. To them, the US healthcare system has a sterling reputation for having highly trained physicians, state-of-the-art medical equipment and facilities, high customer service standards, and expeditious access to treatment. Canada and Mexico, for example, provide a steady flow of patients to US hospitals and other providers.

Many parts of the world, such as Europe, Asia, and the Middle East, are a rich source of healthcare customers. The fast-growing economies and populations of China and India, for example, are creating a demand for health services that is exceeding these countries' ability to provide. Given the growth of the global economy and the sterling healthcare reputation of the United States, more and more American healthcare businesses are marketing to international consumers. American healthcare organizations that serve foreign nationals can benefit in a number of ways, such as

- attain national and international recognition;
- earn the loyalty of certain consumers from countries, regions, and referral sources;
- gain experience in treating medical cases of great severity and complexity; and
- receive maximum reimbursement.

These are strong incentives for healthcare providers to take advantage of medical tourism.

Medical tourism—now rebranded as *global medicine*—experienced substantial growth up through the first decade of the twenty-first century followed by a presumably temporary leveling off after 2010. In 2009, according

Medical tourism
The practice of traveling to another country to obtain medical care; also known as *global medicine*

to the Organisation for Economic Co-operation and Development (2011), Americans spent an estimated $600 on medical care overseas. This represented a 13 percent increase over the 2004 estimate. By the end of the 2000s, however, the worldwide economic downturn—coupled with the high cost of travel—slowed the growth of medical tourism. The industry also experienced some shakeout of competitors, leaving to the wayside those organizations less prepared to serve this market. (Medical tourism is discussed further later in this chapter.)

Establishing a Business or Partnership Overseas

Many US hospitals and health systems have developed institutional affiliations with facilities abroad or established independent operations in foreign countries. These relationships take a variety of forms—from a US organization's investment in a foreign-owned-and-operated healthcare system to a partnership between an American entity and a foreign entity to a US corporation's ownership of a facility or group of facilities abroad. Other forms of interaction include clinical consultation, organizational management consultation, architectural design and engineering, regulatory and accreditation support, and staff training and development.

Many US not-for-profits—including Johns Hopkins Medical Center, St. Jude Children's Research Hospital, and Harvard Medical School—have built healthcare facilities in South America, Asia, and the Middle East structured to resemble the hospitals and clinics in these countries. In addition, many large US for-profits—including HCA, Tenet Healthcare, Sun Healthcare, and Integrated Health Systems—have become multinational corporations (to some extent) as a result of expanding their holdings internationally. Some US companies have even been set up exclusively to establish American-style healthcare facilities overseas.

Other US healthcare organizations are discovering investment opportunities abroad. Health insurance, home health, and medical technology companies, for example, have experimented with exporting their expertise in exchange for new sources of revenue and growth. Another area of expansion involves the clinical trials for new drugs. The US pharmaceutical industry is increasing the proportion of its clinical trials conducted overseas to lower costs, expedite approval, and test the drugs in the countries where they will be sold. Approximately half of the industry's spending on human drug testing takes place outside the United States, with nearly 6,500 clinical trials underway overseas in 2008 (Bartlett and Steele 2011). This figure is 23 times the number conducted in 1990. Pharmaceutical companies can reportedly reduce human-testing costs significantly by conducting trials in Eastern Europe, Asia, and Central and South America. Some nations even request that drugs be tested on their populations before approving them for use.

Marketing US Healthcare Products Abroad

American companies have a long history of selling domestically produced healthcare products to other countries. With its strong manufacturing sector, the United States has produced the lion's share of industrial healthcare goods (e.g., medical equipment) and consumer healthcare goods (e.g., baby formula). The country also has been the world's largest producer of pharmaceutical products with $46 billion in drug exports in 2011 (BLS 2013). The share of products produced by American corporations is somewhat difficult to determine, however, because of the practice of outsourcing the production of "American-made" goods to foreign factories.

Overseas markets for healthcare products are considered attractive because of their high growth rates. For example, the demand for medical supplies in China and India is growing three times faster than the demand in countries with mature markets, such as the United States and most European countries. In the US market, competition is fierce and cost containment has driven down margins, but foreign markets are still relatively untapped and underserved.

Medical Tourism

Modern, state-of-the-art healthcare systems in Central and South America, Asia, and the Middle East are a relatively new phenomenon. These facilities were established primarily to meet the needs of increasingly affluent indigenous populations as well as wealthy medical tourists. Even "regular" consumers from abroad (those not necessarily wealthy) may appear attractive to these healthcare operations. Increasingly, US residents who want elective surgeries and procedures are considering and often choosing doctors, surgeons, medical facilities, and hospitals abroad, where costs are a fraction of the costs at home and the quality of care is the same or—some would argue—even better.

Medical tourism pairs a medical experience with sightseeing in a foreign country. This term is something of a misnomer, however, in that few medical tourists consider the recreational part to be as important as the clinical component. Thus, a more appropriate label for this activity might be "global medicine."

India is often considered the premier example of global medicine. It is known for its quality of care, relatively low prices, and the opportunity for a vacation for those who so choose. Private entities have established facilities to cater to foreigners, despite the fact that the country's own healthcare needs outstrip its capacity. Other countries that attract medical tourists include Singapore, Dubai, Thailand, Malaysia, Mexico, Costa Rica, Panama, and

Argentina. Some of these facilities may specialize in certain conditions or procedures, such as cardiac surgery, orthopedic surgery, and cosmetic surgery.

Expected Growth

Despite a recent slowdown in the level of activity, some important trends guarantee that the market for medical tourism will expand in the years ahead. First, patients on a waiting list for major surgery (e.g., organ transplantation) and living in countries with a national healthcare system are eager to take advantage of foreign healthcare options. Second, the health of more than 220 million aging baby boomers in the United States, Canada, Europe, Australia, and New Zealand is expected to decline in the near future; this will create a significant market for inexpensive, high-quality medical care. Other factors that will contribute to the rise of medical tourism are as follows:

- Massive investment in private-sector health infrastructure in certain developing countries, resulting in significant improvements in health standards and greater availability of the latest medical technology and treatments
- Increasingly prohibitive medical costs in many European and American countries (See Exhibit 12.1 comparing the costs of medical procedures in the United States with those in some countries abroad.)
- The growing level of expertise of doctors, nurses, and other medical support staff who have trained in some of the best centers in the world, coupled with the continuing shortage of primary care physicians and specialists in developed countries
- Deficiencies in the public health systems in many countries, including long delays for services and bureaucratic hurdles to obtaining care
- The positive experiences of US-based patients who have received excellent care overseas and experienced a level of personal service rare in the United States
- A well-organized medical travel industry supporting the development of attractive packages of services and amenities and offering extensive support for those interested in medical tourism
- For some patients, the opportunity to experience a foreign culture and visit tourist attractions

Misconceptions Concerning Medical Tourism

Marketers who promote medical tourism must address three common misconceptions. The first is that global medicine is something of a gimmick, that the idea of obtaining health services at a 30 to 80 percent discount seems too good to be true. Many people think that either the care will not be as good or the service will be provided in a primitive setting. These misconceptions suggest that many Americans are not familiar with other cultures and have a hard time believing that healthcare delivered elsewhere could be comparable to US healthcare, which they perceive to be the best in the world.

A second common misconception is that it is about fun and sun. In the early years, medical tourism was promoted by health travel brokers as getting cosmetic surgery (e.g., liposuction) for one day and then lying on the beach for the next ten days. This aspect is not touted as often today as the industry has matured. Instead, marketers and the media discuss the important issues of quality of care, clinical outcome, and personalized service.

A third misconception is that medical tourism outsources US services to foreign entities, siphoning off customers from American healthcare providers. In reality, facilities (whether or not established in partnership with US businesses) in Asia, South America, and the Middle East were not built to attract the medical tourists from the United States but rather those from Europe, the Middle East, and Africa.

Categories of International Medical Travelers

US customers who are interested in or become international medical travelers typically fall into one of four categories, most of which are financially driven. The first category comprises those who lack insurance coverage but need a major operation; this category is likely to change as a result of the implementation of the Affordable Care Act (ACA). A patient without insurance has to pay out of pocket for the required procedure, and going overseas could save the patient a tremendous amount as the costs are lower in foreign facilities. For example, by undergoing a total hip replacement in India rather than in the United States, the patient would realize $47,000 in savings—minus the cost of the trip (see Exhibit 12.1).

EXHIBIT 12.1 Comparative International Pricing by Procedure, 2013

Medical Procedure	Price (in US dollars)				
	United States	Colombia	Thailand	India	Mexico
Heart valve replacement	170,000	18,000	21,212	5,500	18,000
Coronary artery bypass graft	144,000	14,802	15,121	5,200	27,000
Gastric bypass	32,972	9,900	16,667	5,000	10,950
Hip replacement	50,000	6,500	7,879	7,000	13,000
Knee replacement	50,000	6,500	12,297	6,200	12,000
Facelift	15,500	5,000	3,697	4,000	4,900

Source: Data from Medical Tourism Association (2013).

The second category is composed of those who are underinsured; even with wider coverage under the ACA, many patients will still face significant uncovered costs. Despite having some level of insurance coverage, underinsured patients face high deductibles or are unable to pay for the portion of their medical expenses not covered by their existing insurance plan. As shown in Exhibit 12.1, if a coronary artery bypass graft costs $144,000 in the United States and insurance pays only 80 percent of the cost, a US patient will still owe $28,800; thus, the patient is better off undergoing this procedure in India, where the total cost for the procedure is $5,200.

The third category consists of those who are seeking elective surgery, following the example of Hollywood celebrities who routinely go abroad for cosmetic surgery. Because the US healthcare system does not consider elective procedures such as facelifts, tummy tucks, and hair transplants as medically necessary, patients have to pay for them out of pocket and thus look for alternative ways to cut costs—including medical tourism. Even some procedures that would improve mobility (e.g., correction of tennis elbow) may not be considered medically necessary if the person's functional limitation is not deemed to be significant.

The fourth and final category includes those who are seeking services not available in the United States—perhaps the most publicized of which are certain treatments for cancer. Some of these procedures may fail to meet US standards, while others may still be under review but will likely be approved at some time in the future. Although the use of such services involves some risks (e.g., lack of recourse in the case of malpractice), the potential risks do not appear to prevent thousands of healthcare consumers from taking advantage of treatments offered in other countries.

A new category may be composed of those who are being encouraged by their health insurance companies or employers to partake in medical tourism. US insurers that are at risk for the cost of care may profit from referring their plan members to overseas medical facilities; some even enter into formal relationships with foreign hospitals. Similarly, some employers—concerned about rising healthcare costs—are using financial incentives (e.g., subsidizing the cost of travel) to encourage employees to use less costly services abroad. This practice is especially common in large firms that self-insure and pay directly for their employees' medical expenses.

Some level of backlash has occurred in the United States in response to the increase in medical tourism. Realistically, the proportion of US healthcare consumers traveling overseas is still small, and American facilities have enough of a challenge dealing with existing patients. Employee unions have raised concerns over the fact that their members are encouraged by their health plans to go to foreign countries for care, which is in apparent violation of "buy American" restrictions. These types of reactions are to be expected as people adapt to the globalization of healthcare.

Keys to Successful Adoption

Consensus in the medical tourism industry points to four critical factors that make a health facility successful at attracting and effectively serving medical tourists. These healthcare organizations must do the following:

1. Assure prospective customers that the facility and the skill levels of its practitioners meet or exceed the standards in the country.
2. Partner with representatives in targeted countries who can help provide assurance and support to prospects.
3. Develop a complete package that addresses all aspects of the experience—travel documents, lodging and meals options, medical and cost information, rehabilitation needs, sightseeing services, financial aid or plans, and other resources.
4. Offer personalized, customer-focused attention.

Research suggests that 15 percent of Americans who received care overseas had less-than-positive experiences, a figure that would not be acceptable among US healthcare providers (*International Medical Travel Journal* 2011). Still, an 85 percent approval rating for services that have a lot of potential to go wrong does not appear unreasonable. With word of mouth being such a critical means of promoting medical tourism, healthcare organizations must strive to provide a positive experience every time.

Scarce Market Research Data

Limited research has been conducted on medical tourism, and few official statistics are available on the number of foreign nationals treated in US hospitals or the number of Americans who travel to facilities abroad for medical procedures. Some US healthcare organizations do track their international patients and study their characteristics and motives, but this information remains fragmented. Little progress has been made toward a national means of tracking these data.

The US federal government and certain trade organizations track the country's export of medical products to other countries. Some research companies study trends in the sale of US healthcare products around the world, and some associations (e.g., Medical Tourism Association) promote international medical travel and/or collect related data from their member organizations (e.g., Joint Commission International). Much of these data and information are collected at the country level and do not necessarily provide a comprehensive account of the actual volume of medical tourism. Even within a country, tracking all of the related activity is difficult.

The Applicable Four Ps

As noted in previous chapters, the four Ps of the marketing mix—product, price, place, and promotion—do not apply easily to traditional healthcare. Healthcare products, except for some elective procedures, are highly standardized. Healthcare price is so controlled by third-party payers that it seldom serves as a basis for differentiation between service providers. *Place* became more relevant in healthcare when providers started taking health services to where the customers live. Healthcare promotion is the most applicable to healthcare because most organizations must compete for customers.

The product dimension requires a tailored approach. Obviously, US-based healthcare systems want to package the product in a manner that reflects the high quality associated with US healthcare. Thus, these systems emphasize the use of state-of-the-art technology and assure consumers that only the most up-to-date treatment and diagnosis processes are used. Health facilities overseas, meanwhile, tout the personal attention and concierge services they offer that may be lacking from the US healthcare packages. Large tertiary medical centers and teaching hospitals always have a competitive advantage when it comes to the product, as do health systems that have built national and international reputations.

The price dimension is the most salient aspect in marketing to medical tourists. As noted, the primary draw of going abroad for a procedure—for US patients at least—is to take advantage of the lower overall cost. Of course, the price differential is meaningless unless the services are equivalent in quality and outcomes. Price may be an important consideration to patients from other countries as well, but price is not as paramount to them as the availability of these services. Foreign consumers—most of whom are well-to-do—are likely to pay any price just to receive the treatment, diagnosis, or procedure not offered in their own countries.

The place dimension is intrinsic to the concept of medical tourism. In this regard, the United States has an advantage over other countries for several reasons. First, the states and their many world-renowned attractions are desired destinations for foreign visitors. Second, major US cities, hubs, and ports make entering and leaving the country relatively easy. Third, the country is modern, diverse, and relatively safe and peaceful, which encourage medical tourists to feel welcome and relax. With civil wars, revolutions, or other military conflicts taking place in many parts of the world, healthcare facilities in other countries may highlight the hospitable setting in which a medical traveler can recuperate.

The promotion dimension (described in more detail later) of marketing for both US and foreign entities is similar. They all prepare standard promotional materials and present these promos at professional meetings and exhibitions. Beyond these basic activities, foreign-based facilities rely more heavily on word-of-mouth marketing than do US-based facilities. In addition, foreign healthcare organizations typically maintain an office and some agents in countries they are targeting; these agents serve as liaisons, informing prospective customers of the benefits of the facilities, their services, and traveling amenities. Of course, as with most aspects of healthcare today, the Internet has become the first promotion point for reaching potential customers.

Strategies and Techniques for International Healthcare Marketers

Whether an organization already enjoys a large base of international business or is currently building an international program, its success depends on a detailed business strategy and a solid marketing plan. World-class institutions do not have to advertise aggressively but can rely instead on their reputations and established brands to attract international referrals and customers. Small medical centers that are less well known (the bulk of the institutions in the United States) must make a greater effort to generate awareness and referrals to their programs and carve out a niche in the shadow of the established hospitals or systems.

The marketing strategy that an organization decides to pursue depends on the types of goods or services it offers and its location. Thus, the approach taken by US healthcare providers catering to medical tourists differs from the approach taken by overseas facilities soliciting Americans and customers from other countries.

Marketing staff of US healthcare organizations can capitalize on and promote the following attributes:

- *Brand recognition.* A highly revered, internationally popular name makes a facility prominent in the minds of potential customers and, perhaps more important, in the minds of opinion leaders in the target country. For example, Mayo Clinic has global brand recognition, serving patients from 150 countries.
- *Physician acclaim.* Although prospective customers may not be knowledgeable about individual physicians, their local medical

contacts might be. Doctors who have developed cures or treatments, who have won international awards or earned prestigious honors, who are leaders in their specialty, or who have a loyal following are highly sought after—especially by high-end, deep-pocketed customers.

- *Clinical expertise in a specialty.* When someone is considering treatment for a particular condition—such as cancer, heart disease, or liver disease—that person will think first of the provider (individual or organization) that is synonymous with that clinical area. For example, Johns Hopkins Hospital has consistently appeared at the top of *US News & World Report's* annual best hospital list. The hospital is well known for its expertise in five specialties: neurology; ear, nose, and throat; rheumatology, geriatrics; and urology.
- *Medical reputation.* US marketers can capitalize on the premium people from other countries place on all things American—including its high-tech, high-care, high-quality medical reputation.
- *Distinctive or unique assets.* As increasing numbers of competitors enter the global medicine arena, it will become important for a healthcare organization to differentiate itself from other players in the market. Medical specialty, building design and location, in-demand equipment or technology not widely available, amenities package, patented procedures, or innovative healing approaches—each serves as a point of differentiation and a competitive advantage.

In addition, US healthcare marketers might adopt one of the following strategic frameworks:

- *Relationship-based strategy.* This approach takes advantage of existing relationships between domestic health systems and foreign individuals, groups, and organizations. Ideally, a new facility abroad could be presented as a tangible extension of an existing relationship between health professionals.
- *Needs-based strategy.* This approach focuses on gaps in existing services in other countries and seeks to fulfill an unmet need.
- *Product-oriented strategy.* This approach emphasizes the expertise, high quality, and technological sophistication associated with US medicine and American-made healthcare products.
- *Partnering strategy.* This approach recognizes the importance of involving local entities to facilitate customers' entry into what they might perceive as an alien culture.

Marketers who work for foreign-based healthcare organizations may pursue one of these strategies:

- *Service-based strategy.* This approach emphasizes high-quality services that take advantage of the best specialists and the latest biomedical technology to provide a superior experience comparable to that provided in US medicine.
- *Price-based strategy.* This approach capitalizes on the significant cost differential between most foreign health systems and the US system and promises a level of quality that is equal or better.
- *Patient-centered strategy.* This approach emphasizes the personal attention accorded the customer who chooses to use a foreign-based healthcare facility, contrasting this approach to the more impersonal care often provided in US institutions.
- *Collateral benefit strategy.* This approach promises not only a positive healthcare experience but also an opportunity to experience a different culture.

Any international healthcare marketer must recognize that, for a marketing campaign to be successful, offering some information in another language on the organization's website does not suffice; the marketer must implement an integrated marketing strategy. Specifically, the campaign must include these activities:

- Design a website that provides a point of first contact; this contact then engages the customer from first exposure through completion of the treatment program.
- Employ experienced call center and support staff who can coordinate all aspects of a customer's care, including travel, cross-cultural considerations, and personal needs.
- Establish field offices and base sales representatives abroad to ensure continuity with marketing contacts and referral channel management.
- Offer tours to business, consumer, civic, and medical groups to showcase the facility and its services to potential healthcare audiences.
- Maintain relationships with physicians and other health professionals who are active in medical tourism circles; support exchange programs, mission trips, and educational conferences.
- Take advantage of relationships with medical schools and residency programs that train foreign physicians.
- Cultivate relationships with US companies that have overseas operations and with foreign companies that have US operations; these organizations could serve as venues for marketing to international customers and sources of referrals.
- Work with the health ministries of foreign governments, American embassies, and other overseas government offices to gain access to

referral lists and identify potential partners for ventures in other countries.

- Partner with organizations involved in international programs (e.g., Sister City programs) as well as the local chamber of commerce to promote hometown health facilities.
- Initiate carefully thought-out international advertising as part of a coordinated marketing and communications effort.
- Maintain ongoing public relations efforts to highlight recent successes, medical breakthroughs, new technology, and exceptional physicians.
- Maintain listings in international medical directories, both print and online, even if some cost is involved.
- Take advantage of social media to maintain a worldwide presence and real-time communication capabilities.

Case Study 12.1 provides an example of one country's global medicine marketing efforts.

CASE STUDY 12.1
Marketing Medical Tourism in Asia

In 2013, Ballistan—a fictional country based on a small Asian nation with a modern healthcare system and a strong economy—recognized that its healthcare system had features that would be attractive to medical tourists. The potential revenue that medical tourism could generate was large enough for the national government to take a vested interest in ensuring the success of this endeavor. To this end, Ballistan established an agency to attract international business and promote medical tourism. Funded by the national government, the agency was a ministry operated with the full cooperation of the country's healthcare organizations and directed by a high-ranking government official.

One of the first steps the agency took was to assess the current domestic need for health services and the availability of local facilities. It identified existing capacity, took an inventory of medical equipment, and determined the number and qualifications of existing clinical personnel. It also evaluated the system's ability to meet domestic needs and to serve an international clientele. Further, it estimated the size of the international market and calculated potential revenue.

Having determined that there was a large and growing market with substantial resources to spend on healthcare and that the system would be able to absorb a substantial number of international patients, the agency developed a multipronged marketing initiative. The first campaign raised awareness about available services for the countries that had the most potential customers (i.e., elsewhere in Asia, the Middle East, and the United States). The follow-up campaign promoted Ballistan and its healthcare resources. Related articles were written and published in newspapers, magazines, and journals. These print materials were supplemented by a website with interactive features, including not only a blog, a cost calculator, and a map of the country's health facilities but also colorful infographics about medical tourism. A Facebook page, a Twitter feed, an Instagram account, and other social media platforms were used to connect to prospects. Although some paid advertising was used, the agency felt that paid advertising was the least effective means of reaching the target population.

The agency put together comprehensive medical tourism packages with the help of the country's travel and hospitality industries. These packages had a fixed price and were all-inclusive, covering charges for air or train travel; room and board; medical, rehabilitation (if needed), and follow-up care; and local tours.

The agency installed liaison offices and staffs in several foreign countries to ensure that someone in-country was available to answer questions and coordinate arrangements for incoming customers. In addition, these satellite offices forged a relationship with medical practitioners in these countries to establish legitimacy and ensure a steady source of referrals. Negotiations were carried out with health insurance plans that agreed to refer some of their cases to these countries' practitioners.

In convincing potential customers to travel to Ballistan to obtain health services, the agency highlighted the following benefits:

- One fixed, competitive price
- State-of-the-art facilities staffed by English-speaking clinical experts who had been trained in the United States
- Care and services whose quality is equal to or better than that found elsewhere
- Personalized attention before, during, and after the treatment or procedure
- Various cultural and sightseeing opportunities available to visitors and their families

(continued)

The campaign to promote medical tourism in Ballistan was highly successful, particularly among consumers from the United States. People with medical needs or wants have been flocking to its cities since. Customers with commercial insurance have been able to cover either the full or partial cost of care, but those who pay out of pocket are delighted to pay only a fraction of what the same care would cost in the United States. Notably, the agency's market research revealed that a high number of these medical tourists were satisfied with the outcomes of care and the manner in which the services were delivered—a critical finding that marketers can use and considering the importance of word of mouth to growing medical tourism.

Case Study Discussion Questions

1. What prompted officials in Ballistan to consider entering the medical tourism business?
2. What steps were taken to identify the current status and future potential of medical tourism?
3. What factors encouraged government officials to develop a marketing campaign to attract medical tourists?
4. What marketing techniques did the agency use to promote medical tourism?
5. What role did relationship development play in implementing the promotional strategy?
6. How effective was the campaign to Ballistan's thriving medical tourism?

What Is Most Important to International Healthcare Consumers?

Different types of consumers have differing motivations when using new and innovative services. Both US- and foreign-based healthcare organizations have identified the following as prerequisites for attracting an international clientele:

- *Excellent care.* High-quality service is a must for those hoping to compete in this arena. Consumers will travel to another country for services only if they are assured that they will receive the best services possible and their needs will be fulfilled.
- *Physician skill set.* Most healthcare consumers, regardless of nationality, are looking for a physician who is capable of performing

the basics of the job, is knowledgeable, has good bedside manner, is willing to answer questions and explain procedures, and personally guarantees the customer's satisfaction. All of these signify that the doctor cares about the outcomes. This factor may be less important to US patients, who are not used to this consumer-driven orientation from clinicians.

- *Word-of-mouth reputation.* Word-of-mouth recommendations carry a lot of weight in the absence of objective information about a provider or an organization that has not yet established itself or built a good reputation. This type of publicity is essential in the marketing of an unfamiliar service.

- *Physician recommendation.* Most people are not likely to be familiar with the medical facilities—or even the world-class hospitals or centers—in another country. For this reason, few people will travel overseas for health services without a referral by a medical professional in their home country.

Summary

In the United States, globalization of healthcare began with the need to accommodate the growing foreign-born patient population and has been spurred by advances in communication technology, the growth in immigration, the success of multinational corporations, the expanding middle class worldwide, and high supply and low demand in the United States. Today, both lesser-known and world-class American medical facilities have established branches in foreign countries, and the flow of healthcare consumers across international borders continues. US healthcare organizations are competing for medical tourism revenues with foreign provider organizations that can deliver the same (or better) quality of care using advanced technology and highly trained physicians. In this global healthcare environment, organizations have to work harder to differentiate themselves and to understand the needs, wants, and expectations of medical tourists.

The approach marketers take to promote a medical tourism program depends on the organization's attributes and goals. For example, a US healthcare facility soliciting an Asian consumer's business would capitalize on the cachet of all things American, while a Thai facility soliciting an American consumer may tout its exotic but modern setting and its US-trained clinicians. Medical tourists, however, are attracted to a whole list of benefits, such as lower cost (for US consumers at least), attractive location, physician expertise, state-of-the-art technology, organizational brand, provider reputation, and a comprehensive package. Comprehensive packages that include the cost and arrangements for the clinical procedure, travel, lodging, sightseeing, and follow-up care are highly desired.

Despite the current political, military, societal, and economic turmoil in the world (which has reduced international traveling a bit), medical tourism is expected to continue to grow. Provision of outstanding medical care and sensitive service to patients, regardless of their nationality and location, is the most productive marketing strategy.

Key Points

- Healthcare has undergone globalization in much the same manner as have other industries.
- The Internet, computers, and other technologies have shrunk the world, so to speak, and made information more accessible. This has enabled healthcare consumers to cross healthcare borders as well.
- The populations served by US healthcare organizations over the years have become increasingly diverse. Some healthcare systems have catered to foreign-born patient populations for decades.
- As long as the US market for inpatient services remains flat, more attention is likely to be paid to the growing pool of patients in other countries.
- US medical supply and equipment companies, as well as pharmaceutical companies, have a long history of selling US healthcare products overseas.
- Foreign-based healthcare facilities have emerged primarily to address the needs of local and regional patients, but they also have a growing interest in international patients.
- Market research on international patients has been limited to date. There is a lot more to be learned about the subject. The more information marketers have, the more effective their promotion will be.
- Several countries in Asia, the Middle East, and Latin America have developed facilities (often with American input) to rival those in the United States and are attracting a worldwide clientele.
- Foreign health facilities compete in terms of price and quality and often distinguish themselves by emphasizing the personal service they provide.
- Product, price, place, and promotion have implications and applicability for medical tourism that are different from those for traditional US healthcare services.

- Both US- and foreign-based healthcare facilities should implement a multipronged marketing strategy that emphasizes personal interaction between health professionals and prospective patients.

Discussion Questions

1. What factors contribute to the globalization of healthcare?
2. What developments have allowed foreign facilities to compete with US facilities for customers, including US citizens?
3. What attributes of US facilities have historically attracted foreign customers?
4. What factors lead to Americans traveling abroad for medical care?
5. Does the migration of American medical tourists negatively affect the US healthcare system and economy? If so, how?
6. What factors should marketers be sensitive to when seeking to attract foreign patients to a US facility?

Additional Resources

Bartlett, D. L., and J. B. Steele. 2011. "Deadly Medicine." *Vanity Fair*. Published January. www.vanityfair.com/politics/features/2011/01/deadly-medicine -201101.

Bookman, M. Z., and K. R. Bookman. 2007. *Medical Tourism in Developing Countries*. Basingstoke, UK: Palgrave Macmillan.

Bureau of Labor Statistics. 2011. The Pharmaceutical Industry: An Overview of CPI, PPI, and IPP Methodology. www.bls.gov/ppi/pharmpricescomparison.pdf.

Derose, K. P., J. I. Escarce, and N. Lurie. 2007. "Immigrants and Health Care: Sources of Vulnerability." *Health Affairs* 26 (5): 1258–68.

International Medical Travel Journal: www.imtj.com

International Medical Travel Journal. 2011. "Medical Tourism: Trends for 2012 and Beyond." www.imtj.com/articles/2011/medical-tourism-trends/.

Medical Tourism: www.medicaltourism.com

Organisation for Economic Co-operation and Development. 2011. *Health at a Glance: 2011*. Paris: OECD.

THE MARKETING EFFORT

It is one thing to come up with a marketing idea but another to develop and implement a marketing plan or coordinate a marketing campaign. To carry out these activities, marketers must understand the entire marketing process and must exhibit campaign management skills. The chapters in Part IV address the nuts and bolts of organizing, developing, and implementing marketing initiatives. The marketing process is described from beginning to end, and the support activities that make effective marketing possible—such as market research, marketing planning, and marketing data management— are explored.

MARKETING MANAGEMENT

13

Numerous activities are involved in developing and implementing a marketing campaign. The process begins with a decision to carry out a marketing effort and ends with an evaluation of that initiative. This chapter provides a guide through the steps involved in this process. It identifies the players involved and describes the manner in which the many components of the process come together to create a marketing campaign.

The form that the marketing initiative takes depends on a number of factors. First, is the intent to develop a comprehensive plan or a specific marketing campaign? Second, is it supposed to represent an ongoing framework for various efforts or is it a one-shot campaign? Third, is it meant to influence the general public (or at least a broad swath of it) or a narrowly defined target population? The answers to these and more questions are reflected in the design of the marketing campaign.

Steps in a Marketing Campaign

Although circumstances vary from situation to situation, all marketing campaigns should operate under the assumption that the following conditions are in place:

- The organization is promoting well-defined products that lend themselves to marketing.
- The initiative fits within an established overarching strategic plan.
- Adequate information is available on the potential target audiences.
- The marketers have an in-depth understanding of consumer behavior.

Marketing is not an act, but a process. As such, it involves a series of activities or steps that are integrated and appropriately sequenced. These steps must be followed, regardless of who is responsible for the marketing function:

1. Organize the campaign.
2. Define the target audience.
3. Determine the marketing objectives.

4. Determine the resource requirements.
5. Develop the message.
6. Specify the media plan.
7. Implement the marketing campaign.
8. Evaluate the marketing campaign.

This section discusses each of these steps and considers their relevance for both plan development and campaign implementation.

Step 1: Organize the Campaign

The first step is the planning phase, the foundation on which the rest of the process is built. It typically involves pulling together appropriate personnel both inside and outside the marketing department. This team is responsible for conceptualizing the campaign. In general, marketers are not knowledgeable about a particular clinical area being marketed, so they need input from administrative and technical staffs. Further, whether the campaign is long-term or short-term, a campaign *champion*—someone who understands the value of and ideas behind the initiative and thus supports it in the face of obstacles and opposition from within the organization—must be identified.

To create an effective marketing plan, marketers must understand the problem being addressed, the audiences being targeted, and the environment in which the campaign will be implemented. Market research is used to analyze these factors and to develop a workable strategy for effecting behavior change. As noted earlier, marketers are assumed to already have a body of relevant knowledge on the service area and its population.

Step 2: Define the Target Audience

A marketing campaign has, at its core, the wants and needs of its consumers. As discussed in previous chapters, these wants and needs are determined through market segmentation analysis and market research, which identify the target audience and its thoughts, feelings, and behaviors about the service being offered. These methods include quantitative research (which generates objective data on the target population) and qualitative research (which provides insight into why people think what they think or do what they do). The actions taken to complete this step depend on whether an overall marketing plan or a specific marketing campaign is being pursued.

As noted previously, the healthcare marketer faces a challenge unknown to marketers in other industries. To wit, not all customers are created equal. Realistically, some have greater ability to pay for health services than others. Thus, any effort to identify a target audience for a marketing campaign must be tempered by the need to *not attract* certain types of customers. Obviously, this is a tricky situation because many healthcare organizations have a not-for-profit status that requires them to provide a certain amount of charity care.

Further, all hospitals and medical facilities are ethically required to treat any individuals who present themselves for care. While this is not always observed in actual practice, the marketer has to be aware of the danger of appearing to court some patients at the expense of others.

Step 3: Determine the Marketing Objectives

The objectives of a marketing plan should be determined within the broad context of the organization's strategic plan. If the focus is on a specific marketing initiative, the objectives that are set should be in keeping with those of the overall marketing plan. Here, as elsewhere, the objectives established should be specific, should include quantifiable concepts, and should be time limited. The marketing objectives should be based on the stage at which the consumers are located in the purchase decision-making process and/or the point in the product lifecycle at which the particular service is located. The introduction of a new innovative service illustrates both points—that no one is familiar with the new service and that everyone needs to be educated. At the same time, consumers are at the point of information search and nowhere near making a decision about utilization because they are as yet unfamiliar with the new service.

Step 4: Determine the Resource Requirements

A well-thought-out marketing budget is critical. The marketing budget is the section of the overall marketing plan or project plan that indicates projected revenues, costs, and profits. The marketing budget for a specific initiative should consider such direct costs as personnel expenses, market research costs, creative costs, production costs, media expenses, and other resource requirements. For initiatives built around advertising, media costs are likely to be the main expense and include the cost of advertising through various channels of communication, such as print, electronic, outdoor, and direct mail. The resources required for marketing include the dollars necessary not only for their direct contributions (e.g., creative development, media time) but also for personnel, production facilities, and other resources required to carry out the campaign.

Indirect costs may also be significant, although often difficult to determine. Even if the campaign is outsourced, the marketing agency requires some time with internal staff, and some overhead costs are involved. (Budgetary issues are covered later in this chapter.)

Step 5: Develop the Message

The message is a combination of symbols and words that the **sender** transmits to the **receiver**. It is typically based on the results of the research conducted in the planning stages of the campaign. The message embodies the campaign *theme*—the primary topic, motif, or idea around which a promotion is

Sender
In communication theory, the party that generates and disseminates a message to the target audience

Receiver
In communication theory, the target audience of a message

organized—as well as the campaign slogan that the sender wants the receiver to identify with the good or service.

The concepts and materials of a message are usually tested on a group of target consumers to learn how well they resonate and determine the best approach for achieving the campaign's objectives. Focus groups, consumer panels, and other methods can be used to test messages, materials, and proposed tactics. Marketers may have to go back and forth several times between development and testing before the message is finalized.

Positioning (the way in which the product is perceived by the target audience relative to similar products) concepts must be developed by the marketing staff and evaluated by members of the target audience. Generally, positioning is based on the product's key selling point(s). Marketers typically select the best positioning statement that emerges after testing different concepts in focus groups or in-depth interviews.

Using the information obtained from concept testing, marketers then create the "final" materials—such as slogans, posters, news clips, videotapes, brochures, public service announcements, and product packaging—and then test them through different executions. Members of the target audience can test the materials for memorability, impact, communication effectiveness, comprehension, believability, acceptability, image, ability to persuade, and other key attributes.

With printed materials, the readability of the text is crucial, particularly for audiences with low health literacy. Sentence length and the number of polysyllabic words should be checked, and word processing programs with built-in readability calculators can simplify this task. Readability testing is generally recommended for materials that include a lot of text, such as long print advertisements, brochures, and information kits. Asking health communication peers and representatives of intermediary organizations to review the text as well is often helpful.

Marketing brief
A short document that presents the specifics of a marketing campaign

After a certain point, marketers develop a **marketing brief** to present the specifics of the campaign (see Exhibit 13.1 for an example). A brief is essential if the organization is going to seek bids from external marketing agencies, as they base their proposals and presentations on the brief. Even if most aspects of the campaign are to be handled in-house, a brief is critical in getting every organizational stakeholder to buy into the initiative and its objectives.

Step 6: Specify the Media Plan

Campaigns differ in the extent they use media. Some initiatives do not even plan on a media component. However, even those that do not involve advertising are likely to distribute press releases or other communiqués that end up in the media (especially in the era of the Internet and social networking).

EXHIBIT 13.1
Developing a
Marketing Brief

A marketing brief contains the details of the campaign to the extent that they are known. The marketing sophistication of the healthcare organization determines the sophistication of its marketing brief. However, even a bare-bones brief gives a marketing agency (if the organization opts to hire an external firm) something to which it can respond.

A brief typically includes the following components:

- Description of the good or service to be marketed
- Situational information on the organization and the product
- Objectives of the marketing campaign
- Proposed marketing strategy
- Anticipated marketing budget
- Campaign timelines or target schedule
- In-house personnel involved and their potential contributions
- Planned methods of evaluating the campaign's effectiveness

An agency bidding for a campaign will address each of the components listed in the brief. It will offer insight into the marketing challenge, suggest creative and media strategies, indicate the control mechanism it will use, and show how it will assign responsibilities. Further, it will state the terms and conditions under which it will carry out the campaign.

Thus, a media plan is essential. The media plan outlines the objectives of the advertising campaign, the target audience, the media vehicles for reaching that audience, and the schedule for communicating the message.

The steps of the media planning process are as follows:

1. Define the objectives
2. Identify the audience
3. Establish a media budget
4. Evaluate media options
5. Select the type of medium
6. Determine the specific form of that medium
7. Negotiate media relationships
8. Develop the media schedule
9. Implement the plan
10. Evaluate the plan

This step applies more directly to a specific marketing campaign than to overall plan development. For example, if the intent is to advertise, the marketer needs to consider whether print or electronic advertisement will work best. If electronic, will radio, television, or the Internet be used? If television, will the advertisement appear on network or cable channels? If cable, which channel(s) and time slots will be appropriate?

In addition, the media plan must consider—and balance out—the reach, frequency, and waste involved. *Reach* refers to the number of people exposed to an ad. *Frequency* refers to the number of times a person sees the ad within a defined time frame. *Waste* refers to the number of people the ad reaches who are not part of the target audience. This last issue is particularly important in healthcare marketing, given that the healthcare organization may not want to encourage the patronage of patients with limited ability to pay for care.

Step 7: Implement the Marketing Campaign

Campaign implementation turns strategies and plans into actions to accomplish objectives. This is when the initiative is introduced to the target audience and when the process shifts from the planning function to the implementation function and from the concept people to the operational staff. (Note that marketing planning is different from other types of planning in that the same people are likely to be involved in both planning and implementation.) The implementation must be monitored to ensure that every element proceeds as planned.

A systematic implementation requires marketers to develop a project plan and an implementation matrix. The *project plan* details the steps in the process and the exact sequence they should follow. It also indicates the relationships between tasks and the extent to which completing some tasks is a prerequisite to accomplishing others. The *implementation matrix* lists every action and breaks down each action into tasks, if appropriate. For each action or task, the responsible party is identified, along with any secondary parties involved in the activity. Resource requirements (e.g., staff time, money) and the start and end dates for each activity are specified as well.

The resource requirements listed should be priced and combined to determine the total resource requirements of the campaign. This information feeds back into step 4, where required resources are estimated. Once identified, the extent of the resource requirements may have to be addressed in relation to available funds and any other fiscal constraints. (See Chapter 15 for an additional discussion of marketing plan implementation.)

Step 8: Evaluate the Marketing Campaign

Evaluation of the initiative should be top of mind from the outset of the process and, in fact, should be built into the process itself. Campaign evaluation should include ongoing monitoring, using benchmarks and/or milestones along the way. Although evaluation is important for all types of planning, it is particularly important in marketing planning. Because the objectives of a marketing campaign are usually highly focused and there is likely to be concern over the return on investment, measures of marketing effectiveness are essential.

Marketing campaigns may be evaluated using two types of techniques: process evaluation (or formative analysis) and outcome evaluation (or summative analysis, which is particularly important for the marketing process.) **Process evaluation** assesses the efficiency of the marketing effort, and **outcome evaluation** addresses effectiveness. Effectiveness can be measured in a variety of ways, and most campaigns involve more than one means of evaluation—particularly in healthcare, where the intangible benefits of a marketing initiative may be as important as the tangible benefits.

While the campaign is under way, process evaluation should take place intermittently during each step. It involves media monitoring and analysis as well as assessment of program activities. The key indicators to track include consumer knowledge of the product being marketed, advertising awareness and recall, attitudes and perceptions, images of the product and users, experience with the product, and behaviors (trial and repeat). The target audience should be asked specific questions about the product or campaign (on top of general questions about attitudes and behaviors regarding the marketing approach) to determine the message's level of penetration. For example, how many consumers can recall seeing the television commercial or reading the newspaper ad? How often have they seen it? What image did the ad convey? While some of these factors will be revisited during outcome evaluation, they serve as markers for process evaluation itself.

Outcome evaluation measures the extent to which the campaign induced the desired change (e.g., an increase in consumer approval or greater patient volume). Impact is often difficult to assess accurately, however. For example, can one public service announcement cause a drop in morbidity and mortality from heart disease? Probably not, but several such efforts may combine synergistically to become a contributing factor in health status improvement. Because campaigns are relatively short lived, the effect of a particular spot on overall trends cannot be determined. However, one can at least compare mortality and morbidity rates before and after the implementation of, say, a social marketing initiative.

When marketers seek mass media coverage for their promotional activities, they need to be able to evaluate the outcomes of these activities. The most effective way to determine media "hits" is by subscribing to a clippings service. In addition, a media monitoring service—Nielsen Audio, for example—may be used to track the frequency with which a program's public service announcements are broadcast on radio or to monitor television

Process evaluation
An assessment of how efficiently a marketing initiative is carried out

Outcome evaluation
An assessment of how effectively a marketing initiative reached its objectives

viewing patterns. Today, access to the Internet makes tracking media attention much easier, and monitoring social media activity has itself become a business (e.g., customscoop.com).

The most effective way of establishing a cause-and-effect relationship between healthcare marketing campaigns and changes in behavior and health outcomes is to conduct an intervention study in one or more communities, using matched communities as controls. Assuming that no significant differences exist between the intervention and control communities, marketing activities may be linked with precision and reliability to changes in the communities.

A factor that makes healthcare campaign evaluation particularly problematic is the difficulty of isolating the campaign's effects. In most industries, changes in knowledge, attitudes, or behaviors can be linked or attributed, with a certain level of confidence, to the introduction of a campaign. For example, an increase in the number of people signing up for the National Do Not Call registry is the direct result of a multichannel promotional effort. This is not typically the case in healthcare, because so many factors are at play that are outside the control of the marketer or even the healthcare organization. For example, a decrease in the number of obese children in one community does not necessarily mean that a hospital's family-fitness-and-nutrition campaign was effective, but rather it could be the result of a health insurance plan's new restrictions on coverage, inaccurate reporting, changes in the national body-mass-index standards, parental and/or physician interventions, school district incentives, competitors' weight loss programs, and so on.

Players in the Marketing Function

The extent to which staff members of the healthcare organization participate in the marketing function or a marketing campaign reflects the extent to which marketing is internalized within the organization. This participation influences how the marketing initiative is carried out. If the function is not internalized, an organization has a number of marketing arrangements options, each with different implications.

One option is to outsource the marketing function. Outsourcing was typical in the early years of healthcare marketing and is still common among small organizations—such as physicians' offices—that cannot support an in-house marketing resource. In this case, all of the activities related to the marketing process are handled by an external entity or entities. The process can never be fully outsourced, however; the organization still must provide information on the product to be marketed, offer feedback on marketing strategies, and approve the concepts and materials developed by the marketing agency. Even with totally outsourced marketing, the organization has to invest time, energy, and money in the process. For example, if key internal staff members have to spend two person-days explaining a complicated service to an external marketer, the organization incurs considerable direct and indirect costs. Unanticipated opportunity costs may also result when an organization diverts resources to participate in the marketing campaign.

A second option is to outsource most of the marketing function and carry out some activities in-house. Organizations that choose this arrangement typically have a marketing professional (a marketing director) on staff but no one else who can perform the required marketing tasks. In this case, the marketing director is responsible for coordinating the process and overseeing the tasks delegated to the contracted agency. Conversely, a large hospital may have full-time personnel to perform marketing tasks in-house but no formal marketing function. The in-house staff may consist of copywriters, designers or graphic artists, website developers, printers, and support personnel but no director to guide the work.

A third option is to occasionally farm out some aspects of the process that require specialized skills. For example, the in-house marketing department may not have the know-how or experience in negotiating media purchases or implementing a direct-mail campaign. Few organizations can support nearly all of the marketing tasks. Most multifacility health systems, for example, have a centralized marketing department. This department coordinates the marketing activities and ensures that all corporate entities convey a consistent message. Even these organizations, however, may rely on outside parties for certain specialized functions like film production.

The marketing process involves a variety of personnel and departments, depending on the extent of outsourcing. If marketing is fully internal, most of these marketing players are in-house. If it is partially outsourced, some are in-house and others are contractors. If it is entirely outsourced, nearly all are external.

This section discusses some of the entities involved in the marketing process.

Agencies

The term **agency** covers many different entities in the marketing industry. It could refer to a full-service marketing firm; specialty shop; à la carte operation; or any other entity that offers the creative, production, media, account management, or planning services needed to support marketing. It could even apply to an in-house group that carries out agency functions. Although an agency may be referred to informally as an *advertising agency*, it usually provides a wide range of services beyond generating ads. A full-service agency delivers start-to-finish marketing; a specialty agency performs a certain function like social media branding or Internet marketing; and an *à la carte*

Agency
An independent organization that supports one or more marketing functions on behalf of a client

agency offers an on-demand menu of services customized for the client and provided by separate, independent sub-agencies.

Some of the functions that marketing agencies perform are as follows:

- Plan marketing campaigns
- Design creative components
- Schedule and buy media
- Design and produce promotional materials
- Provide administration and accountancy functions
- Implement marketing campaigns
- Monitor and evaluate marketing campaigns

Choosing the appropriate agency is an important step and thus should not be taken lightly. Healthcare organizations that want to outsource all or some of their marketing functions must conduct meaningful research on available options. Exhibit 13.2 presents guidelines for selecting an agency.

Clients

The healthcare organization is typically the *client* in the marketing process. If the marketing function is internal, the client is typically another department in the organization. The client should not be considered a passive customer and should play an important role in the following:

- Stating the justification for the marketing campaign
- Selecting and briefing the marketing agency
- Providing input into and approving campaign plans
- Integrating promotional planning into marketing planning
- Evaluating and controlling the campaign
- Financing the campaign

Media Suppliers

Media supplier
An entity that provides communication channels for marketing campaigns

Media suppliers include commercial television companies, commercial radio companies, newspaper and magazine owners, creators of posters and other artwork, and other organizations that make media available to the campaign. A complex marketing campaign may require the marketing team to coordinate the activities of a variety of media suppliers.

Promotional Materials Suppliers

A number of other specialty suppliers exist, including printers, promotional gift makers, exhibition organizers, and corporate event planners. These specialty services are bought directly by client companies or managed through the advertising agency.

EXHIBIT 13.2
Guidelines
for Selecting
a Marketing
Agency

Many healthcare organizations and their staffers have limited experience dealing with—let alone searching for and then hiring—marketing agencies. Although much of the decision involved in selecting an agency is a matter of common sense, the unique aspects of healthcare make this decision a critical one. Following are some suggestions that may help in this regard.

- *Prepare to engage in an informative discussion with prospective agencies.* The client (the organization), at the very least, must be able to describe the product to be marketed, articulate the ultimate goal of the campaign, and talk about other organizational components involved. Some health professionals might argue that they know little about marketing and thus rely on the agency to propose guidelines for the campaign. Even so, the client should drive the marketing process and be able to ask and answer any pertinent questions from agencies.

  Specifically, the client should present prospective agencies with a marketing brief. This brief, as discussed earlier, contains situational details, objectives, proposed strategy and tactics, target market data, budget and time frames, and evaluation plans. Conversely, the client should request qualified agencies to present their credentials—including examples of current or past projects and descriptions of staff or company experience and capabilities—and other information for the client's review.

- *Consider only agencies that have experience in healthcare marketing.* Remember that the healthcare marketing function is different from that in other industries. If an agency does not understand how healthcare operates, the likelihood that it will cause a highly visible marketing gaffe is great. In addition, the client is very likely to spend precious time and use busy staff members to explain basic concepts about health services, payers, and regulations to an uninformed marketing professional.

- *Seek agency recommendations from other healthcare organizations.* Healthcare organizations tend to be followers rather than leaders, and in this situation it is warranted because so few agencies have healthcare experience. Approaching tried-and-true agencies is more beneficial than vetting inexperienced ones. The client should solicit ideas and recommendations from other organizations because their positive previous experience with an agency may be the best indicator that the agency could work well with the client.

(continued)

Considering several qualified agencies before selecting the best one is ideal. However, given the nature of healthcare and the services being marketed, this practice seems like a waste of everyone's time. Nine times out of ten, the healthcare client does not need the best agency but a good one that can meet its needs. Here again, recommendations from other organizations ought to assist in the decision. Because healthcare marketing resources are likely to be limited, the client should broach the topic of costs as soon as possible.

- *Develop an agency want list.* Some of the traits a healthcare client should want (maybe even require) from an agency include
    — an understanding of the client's product and market,
    — strong research and planning skills,
    — knowledge of the current media landscape,
    — creativity,
    — adequate internal resources, and
    — ability to develop effective campaigns.

  For health professionals in particular, the agency must be "easy" to work with. Easy, in this case, means the agency's willingness to accommodate the constraints of healthcare marketing, to be considerate of the time demands on health professionals, and to appreciate the client's overall mission.

  Some agency characteristics may be more important in healthcare than in other industries. A number of concerns apply here. One is how the agency's culture and management style (which are typically corporate or business driven) might fit with that of the client (which are typically nonprofit and service oriented). Another is the potential conflicts that might exist between the client's business and the business of the agency's other clients. For example, a hospital that incurs significant costs as a result of treating smoking-induced health problems may not find a comfortable fit with an agency that promotes cigarette manufacturers.

- *Negotiate contractual terms.* A variety of factors must be considered in developing the project budget, and this net should be widely cast. The client needs to be aware of any hidden costs, especially if it is new to the marketing arena. Agencies without healthcare experience may assume that all organizations already know about hidden or unanticipated expenditures, but that may not be the case with healthcare entities (which cannot easily adjust their budgets). The contract should cover not only the amount of remuneration but also the terms and timing of payments, issues of nonperformance and termination, and ultimate decision-making authority. In most cases, a confidentiality agreement is also a critical component of the contract.

Marketing Consulting Firms

Marketing consulting firms vary in the services they offer. Some handle one or a few specialty services (e.g., market research, media planning, evaluation), while others perform a comprehensive set of activities. Their input may be narrow (e.g., providing a targeted mailing list) or broad (e.g., determining the overall strategic plan).

For a healthcare organization that is new to marketing, hiring a consulting firm should be a foremost consideration. Such a firm will help the organization understand its marketplace, marketing planning capabilities, evaluation skills, and ability to marshal the various resources required for a marketing campaign.

Marketing consulting firm
An external agency that provides various services to support an organization's marketing function

Departments in the Marketing Function

Even if the healthcare organization outsources its entire marketing function or a marketing campaign, it should familiarize itself with the common departments of an agency. This section briefly describes the responsibilities of each department.

Creative

The **creative department** houses the "idea people" who write the words (or copy), design the visuals (e.g., pictures, logos, spatial and color placement), and conceptualize all the artistic elements of a campaign or brand. Slogans, promotional websites, catalogs and brochures, jingles, print and electronic posters, interactive computer games and apps, product labels, viral images and videos, TV and radio commercials, and multimedia displays are just among the myriad creations of this department. Typically headed by an art or a creative director, this influential department employs both full-time and freelance copywriters, web designers, graphic artists, and other professionals with relevant skills and training. It works closely with the production department (either in-house or contract) to bring some aspects of its artistic vision to fruition.

Creative department
The function that generates ideas for a campaign and translates them into words, images, and other artistic content

Production

The production department is responsible for producing the creative department's ideas, whatever form they may take. Its tasks range from laying out posters to printing catalogs to photographing a scene to filming a video that features musicians or actors to building a website. Like media buying, production is difficult and expensive to fully implement in-house because of the specialized equipment and expertise the function requires.

Media Planning and Buying

Media planning and buying department
The function that researches, selects, and negotiates with media channels to increase a campaign's media exposure

The dual job of determining media needs and negotiating for ad placement is an industry in its own right. This area is fairly specialized and thus may be difficult to effectively bring in-house. The **media planning and buying department** knows the landscape and makes arrangements for the most suitable type of medium, the best time slots, and the fairest prices for all forms of advertisement. The more central media are to the campaign, the more important this function becomes. If most of the marketing eggs for a particular campaign are placed in the advertising basket, then identifying the appropriate medium, determining how to best use it, and negotiating a favorable contract are critical tasks.

Account Management

Account management department
The function that interacts and builds a relationship with a marketing client throughout a campaign

The **account management department** consists of account managers, each of whom serves as the primary contact for an internal or external client during a marketing campaign. Account managers attend all planning meetings, write activity reports, coordinate tasks, present market research findings, and communicate feedback or comments to their clients. They are ultimately responsible for the client's satisfaction with the agency or the process.

Traffic

Traffic department
The function that delivers promotional content to the appropriate media channels on time

The **traffic department** is responsible for delivering the copy, image, film, audio, poster, and other promotional content to the media channel (e.g., radio station, movie or television studio, website, publishing office, printer) on time. When the campaign is distributed through multiple types of media, traffic coordination becomes complicated, requiring several modes of transmission or transportation.

Marketing budget
The itemized allocation of financial resources to the department or a campaign

Marketing Budget

Budgeting is tricky in marketing because all the costs of achieving marketing objectives can be difficult to determine accurately and fully. Numerous factors affect the **marketing budget**. Many of them are obvious, but others are not and thus may be overlooked by those not familiar with marketing planning. In addition to direct costs, indirect costs and opportunity costs are likely to be incurred.

Two types of marketing budgets need to be set: annual and campaign specific. The annual budget comprises the expected expenditures for the entire fiscal year on *all* marketing activities. The campaign-specific budget includes the expected expenses for just one campaign. The cumulative campaign budgets for the year should approximate the annual budget amount. Both budgets help in

- setting milestones for accomplishing tasks;
- putting all activities in financial terms;
- keeping activities on budget;
- motivating staff members to control their spending;
- making managers accountable for their actions;
- communicating objectives; and
- increasing coordination among all business units, departments, and relevant staff members.

In general, a healthcare organization or an agency budgets for the following marketing expenses:

- Salaries and benefits for marketing personnel
- Market research
- Creative development
- Production of promotional materials
- Printing (if applicable)
- Postage (if applicable)
- Promotional giveaways (if applicable)
- Media time/space purchase
- Evaluation

Expenses that are indirectly attributable to a campaign may include the following:

- Administrative (management, secretarial, accounting, and other similar services):
  — Salaries of directors, managers, and office staff
  — Rent and associated costs
  — Insurance

- — Telephone and postage
- — Printing and stationery
- — Heating and lighting
- Distribution and selling:
  - — Salaries of marketing and sales directors and managers
  - — Salaries and commissions of sales staff
  - — Travel and entertainment used by salespeople

As noted in previous chapters, nonmarketing staff devote a considerable amount of their time working with marketing personnel to develop the marketing plan or marketing campaign. As a result, the organization not only incurs direct costs of nonmarketing staff's involvement in the marketing function but also experiences considerable disruption in its operations.

Other factors that could affect the size of the marketing budget include the following:

- Geographic market to be covered
- Type of product (e.g., industrial, consumer durable, consumer convenience items)
- Distribution of consumers
- External factors (e.g., competitors' promotional budgets)

Return on Investment

Return on investment (ROI)
The value and benefit received in exchange for the resources given

Healthcare administrators have been concerned about the costs and perceived benefits of promotional activities since marketing was introduced into healthcare. Of particular concern is the **return on investment (ROI)** for marketing dollars. This concern heightens when a national economic downturn (such as the 2007–2009 Great Recession) is heaped on the ongoing financial pressures facing healthcare organizations. In fact, the 2013 results of the annual survey by the American College of Healthcare Executives (ACHE) indicate that finance-related challenges have been top of mind for hospital and system leaders for a decade now. The report listed the first few financial issues in order of importance: government funding cuts; problems with Medicaid and Medicare reimbursement; bad debt; decreasing inpatient volume; and increasing costs for staff, supplies, and other necessities (ACHE 2013).

ROI is the value received in exchange for the marketing dollars and other resources invested. It is typically calculated as a percentage return on the use of specific assets (financial or otherwise). Consider, as an example, the concept of depositing money in a bank account and receiving interest for that deposit. If the annual interest rate paid by the bank is 5 percent, a deposit of $100 accrues $5 in interest by the end of the year. Thus, the ROI is 5 percent.

Of course, ROI calculation is much more complicated in healthcare marketing. For example, consider the ROI of a direct-mail campaign for an urgent care center. Here, ROI is calculated by subtracting the direct costs of implementing the campaign (e.g., advertising agency fees, printing charges, postage and handling expenses) from the value gained from the campaign (e.g., revenue increase, patient volume growth). Thus, if the campaign cost $10,000 and generated $20,000 in new business, the ROI is 100 percent. Remember that, in some cases, the return may be less than the investment, resulting in a negative ROI. This straightforward example, however, involves a number of ambiguities and thus reflects the complications of determining the ROI in an actual healthcare setting.

First, the calculation includes the direct costs but not the total investment, including indirect costs. Indirect costs are expenses associated with market research previously conducted, the time and salary of staff who worked with the agency to design promotional materials and profile the target audience, the time of staff who evaluated the effectiveness of the campaign, the overhead of the office space and equipment used, and so on. Typically, the full costs allocated to a campaign greatly exceed the direct costs.

Second, the time frame in which the ROI should be calculated is not defined. Should the marketer wait to measure changes in revenue or other proxy of revenue until the end of the campaign, do so regularly during the campaign, or allow some time to pass after campaign implementation? The latter suggests that the promotional piece will likely attract only a few consumers immediately after the mailing, but it could spread and attract more people nine months down the road and thus its effect might be better measured then.

Third, the ROI of a healthcare marketing campaign is difficult to isolate. If the urgent care center recorded an increase in revenue after the direct-mail campaign, how much of that increase could be attributed to the campaign? Many factors influence a healthcare consumer's choice of a provider (and thus patient volume and revenue), such as changes to health plan provisions, an increase or a decrease in competition, or even demographic changes within the service area.

The indirect benefits of a marketing campaign are additional factors to consider in calculating ROI in healthcare. At first, the urgent care center may concede that, at best, it will break even as a result of the campaign. However, in looking at the bigger picture, the hospital that owns the urgent care center may be counting on the facility to make referrals to hospital specialists, which would result in subsequent hospital admissions by these specialists. Thus, a considerable amount of time may pass before the effects of the campaign unfold. Case Study 13.1 illustrates ways in which ROI might be determined for a marketing campaign.

In summary, the following factors affect the marketer's ability to calculate ROI in healthcare:

- Often, significant time elapses between implementation of a marketing campaign and utilization of the service promoted in the campaign.
- Routine checkups aside, most utilization of services is not planned but is a spontaneous response to an unanticipated event.
- The accounting systems many healthcare organizations use are not designed to generate the type of data necessary to accurately measure ROI.
- Healthcare marketers typically have limited knowledge of financial management and accounting systems.
- Because of the complexity of healthcare, the impact of marketing on operations and utilization is almost impossible to isolate.
- Healthcare involves so many intangibles that traditional measures of ROI may not be applicable.

Marketing Management

Marketing management is an art and a science and is particularly challenging in healthcare (see, for example, Kotler and Keller 2011). It can be defined as the analysis, planning, implementation, and control of programs designed to create, build, and maintain beneficial exchanges with target buyers for the purpose of achieving organizational objectives; in short, it is about overseeing the marketing process from start to finish. Control includes, among other things, measuring and evaluating the results of marketing strategies and plans.

Strong marketing management is particularly important in healthcare because most organizations have limited marketing experience. They often have diffuse objectives and a range of customers, and they may have a variety of stakeholders with competing agendas. Because healthcare administrators may be skeptical about the efficacy of marketing, strong controls are required.

The negative potential of marketing is also a growing concern in healthcare. Organizations must be careful not to convey the wrong image or appear to be recklessly expending resources on marketing. The damage done by a poorly conceived, targeted, or implemented campaign may be hard to rectify.

CASE STUDY 13.1
Measuring ROI for a Marketing Campaign

Southwest Regional Medical Center (SRMC) believed it could boost its orthopedic presence by establishing a service line called the Orthopedics Center of Excellence. To support the center, SRMC recruited three new physicians; bought state-of-the-art equipment; renovated a nursing unit; added nurses and technicians; developed a dedicated web page and linked it to the enterprise website; conducted educational programs for referring physicians; made sales calls to primary care physicians; published articles in local publications; and advertised on radio, on television, in newspapers and magazines, and on the Internet and social media. The total investment in the first year for programmatic changes and marketing was $1.6 million.

To determine ROI for the center, SRMC compared the increase in the center's first-year income with the incremental revenue the orthopedics services generated. In the 12 months before the center was established, orthopedics-related services generated $4.5 million in net revenue. In the 12 months after the center's launch date, the center generated $7.9 million in net revenue. On the basis of incremental gain and net revenues, SRMC realized ROI of 76 percent. This figure assumes that the gain resulted from the center's creation and would not have occurred otherwise.

Some argued that, in addition to direct investment in the service line, indirect contributions (e.g., spillover services provided by other departments) should be figured into the calculation and added to the total cost. SRMC's administrators asked the marketing team to isolate ROI for the programmatic investments and marketing expenditures. The team found this task to be extremely difficult, given the extent to which the different aspects of the service line were intertwined. The marketing team determined that it would need to employ more sophisticated accounting processes to factor out ROI for specific components of the service line.

This case highlights the potential pitfalls of taking ROI analysis too far. Calculating ROI for the entire investment makes sense, but attempting to calculate ROI for every individual element probably does not. SRMC concluded that its evaluation efforts would be better spent developing other indicators of tangible and intangible benefits of the service line initiative, such as the public's top-of-mind awareness of the center, new referral sources, consumer inquiries, and so forth. Although

(continued)

SRMC was pleased with the overall ROI generated through enhanced operations and the multipronged marketing effort, it was justifiably cautious about carrying ROI analysis too deep into the program.

Case Study Discussion Questions

1. What factors influenced SRMC to consolidate its orthopedic services under the service line model?
2. What programmatic changes were made to establish the center?
3. What marketing options could SRMC have considered, and why do you think it chose the options it did?
4. Aside from net revenue, were there other tangible and intangible measures that SRMC could have used to evaluate the campaign?
5. What caveats must be observed when trying to isolate ROI for program components?

Marketing management has two aspects: (1) managing the process (e.g., forecasting, planning, monitoring, and controlling) and (2) managing the people inside and outside the organization who are involved in the process. The first aspect emphasizes oversight of the structures and resources that support and carry out the functions of the marketing campaign. The second aspect focuses on the direct management of the personnel who perform these functions. Neither of these aspects is likely to be in place in most organizations, but they are both necessary for marketing to be integrated into the corporate structure.

Marketing management usually is better carried out by a marketing consulting firm or a full-service agency. While specific aspects of a campaign may appear doable, the absence of an overarching management entity could lead to a marketing disaster.

Summary

Many steps are involved in developing and implementing a marketing campaign. This process begins with a decision to embark on a marketing initiative and ends with the evaluation of that effort. The extent to which the staff members of the healthcare organization are involved in the process depends on the extent to which the marketing function is internalized.

A healthcare organization has a number of options when faced with having to perform marketing, ranging from total outsourcing to developing the full range of marketing capabilities in-house. Each option has different implications. The organization's circumstances determine the extent to which these tasks are internalized. The extent to which the process is incorporated into the operations determines the amount of control and responsibility the organization retains. Even in the case of an outsourced marketing function, staff can expect to spend substantial time interacting with marketing personnel.

The marketing function and campaign involve a variety of personnel and departments, depending on the extent of outsourcing involved. Health professionals and organizations should become familiar with marketing agencies, marketing consulting firms, and marketing departments and their responsibilities. Every marketing initiative requires interaction with at least some of these entities.

Managing a campaign requires coordinating a sequence of activities; this includes establishing a planning team (and identifying a champion), defining the product, identifying the target audience, specifying marketing objectives, and developing a marketing strategy. Subsequent steps include developing the message and identifying the mechanism for delivering it. Finally, the marketing concept needs to be pretested and modified as appropriate before the campaign is implemented.

Evaluating the marketing initiative should be top of mind from the outset of the process and, in fact, should be built into the process. There are two primary evaluation functions: process evaluation and outcome evaluation. Both have a role to play in the project, although outcome evaluation is particularly important in that it assesses how the campaign induced the desired change.

The organization sets two kinds of marketing budget: an annual budget for the general function and a campaign-specific budget for a single initiative. Both budgets should consider direct, indirect, and hidden costs. In healthcare, indirect costs are often significant, especially if personnel are pulled away from their core functions to work on the marketing campaign, thereby disrupting the regular operation of the organization.

Campaign effectiveness can be measured in a number of ways. Most projects need more than one means of evaluation—particularly healthcare projects, in which evaluation of the intangible benefits of a campaign is often as important as evaluation of the tangible benefits. The ability to measure ROI has become increasingly important in today's financially challenged environment. Healthcare marketers must be able to demonstrate the value and benefits (both tangible and intangible) that result from marketing activities.

Key Points

- The marketing of any product is not a single activity but involves a complicated set of sequential activities.
- Healthcare organizations have a variety of marketing options—from outsourcing the entire function to developing an in-house capability to outsourcing certain aspects of the function. Because the organization's staff must be involved in designing and implementing a marketing campaign, the function can never be fully outsourced.
- The eight steps in a marketing campaign include organizing the campaign, defining the target audience, determining the marketing objectives, determining the resource requirements, developing the message, specifying the media plan, implementing the marketing campaign, and evaluating the marketing campaign.
- During the implementation step, the marketer should develop a project plan to integrate the disparate activities of the campaign and an implementation matrix to facilitate the effort.
- Campaign evaluation is an important but often neglected aspect of the marketing process.
- Process evaluation assesses the campaign's efficiency, while outcome evaluation assesses the campaign's effectiveness.
- The healthcare organization and health professionals must interact with a variety of marketing personnel and departments, so they must familiarize themselves with these players' responsibilities.
- An in-house marketing function should have capabilities that are similar to the departments of a marketing agency or consulting firm.
- The marketing budget—whether for the overall marketing function or for a particular campaign—should be carefully thought out and managed.
- Marketing activities typically involve considerable direct, indirect, and hidden costs.
- Marketers should be familiar with the concept of calculating ROI and the factors that could affect ROI.
- Marketing management involves managing both the marketing process and the people involved in this process.

Discussion Questions

1. Why is the careful planning of a marketing campaign considered so important?

2. What is a marketing brief, and why is it important to the marketing process?

3. What role might the marketing agency play in developing and implementing the marketing plan?

4. How active a role should the healthcare organization play in the marketing process if the actual marketing is outsourced?

5. What departments are usually included in a marketing function, and what responsibilities do they have?

6. What indirect costs must an organization factor into its marketing budget?

7. Why is strong marketing management probably more important in healthcare than in other industries?

8. In what ways are process evaluation and outcome evaluation in healthcare somewhat different from those in other industries?

9. Why should marketers use a variety of means to evaluate a marketing campaign? To evaluate different marketing techniques?

10. Why is measuring ROI more of a challenge in healthcare than in other industries?

Additional Resources

Marketing Management: www.ama.org/publications/MarketingHealthServices /Pages/About.aspx

Armstrong, J. S. 2000. "How to Select an Advertising Agency: A Structured Approach." http://advertisingprinciples.com/evaluate-proposals#sthash .Kwpm6F2x.dpbs.

Boundless. 2013. "Create a Media Plan." www.boundless.com/marketing /advertising-and-public-relations/the-advertising-campaign/create-a-media -plan/.

Lake, L. 2013. "Understanding the Media Buying Process Step-by-Step." http:// marketing.about.com/od/plantutorialsandsamples/a/mediabuying.htm.

Weinberger, R. 2003. "These Five Steps Can Lead to a Successful Marketing Campaign." www.bizjournals.com/boston/stories/2003/09/01/smallb2 .html?page=all.

CHAPTER

14

MARKETING RESEARCH

Any marketing effort inevitably involves marketing research (also called *market research*). It encompasses market, product, pricing, promotional, and distribution research, and its purpose is to identify the nature of the product to be marketed, the characteristics of consumers, the size of the potential market, the nature of competitors, and other relevant factors. This chapter discusses the marketing research process and its role in healthcare.

The Scope of Marketing Research

Those who remember past attempts to introduce marketing research into healthcare would be impressed by the breadth of today's healthcare marketing research. The scope of research broadened just as health professionals expanded their narrow (and naïve) perception of marketing as merely advertising. In the past, a qualified researcher needed to be only somewhat familiar with demographic data and able to conduct a patient satisfaction survey. That is no longer the case, however; modern researchers now have to know the extensive array of tools, techniques, and technology needed to carry out a broad range of research activities. Researchers today are asked to address issues that would have been considered beyond their expertise and purview decades ago.

Marketing research is intended to answer a range of questions, from a focused query such as "How will customers react if we raise our monthly fitness program fee from $40 to $60?" to a diffuse query such as "How will the integrated delivery system planned by a competitor affect our market share?" Research is expected to contribute to various narrow and broad marketing functions, such as the following:

- Determining the appropriate location for a facility
- Identifying employers' needs for the healthcare of their employees
- Discovering whether a particular market could support a certain service
- Evaluating the level of demand among providers for a new type of equipment

- Measuring patient or customer satisfaction with a health plan or service
- Identifying appropriate market niches for a facility in a highly competitive market
- Ascertaining the potential business for a national chain on the local level
- Discerning the types of services desired by a community
- Determining the size and characteristics of the audience amenable to marketing
- Determining the impact of the Affordable Care Act (ACA) on the local market

Today, it seems that most (if not all) components of healthcare can benefit from the application of marketing research. Exhibit 14.1 presents contemporary examples of healthcare marketing research initiatives.

Related Changes

The expansion of the scope of healthcare marketing research brought about changes in other related activities. First, the "customers" for marketing research have grown in number and type. Historically, the main users of health-related data and information have been hospitals, health systems, and some for-profit entities (e.g., pharmaceutical companies). Today, any group that provides or is involved in direct patient care—such as clinics, physician practices, home health agencies, urgent care center networks, and managed care organizations—can be considered users.

Demand for market data has soared; for example,

- human resources departments need information on the future labor pool,
- finance departments need demand projections to forecast future revenue,
- managed care departments need detailed data to negotiate contracts with employers,
- patient care departments need anticipated future volumes for planning purposes,
- facilities planning departments need future demand estimates to allocate floor space appropriately, and
- physician relations departments need information for medical staff development purposes.

Second, the scope of strategic planning has broadened. Gone are the days when marketing research focused primarily on measuring the corporate

EXHIBIT 14.1
Healthcare
Marketing
Research
Vignettes

The following are snapshots of the types of research activities undertaken in today's healthcare environment.

Identifying Unmet Healthcare Needs

To plan its services, a faith-based clinic engaged a market researcher to identify segments of the population affected by untreated health problems. The researcher collected demographic data and health-related statistics on the service area to identify high-risk populations and their healthcare needs. On the basis of this information, the researcher determined the level of health problems among the sample and the extent to which the problems were being treated. (Today, of course, the impact of the ACA would have to be taken into account.)

Evaluating a Market's Potential

A clinical psychologist was interested in establishing an outpatient eating disorders program. She engaged a marketing researcher with expertise in behavioral health to explore the market potential for such a program. The researcher identified the characteristics of the people most likely to be affected by eating disorders, developed an estimate of the number of potential cases in the community, and assessed the strength of competitor programs.

Monitoring Changing Market Characteristics

Physicians in an obstetrics/gynecology practice noticed a decrease of younger obstetrics patients but an increase in older gynecologic patients, so the practice engaged a market researcher to identify the reasons. The researcher found that the community demographics was changing along with the national trends: The birth rate among people of child-bearing age (millennials)—within the community and nationally—was the lowest in decades, and more aging baby boomers were moving into the practice's service area. The researcher provided the information that helped the physicians determine the feasibility of switching from an obstetrics-oriented to a gynecology-oriented practice.

Conducting a Feasibility Study

Many members of a hospital's medical staff had relocated to a distant suburb to take advantage of an emerging market there. The hospital's administrators began to consider establishing a satellite facility there, so they requested the market research department to assess the feasibility of this idea. Using computer-based algorithms to project demand,

(continued)

the researchers were able to determine the numbers and types of physicians this population required and the potential business a new facility could bring in.

Predicting the Changing Demand for Inpatient Care

The inpatient census at one hospital had been steadily declining, and some nursing units had already been closed. The hospital's administrators wondered whether the downward trend would be short term or the "new normal," so they engaged the market research department to review past utilization patterns. The data indicated a short-term decline in inpatient demand but projected a steady increase in the near future as the population ages and develops chronic conditions.

Determining a Social Media Tactic

A local public health agency wanted to use social media to reach out to youth aged 13 to 21 in an effort to reduce the rate of HIV infection among that population. The agency hired an expert in market research to determine the extent of social media use and the specific types and platforms preferred by young people in the community. Results of this research would dictate what the message should be and how it would be transmitted so that it could quickly spread and resonate with the target population.

image or supporting advertising campaigns. Research now covers analysis of human resources, assessment of managed care, evaluation of facilities for acquisition, assessment of the impact of competitor activities, and justification of the organization's tax-exempt status among others. Involvement of researchers is limited only by the organization's range of services.

Third, the subjects for healthcare marketing research have multiplied. At one time, patients and the general public were the primary targets of market researchers. Today, the subjects include patients or end users, families, employers, employees, medical staff, other clinicians, caregivers, and so on. Almost every segment of the service area is relevant to researchers in one way or another.

Fourth, new research techniques continue to be developed and rolled out, while old techniques are constantly revised to keep up with industry developments and technological advances. Contemporary geographic information systems, for example, have transformed the simple mapping of health-related phenomena into increasingly sophisticated spatial analyses.

In addition, social media, data-collection and data-analysis software, online surveys, and myriad other technology-based methods have become available.

Fifth, the disciplines from which market researchers are drawn have increasingly become diverse. Healthcare, more so than other industries, demands a multidisciplinary approach to research. Qualitative techniques often require a broad range of expertise, and as more innovative methods emerge the need for analysts with training in sociology, anthropology, demography, epidemiology, and organizational development (to name a few disciplines) will increase.

Contributions to Healthcare Decision Making

Healthcare has become more market driven, and data generated through market research drive marketing. The characteristics of the market can no longer be ignored. More and more, the market's needs are determining the types of healthcare goods and services offered.

Today's healthcare environment calls for a more aggressive approach to research. Marketers must be constantly on alert for new market opportunities and be aware of threats to the organization's market share or financial viability. In addition, researchers must have monitoring capabilities in place that will flag any out-of-range statistics. For example, if a researcher maintains a database on physicians within the market area, the researcher should be one of the first to identify a community in which a shortage of physicians is emerging.

The growing diversity of US consumers—including healthcare users—has boosted the importance of research. Once the importance of consumers was recognized in healthcare, they came to be subjected to the same segmentation processes as consumers in other industries. The US population has become racially and ethnically diverse, has maintained and enhanced regional differences, and has adopted lifestyles disparate enough to be daunting to any marketer (Thomas 2003b). As a result, the characteristics of the healthcare customer have changed and health behavior has become less predictable.

For many types of services, the market is no longer growing. A good example is the slumping demand for inpatient care and the rise of outpatient care (Kutscher and Evans 2013). The success of inpatient programs, therefore, will rely on retaining existing customers, requiring providers to know about them more than ever before. However, anticipating future demand is also important. For example, newly insured individuals (as a result of the ACA) who may not have had previous primary or preventive care are entering the healthcare system. The needs of these healthcare consumers should be factored into the marketing equation.

Other factors also make research an essential fixture in healthcare decision making. Organizations can incur tremendous costs if they locate a facility at a problematic site, undertake a marketing initiative at the wrong time, overlook a key niche market, or develop misleading product packaging. The costs involved in building and outfitting a clinic, mounting a marketing campaign, and developing a product are growing. Losses associated with one bad decision may need to be countered with ten good decisions for the organization to recover.

Even more important in an environment of increasingly scarce resources are the opportunity costs of a wrong decision. Situating a clinic in one place means that other potentially more favorable sites were not selected. Money spent on one promotion cannot be spent on another that may yield higher returns. Product development resources spent on one service could have been spent on another possibly more profitable service. By overlooking a critical niche, an organization may have invited a competitor to outposition it in the market.

As stated in earlier chapters, healthcare decision making relies heavily on accurate, timely, detailed, and complete data. Data supplement the knowledge that the decision maker has acquired through training and experience. Marketing research should be a complement to, rather than a substitute for, an administrator's direct knowledge of the marketplace. The researcher should work closely with the administrator to build the knowledge base for decision making.

Finally, marketing research should drive marketing strategy. Marketing initiatives should not exist in a vacuum but should support an overarching marketing strategy, which in turn supports the organization's long-range strategic plans. If, for example, research indicates that the organization is a niche player (and the public perceives the organization as such), the marketing strategy should capitalize on this positioning. On the other hand, if the organization is perceived as the leader in its service area, the marketing strategy should likewise capitalize on this view.

Steps in the Marketing Research Process

Any type of information gathering on the marketplace constitutes marketing research, so a formal, expensive research process is not always necessary. Although this chapter focuses on a more formal approach, healthcare organizations may also pursue a less formal approach based on observation and data collection via networking.

The type and amount of marketing research undertaken are dictated by several factors, such as the nature of the organization, the objectives of the campaign, the available resources, and the intended use for the findings. A critical skill any marketer should possess is the ability to identify the type and scope of research appropriate for a particular campaign. Other industries (e.g., restaurant, retail, hotel) are more accustomed to heated competition, so they frequently use **mystery shoppers** to collect market intelligence. Although blatant efforts at acquiring intelligence on competitors meet resistance in healthcare, mystery shopping (though the term *shopper* is not quite accurate) can work to reveal interesting insights. Exhibit 14.2 presents one type of market research developed for other industries but that could apply to healthcare as well.

Mystery shopper
An individual hired by an organization to pose as a customer to covertly collect information on its own or a competitor's operations, goods, or services

In an ideal world, marketing research is an ongoing organizational function. It is not practical to initiate discrete research projects from scratch to support each new campaign. By the time an organization implements a data collection process, the campaign period is likely to be over. However, with ongoing monitoring systems in place, the organization could, for example, track changes in physician referral patterns, admission trends, or emerging market niches as they occur.

Marketing research is a multistep endeavor, much like every other marketing activity. While the exact number of steps depends on the campaign and the preferences of the researcher, all research designs include the same basic elements. The process begins with an initial inquiry (e.g., Is the management of eating disorders a service worth pursuing?) and ends with an ultimate decision (e.g., a pilot program for eating disorders should be initiated). No two research experts completely agree on the steps involved, and some of the limitations unique to healthcare (e.g., the sanctity of patient records) distinguish the research conducted in healthcare from that conducted in other industries. The following steps reflect the typical sequence of research activities, although this order is not set in stone. The steps may be iterative and often occur simultaneously and should in any case be modified to fit the circumstances.

Define the Issues

Often, a marketing initiative is triggered by some event or situation. The introduction of a new service in the market area, a competitor's anticipated or unannounced move, or the identification of a new market for an existing service are all examples of triggers. Thus, the main task in this step is to isolate the relevant issues connected to the event by developing a precise statement of the situation. This statement may reveal a concern altogether different from the one that initiated the effort, and it could dictate whether the scope of the market research is broad or narrow. If problems or challenges are not properly defined at this point, the information subsequently generated by the research is unlikely to have much value.

At this point, the marketer should state some assumptions to guide the research design. Are certain audiences more important than others? What

EXHIBIT 14.2
Mystery
Shoppers in
Healthcare

To better understand their processes, products, and other offerings, some healthcare organizations have employed mystery shoppers. These are pseudo-patients or consumers with limited knowledge of the organization or existing employees of the organization, depending on the circumstances. These shoppers may arrive at a facility's front desk, an emergency department (ED), a doctor's office, an outpatient clinic, a cafeteria or gift shop, or some other healthcare setting to observe typical procedures, sample certain services, engage employees and other staff, or perform tasks as ordered by the organization. They may call an advertised phone number, helpline, or hotline to assess the level of customer service and the quality of response. They may visit the organization's website and test its features (e.g., appointment scheduling) and ease of use (e.g., if a person who is not tech savvy can navigate or find information without help). They may pose questions or seek help on the organization's Facebook, Twitter, YouTube, and other platforms to gauge how well social media are incorporated into operations.

Mystery shoppers provide organizations with honest feedback and objective findings regarding the overall service experience, processes, staff skills and behavior, customer service, quality, wait times, technology, and other aspects examined. The organizations then use the data generated to revise procedures, develop orientation and training programs, implement new policies, and institute other changes.

Aggressive organizations engage mystery shoppers to collect information on their competitors, such as operational details, volume of services performed, and sources of customers or patrons. To gather this intelligence, shoppers may pretend to visit a hospitalized patient, call to inquire about a service and its cost, or attend a patient education session offered by the competitor. They may participate in online discussions as well to monitor popular opinions or perceptions.

This type of qualitative data collection is not likely to provide all of the hard data necessary for a thorough market analysis. More often, mystery shoppers provide provisional information on which more formal data collection activities can build. Although the use of mystery shoppers is not widespread and has detractors in healthcare, this method of research has the potential to become common as organizations weigh what works and doesn't work in the era of the ACA. (For a blog post about the Obama Administration's controversial use of mystery shoppers, see http://thehealthcareblog.com/blog/2011/06/28/are-mystery-shoppers-such-a-bad-idea-for-health-care-quality-improvement/.)

issues or questions are off limits? What time constraints are present? These initial assumptions should be refined as more information becomes available.

This step requires a general understanding of the organization and its characteristics, the product, and the market area. Reviewing the existing literature—journals, magazines, newsletters, government reports, technical papers, presentations from professional meetings, annual reports, and other relevant documents—is an obvious place to start. Unfortunately, healthcare marketing has yet to develop a body of literature comparable to that of marketing in other industries. Marketers, however, have access to bibliographic databases, literature reviews, online archives, blogs, and other references as sources of relevant information (with most sources now available on the Internet). One such source is the American Marketing Association, which sponsors special-interest groups that enable its members to come together online and offline for discussions, networking, and other forms of exchange; see www.ama.org/academics/Pages/ama_sigs.aspx.

Set Research Objectives

To determine the objectives of the intended research, a number of questions must be asked. For example, what body of knowledge does the organization want to establish through the research process? Who can provide the information needed to inform this initiative? Answers to these and similar questions determine the research objectives and design.

The objectives that are specified determine the research design. Four general categories of research—exploratory, descriptive, causal, and predictive —should be considered when formulating the design.

1. **Exploratory research** is characterized by a high degree of flexibility and usually relies heavily on reviews of the literature, small-scale surveys, informal interviews and discussions, and subjective evaluations of available data. Its goal is to discern the general nature of the problem or opportunity under study and the associated factors of importance. Exploratory designs are commonly used for initial information gathering at the outset of a marketing initiative. The objective here is to gain insights and information, even if anecdotal, that may reveal the usefulness of other categories of research.

2. **Descriptive research** is the development of a factual portrait of the components of the community or organization. These portraits do not attempt to explain the "why" of the researcher's observations but profile the salient characteristics of the topics under study. Market profiles, community assessments, and resource inventories are products of descriptive research. Any source of information can be used in

Exploratory research
Research that discerns the general nature of a problem or an opportunity to identify factors of importance

Descriptive research
Research that describes (but does not explain) the characteristics of a community or population

descriptive research, although it relies heavily on secondary data sources and survey research. Carefully designed descriptive studies are the bread and butter of marketing research and provide the basis for any subsequent analysis.

Causal research
Research that identifies the specific functional relationship between two or more variables

3. **Causal research** (also known as *inferential research*) identifies the relationship between two or more variables in the situation under study. For example, a cause-and-effect analysis may be used to discover the link between place of medical training and physician referral patterns. Likewise, a study of the market response to a promotional campaign may isolate and identify how increased advertising, for example, fostered the growth of outpatient visits. Causal research designs infer relationships, given that a direct causal relationship usually cannot be demonstrated. Little of the research conducted in healthcare in the past could be characterized as causal. Although this category has contributed to an understanding of consumer behavior and motivation in other industries, it has not reached a level of sophistication to do the same for healthcare.

Predictive research
Research that forecasts future characteristics or actions on the basis of known present characteristics

4. **Predictive research** uses findings from previous research as a basis for forecasting future events and conditions. Predictive modeling is a form of predictive research that has been adopted by some healthcare organizations. For example, health plans and managed care organizations can benefit from identifying at-risk enrollees and predicting (and even influencing) their future utilization of services. Forecasting the utilization of employee health services on the basis of the known characteristics of service users is another example.

Develop the Research Plan

The categories of data to be considered, the means of collecting the relevant data, and the indicators and analytical techniques to be used, among other attributes, are included in the research plan. The research plan specifies the sequence in which tasks (of data collection and statistical analysis) are to be carried out, the responsible party or parties involved, the resources required, and the time frames to be followed.

At this point, decisions must be made regarding which category of data to use—primary, secondary, or a combination of the two. If primary research is deemed necessary, the data collection technique will have to be specified and the questionnaire design, sampling, interviewer training, and other tasks will have to commence.

Because most research is essentially descriptive, the analytical methods used are usually fairly straightforward. Data analysis entails converting a series of observations, however obtained, into information—descriptive statements or inferences about relationships. The type of analyses that can be performed depends on the sampling process, the measurement instrument, and the data collection method. Various analytical approaches can be applied to convert raw data into information that supports the marketing process. An effective marketer is familiar with demographic analysis techniques, epidemiologist-developed methods, and other evaluation approaches.

Estimate Resource Requirements

Time, money, and personnel are required to implement the research plan. If the research is to be performed in-house, resources can be broken down into direct expenses (e.g., the cost of hiring additional interviewers) and in-kind contributions (e.g., staff time, office space, supplies). Time refers to the days, weeks, or months needed to complete the process as well as to the time commitment required of the responsible parties. Money refers to the financial investment and the monetary equivalent of personnel time, materials and supplies, and other tangible and intangible organizational resources to be expended. Personnel, the largest cost item, refers to both internal staff (including those inside and outside the marketing department) and external professionals or contractors who are participants in plan implementation. In addition, research imposes opportunity costs that must be estimated to the extent possible. If the process is outsourced to a marketing consultant or firm, the costs are calculated differently.

Project management tools—such as the program evaluation review technique (PERT) and critical path method (CPM)—help in estimating the resources needed and clarifying the manner in which the process is managed. *PERT* divides the total research plan into its smallest component activities, identifies the sequence in which these activities must be performed, attaches a time estimate for each activity, and presents these details in a flowchart. Marketers can use these same time estimates for the *CPM,* which establishes the critical path for accomplishing the plan objectives. They can then create a chart that indicates the interdependence of the plan's components and the sequence for performing the various tasks.

Collect Data

In selecting the best data collection technique for a particular analysis, the researcher must weigh the advantages and disadvantages of each approach and consider only the methods that will return reliable and valid data. Data collection typically involves both primary data and secondary data research. Primary research is likely to be used to gather data that cannot be acquired through **secondary research**. Secondary data are almost always collected first

Secondary research
The analysis of data originally collected during primary research and for some other purpose

because they are likely to be readily available at little or no additional expense. For example, in collecting data to support marketing for a new health service, a researcher may examine hospital records to see if a similar service has been offered in the past (secondary data), conduct interviews to find out current consumer attitudes about such a service (primary survey data), and launch a pilot study to measure consumer reception of the proposed service (primary experimental data). (The use of secondary data in marketing research is discussed in more detail in Chapter 16.)

Because an unlimited amount of data can be collected on an infinite number of topics, the marketer must ensure that any information collected is relevant to the issues as defined and is actionable, not just interesting. If the data do not contribute to the achievement of research objectives, the time, money, and personnel dedicated to the collection process are wasted. Specifically, the marketer should list the questions that need to be answered by the end of the research period, structure the data collection process accordingly, and determine the actual and potential uses for any information collected.

Analyze Data and Draw Conclusions

The main objective in analyzing collected data is to generate conclusions about the issues defined earlier in the research process. The conclusions drawn rely heavily on the analysis outlined in the research plan. Properly chosen analytical techniques should generate useful findings—whether they are related to market share, utilization trends, or changing market characteristics. These conclusions should provide the basis for subsequent marketing activities. Some of them, in fact, become part of the assumptions stated and restated throughout the process. Acquiring and maintaining a desired share of the patient market are always a top priority for healthcare providers. Market share information not only indicates the position of the organization or a service in the market but also serves as a basis for evaluating the success of a marketing initiative. This critical piece of information is often difficult to calculate in healthcare. See Case Study 14.1 for an example of a market share analysis.

Historically, marketing research was seen as a technical support function. The researcher's role was to turn numbers over to administrators, who would then make the appropriate decision. As marketing issues have become more complex and research methods more sophisticated, decision makers are increasingly asking marketers to offer recommendations (called *recommendation formulation*). Instead of providing the decision maker with three objectively compared options for review, the researcher is likely to be asked to indicate the best choice based on the results of the analyses. Exhibit 14.3 provides some thoughts on interpreting data gathered through research.

CASE STUDY 14.1
Market Share Analysis for a Physician Practice

Southeast Orthopedic Clinic (SOC) had long been the premier orthopedic practice in a middle-sized southern city. Over time, however, competition had become increasingly fierce, and concerns were growing over the perceived erosion of SOC's market share in the community. SOC asked its marketing consultant to analyze the practice's and its competitor's current market share. Because the consultant did not routinely calculate market share, he had to gather data for this task. The calculation of market share is relatively straightforward *if* the required data are available. The formula for calculating market share is as follows:

Volume for the practice ÷ Total volume for the service area
= Market share.

The numerator could be presented as volume (e.g., office visits or hospital admissions), utilization (e.g., number of diagnoses or procedures), or revenue reported for the practice. The denominator could be the combined figure for the numerator selected (e.g., volume, utilization, revenue) for all providers in the service area. The figure for the practice is then divided by the total figure to generate the percentage of the market controlled by the practice.

The consultant did not know whether the data needed for the calculation were readily available. He presumed that SOC had reasonable data on its own volume, utilization, revenue, and so forth. Comparable data on competing practices were not likely to be available, but data on volume for the total service area likely were. Fortunately for SOC, data on hospital admissions were reported to the state annually, allowing the consultant to determine the overall volume of orthopedic admissions for the service area as well as admissions for various types of orthopedic diagnoses. Equipped with data from the state's repository, he was able to determine that 10,000 orthopedic cases were admitted in the previous year. He knew that SOC had admitted 2,000 cases during that time, so its market share of the area's orthopedic patients was calculated to be 20 percent.

For confidentiality reasons, the state would not release data on the hospital admissions recorded by other area orthopedic practices. However, this information was available on individual hospitals, and

(continued)

the consultant was able to develop a reasonable estimate of the market shares of hospital patients for the various players in the orthopedic arena. Had these data not been available, he would have had to assess the relative status of SOC on the basis of the relative size of the various practices (e.g., was the 20 percent market share for SOC commensurate with the size of the practice relative to its competitors?). He was able to further refine the estimate of market share by comparing revenue figures reported to the state by the various practices.

The data acquired from the state were useful for refining the market share estimate of the types of patients treated. The hospital data categorized orthopedic admissions by the types of problems seen (e.g., fractures, back pain, torn ligaments). The consultant was able to calculate the practice's market share for each of the major categories of orthopedic services. The data indicated that SOC maintained a market share of more than 25 percent for traditional orthopedic services (such as hip replacement and back surgery) but controlled less than 15 percent of the market for newer services (such as arthroscopic surgery, sports injuries, and knee replacement).

Despite the usefulness of this information, the consultant was concerned that these data did not capture market share for ambulatory services (i.e., office visits). Office visits for orthopedic services were much more common than hospital admissions, especially because orthopedic care had largely shifted from the inpatient setting to the outpatient setting. In this community, as elsewhere, no repository of data existed for ambulatory services. The consultant was forced to turn to a colleague who provided software-generated estimates of the utilization of various types of services. Using algorithms developed on the basis of known utilization rates, the consultant was able to indicate the *expected* volume of office visits for the community, along with the breakdown of those visits by diagnosis. When these figures were compared to data on SOC volume, he determined that the SOC share of office visits was 18 percent and, as with the hospital data, the share was higher for traditional services and lower for contemporary services.

The consultant reported back to the SOC that, overall, its market share for hospital care was consistent with the size of the practice, but its share of ambulatory patients was lower than anticipated. On both the inpatient and outpatient sides, SOC was more prominent among patients with traditional problems but less prominent among those who sought contemporary treatments.

Case Study Discussion Questions

1. Why do healthcare organizations need to understand market share, and what developments in healthcare are increasing the significance of market share data?

2. What are some of the challenges healthcare organizations face in calculating their market share?

3. Why is it important to go beyond overall market share and disaggregate data by patient type or procedure?

4. How did the SOC market share stack up against its competitors, and in what area was SOC found to be relatively strong? Relatively weak?

5. In the absence of actual data, what approach might be used to develop proxy data as a basis for determining market share?

6. What did the consultant conclude about the position of SOC in its market?

Present Marketing Research Results

Findings are largely useless unless they are presented to the intended audience or appropriate decision makers in an understandable, actionable fashion. Many executives and administrators cannot easily ascertain the quality of the research plan, methodology, or instrument. They can, however, easily recognize the quality of the report presented. Thus, the quality of the report is often used as an indicator of the quality of the research. Visual displays, such as charts and maps, are particularly useful in painting a clear picture. Exhibit 14.4 describes the **geographic information system (GIS)**, a tool for collecting, analyzing, and presenting data that has been used by market researchers in other industries for decades and is now applied to the healthcare arena (for example, see www.cdc.gov/gis/whatis.htm for how the Centers for Disease Control and Prevention applies the technology).

Effective communication of research findings is a challenge for marketers. Typically, they present written or oral reports to hospital leaders (including executives and the board), physicians, department heads, financial analysts, venture capitalists, and a range of other health professionals. These are individuals who are well educated and trained in their respective fields and are at the height of their careers, but they do not necessarily have the research background to discern the nuances in the data presented to them.

Geographic information system (GIS)
A computer application that collects, analyzes, and organizes data geographically for the purpose of spatial analysis and map generation

EXHIBIT 14.3
The Pitfalls of
Interpreting
Research Data

Data interpretation is as much an art as a science, and certain skills and experiences are required to perform it. Interpreting objective data drawn from 1,000 survey forms necessitates an approach that is different from the approach to interpreting observation notes or in-depth interview transcripts. Following are some dangers that analysts should avoid when interpreting data.

First, results are easy to misinterpret. Often, the analysis compares the data from two or more groups or for two or more time spans. For example, the satisfaction of a senior program's members may be compared to the satisfaction of nonmembers, or consumers' awareness of a service before a promotion may be compared to that after a promotion. Accepting *any* difference as evidence that a consequential difference exists or that a change has occurred is tempting. In reality, however, only *some* change may be observed. As statisticians are fond of pointing out, there are many types of change—statistically significant change, meaningful change, and so on. Thus, analysts should first determine if change has occurred, then test for statistical significance, and then assess the meaning of the change.

Second, observed change is difficult to fully attribute to the intervention or initiative applied. Cause-and-effect works well in controlled environments, but in healthcare—even more so than in other industries—many factors are at play (including chance) that influence results. For example, evaluating a campaign to increase admissions for a regional hospital starts out at a disadvantage because audience responses to the promotion are not immediate (i.e., they will not use the hospital right after they see an ad, for example). If this is a six-month campaign, when does the analyst start counting admissions—at the end of the six months, a year after the campaign, two years later? Even when a reasonable time frame is identified, it is not possible to distinguish one factor's effects from another's. Such factors may include the arrival or departure of physicians, the acquisition or loss of a managed care contract, or the opening or closure of a facility in the service area. In addition, determining what constitutes a successful outcome is difficult. Sometimes, simply maintaining the current level of admissions might be considered a success.

Third, failure to qualify the responses generated from a sample survey is equivalent to not getting relevant information. This is a common issue faced by researchers. Take, for example, the overwhelming "yes" response to a proposed hospital-sponsored fitness center. A survey or research initiative that introduces or suggests *any* new service tends to be met with support and agreement. Thus, these responses must be qualified with follow-up questions that give details about the new facility's location, operating hours, amenities, fees, incentives, and so on. When provided some specifics, survey respondents tend to give more practical answers and their level of interest tends to be more tempered.

Fourth, finding that one piece of information that could make or break a decision is complicated. Research yields various findings, some of which are more salient than others. For example, a survey that asks health plan members to rate the attributes and offerings of hospitals in the service area may uncover interesting facts, but ultimately those findings are not relevant. Why? Because plan members usually do not choose the hospitals they use—that is the one piece of information analysts must recognize. Among the hundreds of variables that researchers analyze, only one variable may be deemed useful. For example, a large health system considering the acquisition of an underperforming rural hospital was conducting a feasibility study. Researchers for the system examined all the usual variables: characteristics of the service area population, the state of the facility and its equipment, the referral patterns of the medical staff, and so forth. Researchers found, however, that only one number mattered for the system's purpose: The hospital's market share was more than 85 percent. This variable was crucial because it was not possible to increase that market share and it would be difficult to maintain it in a highly competitive area. In the end, the system decided that the proposed acquisition was not viable.

The marketer's job is to explain, clarify, and illustrate the findings as well as possible, keeping in mind each audience's perspectives, biases, and need for information.

Primary Research Methods

An industry that undergoes constant changes—new regulations, consolidations, technological advancements, service area expansions, demographic shifts, product introductions, to name a few—requires current, accurate, and comprehensive data. This often means the use of primary research.

Primary research is the collection of data for a specific use. One advantage of this type of research is that the data gathered are relevant and current. Another advantage is that the findings can remain proprietary

Primary research
The direct collection of data for a specific use

EXHIBIT 14.4
Using GIS in
Healthcare

Few marketing analyses in other industries would be complete without maps that illustrate the distribution of markets, consumer segments, usage rates, and other essential data. Furthermore, the use of spatial analysis techniques in decision making and developing sales territories is not uncommon in other industries. These functions are made possible by geographic information systems (or GIS, for short). Although this technology has been available to healthcare organizations for more than 25 years, most organizations have failed to incorporate it into their strategies and operations. That is surprising, given the importance of the spatial dimension for many aspects of healthcare.

Unlimited opportunities exist for adopting GIS in healthcare. GIS-generated maps can display a wide variety of health-related information, including distribution of resources (e.g., hospitals, physicians, urgent care centers), patterns of patient flow, demand for health services, and market share. From a marketing perspective, nothing depicts concentrations of potential customers better than a map. Beyond mapping, GIS can track trends in population growth and demographic patterns, determine drive times to various healthcare facilities, compare potential facility sites on the basis of several variables simultaneously, and monitor the progression of disease through the service area. In addition, GIS can be used for specialized applications, such as accessibility analysis for managed care plans.

As GIS becomes more sophisticated but less expensive and easier to use and as the ACA's focus on population health management becomes integrated into providers' operations, the adoption of GIS may increase.

Quantitative research
A data collection technique that uses objective methods, such as experiments and sample surveys

Qualitative research
A data collection technique that uses subjective methods, such as observations, interviews, and focus groups

(i.e., the organization "owns" the results), which is not the case with data collected through secondary research because the instrument used is from another party and for a different purpose. The disadvantages are that it is an expensive and time-consuming process and the administration of the tools requires sophisticated skills that staff members may not have.

Before primary research activities can begin, marketers need to determine the means of collecting the data. Many methods are available (including the ones described in this section) that fall under the quantitative and qualitative categories. **Quantitative research** (e.g., sample surveys) is considered objective and readily lends itself to statistical analysis, while **qualitative research** (e.g., focus groups) is considered subjective and not amenable to rigorous statistical analysis. Exhibit 14.5 compares these two approaches.

In the past, researchers and managers were enamored with quantitative research (surveys) and statistical analyses. Because quantitative research was a well-established science, healthcare administrators deemed (often erroneously) that surveys were easy to conduct. Some administrators even argued against the use of qualitative research, claiming that the data generated were neither scientific nor rigorous.

Quantitative methods present some advantages. Not only can they be subject to statistical analyses, but their findings also can be generalized or applied to other populations. The data they collect are easy to analyze and are definitive (at least within a known range of error), instilling confidence in decision making. The backlash against quantitative methods pushed qualitative approaches to center stage. Some have argued that surveys may yield misleading results, a direct contrast to the reliable data generated through more in-depth qualitative methods (e.g., focus groups, in-depth interviews, and observations). Researchers hail qualitative research for the richness of detail it provides and prefer it (over quantitative) in situations where opinions, choices, and perceptions are sought. Focus groups and interviews with naturally occurring groups are conducted on a regular basis, and observations and content analyses are employed to supplement quantitative research. Qualitative data are analyzed and interpreted through various ways, including specially developed software.

Admittedly, qualitative methods have their limitations. They cannot be subjected to statistical analysis, nor can they be generalized and applied to other populations. Their contributions are limited to generating broad conclusions and hypotheses. In this sense, they can serve as a guide for designing quantitative research initiatives.

Researchers today recognize the value of both quantitative and qualitative approaches. They may be conducted simultaneously to obtain data that supplement each other. Both also have evolved over the years. Surveys, for example, are no longer composed of closed-ended, yes/no questions; they now pose open-ended questions that encourage respondents to volunteer more detail. Often, the use of both qualitative and quantitative data allows the researcher to triangulate the findings for better-informed conclusions.

See Case Study 14.2 on page 409.

EXHIBIT 14.5
Quantitative and Qualitative Research

Observation

In *observational research*, marketers watch and take notes of the actions and attributes of research subjects, who are typically in their "natural" setting (e.g., an employee performing a daily task). In this way, information is not elicited directly from the subjects but captured through structured **observation**—with specified rules based on stated objectives. Three conditions must be met to ensure that observation is a successful endeavor:

Observation
A data collection technique whereby the actions and/or attributes of those being studied are recorded either by an individual or a mechanical device

1. *The activity must be observable*. Motivations, attitudes, opinions, views, and other inclinations are internal and are not visible. Behavior or action, however, can be observed and recorded.

2. *The activity must be generalizable*. Observing one exasperated patient in the physician's waiting room is not a basis for making a generalization about all waiting patients; ten such patients might be. The activity must be one that is repeated, frequent, and predictable.

3. *The activity must not take a long time*. Researchers are usually restricted to observing activities that can be completed in a relatively short time span (e.g., a doctor visit) or short segments of activities that take a long time (e.g., ED wait).

Observations are typically used when data cannot be obtained through interviews or secondary sources and when analyzing a process. For example, a trained observer may sit in the admissions waiting area to watch the intake process, or he or she may follow a patient from an ED bed to the radiology table to an inpatient room. Some organizations, in fact, hire mystery shoppers (see Exhibit 14.2) to carry out observational research. The mystery shopping method often may reveal more information than passive forms of observation could.

Observation is classified as either participatory or nonparticipatory. In *participatory observation*, the researcher becomes part of the group or activity being observed (e.g., mystery shopper). It allows the observer to analyze the group, situation, or process as an insider. By being part of the group, the researcher minimizes the impact of the observation process on the group's behavior; of course, there is still the possibility that the researcher's presence will alter the behavior of the subjects. The drawback to participatory observation is that the researcher typically cannot take notes or otherwise record his or her observations at the time they are made. Thus, the observer must rely on memory to record observations at a later date.

In *nonparticipatory observation*, the researcher is detached from the individuals, situations, or processes being observed. The passive observer may view the subjects from afar or, in more controlled environments, through a one-way mirror in an observation booth. The advantage to this approach is that the researcher typically does not affect the behavior of the subjects because they do not know they are being observed. On the other hand, such an indirect approach makes it harder to interpret the meaning of the observed actions.

Although observational research is good for documenting *what* people do, it does not address *why* people do so. Thus, this method often needs to be supplemented with personal interviews or some other data collection approach.

In-Depth Interviews

In-depth interview, one-on-one interview, and *key informant interview* are terms used interchangeably to mean one person posing probing and often ad hoc questions to another. Complicated questions—those that give the responder pause or that demand more than simplistic explanations—are best asked through an in-depth interview. The interviewer does not necessarily pose a predetermined set of questions in a predetermined order; rather, he or she elicits the information by listening to the responses and asking follow-up questions as necessary. The entire activity typically lasts 30 to 45 minutes, but sometimes it can last several hours. Note the distinction between an in-depth interview and the administration of a survey form: The former takes time because it is meant to be exploratory, while the latter is short both in duration and on content.

Ostensibly, anyone presumed to have knowledge of the topic under study can be interviewed. However, in healthcare, *key informants* are usually interviewed. Key informants are those who have a particular set of knowledge (e.g., technical innovators), have a broad perspective on the study issues (e.g., administrators), hold a position that familiarizes them with the perspectives of many groups of people (e.g., human resources manager), or are opinion leaders (e.g., medical staff members). As discussed earlier, one of the first steps in marketing research is to define the issues the organization is facing; in-depth interviews are an excellent means of accomplishing this task. In fact, typically the survey instruments used in subsequent quantitative research are based on in-depth interviews with key informants.

The in-depth interview method does have some limitations. It must be carried out by a skilled interviewer. The potential for interviewer bias or respondent misrepresentation is great. Key informants or experts may go off on tangents. An opinionated physician interviewee, for example, may be difficult to rein in; valuable time may be wasted discussing irrelevant topics.

Group Interviews

Group interviews have become one of the more popular qualitative research techniques in healthcare. They can be structured (as in the case of focus groups) or informal (as in the case of naturally occurring groups). *Focus groups* consist of people who are assembled to discuss a topic of interest under the direction of a professional moderator. The objective is to have people express their feelings or views on a range of topic components. *Naturally occurring groups,* a subset of focus groups, consist of people who share an interest; in healthcare, such a group may include employees in one department working the same shift or family members of patients admitted at the same time.

Focus groups, and the information they yield, serve several purposes, such as the following:

- *Be the basis for questions in a survey.* For example, generalized perceptions of a hospital's image may be converted into specific survey items.
- *Identify customer needs and wants.* For example, a physician focus group may reveal what programs or services referring physicians would like their health system to offer.
- *Test ideas.* For example, parents of orthopedic patients aged 6 to 18 may assess the feasibility of an orthopedic practice's plan to establish a pediatric sports medicine program.
- *Examine the underlying meaning of survey results.* For example, recent ED users may be asked, as a follow up, why 50 percent of them indicated the ED service they received was unsatisfactory.

Group interviews impart valuable insights that can jumpstart subsequent action steps, research, and other activities. As such, they are a great supplement to other data collection methods. However, they should never be used as a primary tool.

Surveys

Many, if not most, marketing campaigns use surveys for data collection. Some healthcare organizations conduct survey research themselves, while others contract with an outside consultant. Survey data may also be obtained via a syndicated survey or an omnibus survey. In conducting a *syndicated survey*, a number of organizations band together to share the cost of the research. The participating organizations may have the option of including a few custom questions in the survey, but for the most part, all will receive the same information back. *Omnibus surveys* are ongoing (often panel) surveys in which organizations can participate. The survey firm regularly asks questions of a panel of several thousand respondents, and healthcare organizations can submit questions to pose to the pool of respondents.

CASE STUDY 14.2
Applying Quantitative and Qualitative Research to a Community Health Initiative

On the advice of a marketing consultant, a network of faith-based clinics opened a new clinic in an impoverished, predominantly African-American community that had limited access to health services. After one year of operation, the clinic still was not receiving the support it expected from the local community. For some reason, area residents were not taking advantage of the services offered by the clinic, although the health service demand clearly existed. The network's marketing department designed and sent a sample survey to 200 households in the community of 3,000 households. It conducted in-depth interviews with key informants, who either lived in the area or had a long history of working with its residents. It ran focus groups and carried out observational research—all involving local residents.

Findings from the sample survey essentially reinforced the results of the previous market analysis: Respondents reported a high level of morbidity (particularly various chronic diseases), a high level of psychiatric morbidity and substance abuse, and a low level of treatment or medical intervention. Plus, more health problems and greater unmet needs were revealed than anticipated.

Results of the observational research added critical layers of information. While the community had a high rate of home ownership, it was marred by many empty, dilapidated, or abandoned single-family dwellings; trash-filled vacant lots; and crumbling buildings (including the low-rated elementary and high schools). Furthermore, there was little or no social interaction among the residents or even between neighbors. Few adults walked and talked on the streets, and few children played outside. The sight of residents sitting on their porches or puttering around in their yards was rare. Even vehicular traffic was light. Transients roamed the streets, however, along with drug dealers, gang members, and petty criminals. The churches that dotted every corner had low attendance and did little community outreach. Many grocery stores and restaurants had boarded up their doors and moved out, creating a "food desert."

The in-depth interviews and focus groups helped qualify the findings from the sample survey and observations. The observed social dysfunctions were rooted in the decline of the quality of housing, which

(continued)

encouraged detachment from the community. Long-time residents felt marginalized, isolated from their neighbors, and afraid to leave their homes. The community's educational system, once the pride of the neighborhood, faltered partly as a result of young families leaving the area.

The marketing researchers concluded that health problems were symptoms of a bigger problem. Faced with so many environmental concerns, the residents made their medical conditions and general health low priority. As a result of the disintegration of face-to-face interactions and word-of-mouth promotion between neighbors, most people were unaware that a new clinic had been built in the area. Leaders of the network and the clinic realized that at least some of these underlying issues must be fixed before the community could focus on its health problems.

The combined quantitative and qualitative research methods applied in this case, as well as the triangulation of the findings, did not yield a solution. However, they enabled a community health clinic to peel off the layers to reveal social and health issues that need immediate—even urgent—attention.

Case Study Discussion Questions

1. What factors suggested to the network of clinics that an in-depth research (a "deep dive") was required to understand the community's characteristics?
2. Why were both quantitative research and qualitative research needed to get to the bottom of the issues facing the community?
3. How were observation, personal interviews, and focus groups used to gather information?
4. Why did the marketing researchers conclude that health problems were "symptoms" rather than the root of the environmental conditions of the community?
5. Why did community residents place a low priority on their health?

Survey research presents a number of challenges that may not be obvious to healthcare administrators. First, developing an effective questionnaire requires a great deal of professional skill and is not something that just anyone can do. When respondents fail to provide the desired information, often the reason is that they were given a defective survey instrument. Second, the intent of the survey should dictate the population to be surveyed; otherwise, the survey will ask the right questions of the wrong respondents. Thus, an appropriate sampling frame must be established. Third, the set of respondents almost never represents the profile of the originally defined sample. For example, it is almost inevitable that more women and more seniors will respond to a typical survey. The sample may be affected by other factors as well. Although the sample may be statistically adjusted, after a certain point this adjustment could lead to misleading results. All of these complicated considerations reiterate the importance of using professional surveyors.

Survey research typically takes one of these forms: mail survey, personal interview, telephone interview, and online survey. This section describes these four methods for surveying target populations.

Mail Surveys

Mail surveys involve self-administered questionnaires sent to a select sample of respondents; they are often used in healthcare to collect patient satisfaction data. One advantage to such surveys is they are relatively inexpensive. Typically, costs include staff compensation (for survey design and data analysis), printing, and postage (including return stamps). Another advantage is that they allow respondents to remain anonymous and eliminate the potential for interviewer bias. Mail is also an efficient way to contact people who are dispersed over a large geographic area and have no access to electronic communication (e.g., e-mail). Returned survey forms are analyzed according to predetermined analytical techniques.

Mail survey
A data collection technique that uses a self-administered paper questionnaire mailed to and from a sample of respondents

This method has several disadvantages. Response rates to mail surveys are often low and skewed toward certain categories of respondents. The surveys are self-administered, leaving the questions open to the respondent's interpretation. Turnaround time may be lengthy, and the short time frames of healthcare marketing campaigns may preclude the use of mail surveys.

Personal Interviews

Personal (or face-to-face) *interviews* are ideal when the questions are tough or complicated to answer. In contrast to in-depth interviews, face-to-face interviews are completed quickly, involve many respondents, and require respondents to be representatives of the population being studied. If the survey instrument is well designed, interviewers who are not experts on the topics being discussed may suffice, but they still have to have basic interviewing skills. Because marketing research targets specific audiences, on-site interviews are often desirable. Waiting rooms of clinics, EDs, and other public spaces in a healthcare facility can serve as sites for these interviews.

Community surveys—wherein a sample of households is selected and then interviewed in their homes—used to be routinely conducted, but they have been largely replaced by on-site interviews. The costs of community surveys have become prohibitive, and many research organizations are reluctant to use this approach because of the perceived danger of sending interviewers into certain neighborhoods. Potential respondents also are unlikely to be home during the day, and people are now reluctant to open their doors to strangers.

A drawback to the use of personal interviews is the potential for interviewer bias. Poorly trained interviewers may condition responses by their reactions to answers or by their mannerisms, or they may fail to accurately follow the wording of a survey. In terms of cost, the personal interview is the most expensive survey method. Even the most basic surveys involve training and monitoring expenditures—and sometimes travel costs.

Telephone Interviews

Telephone interviews involve the collection of data directly from subjects through the telephone. Generally, telephone interviewers who have a "hook" (e.g., the respondent is a current patient) can obtain a high response rate. They also can do a reasonable amount of probing over the phone. On the other hand, a respondent can terminate a telephone interview more easily (by hanging up, "accidentally" dropping the call, or declining the call altogether) than she can a face-to-face interview.

Sampling bias is inherent in this approach because only people with access to a telephone can participate. Landlines are on the decline: Only 71 percent of households in the United States had them in 2011, according to the Census Bureau (Siebens 2013); that number has been decreasing since, especially among young people. Meanwhile, cell phone ownership has been soaring—up to 89 percent in 2011 from 36 percent in 1998 (Sparshott 2013). In addition, many cell or smartphone owners prefer texting over voice calls, helping to make traditional telephone usage a thing of the past. Prohibitions against accessing cell phones for telemarketing purposes, the National Do Not Call Registry (which now covers cell phones and texts), unlisted numbers, fear of phishing scams, and blocking are additional barriers between potential respondents and telephone interviewers. Software with multiple capabilities has enabled interviewers to bypass some of these barriers, however.

The use of computer-assisted telephone interviewing (CATI) is common among telephone surveyors. CATI is a program that enables the interviewer to read questions on the screen and type in the answers into the system as the respondent speaks. The responses are automatically entered into the database to be analyzed. This software can flag out-of-range answers, adjust subsequent questions on the basis of earlier answers, and lead the interviewer through a series of branching questions.

Online Surveys

Online surveys are self-administered questionnaires that respondents can complete on the Internet. Their use in healthcare is wide-ranging. They could be completed by patients, employees, administrators, senior management, physicians and other clinicians, segments of the service population, vendors, and so on. They could be deployed for many purposes and conducted off-site or on-site. After a doctor's appointment, for example, a patient may be asked to sit at a workstation to fill out a brief survey shown on the computer screen. Each answer to a question item is selected with a touch of the screen, a click of the mouse, or a few keystrokes. When completed and submitted, the responses populate a database for analysis. The questionnaire itself may solicit general feedback, an evaluation of the clinic and its staff, or an opinion on a planned change.

Well-designed surveys are user-friendly; include clear, simple instructions; and require no technical or even Internet proficiency from respondents. More advanced designs may even modify the questions during the course of the survey, auto-correct or edit the responses, and perform immediate analysis. The design possibilities are endless. Many free tools—like Zoomerang and SurveyMonkey—are available to marketers and other staff members who want to create simple online surveys from a template and perform simple analyses. For complicated purposes or large data collection initiatives, however, marketers may purchase a proprietary, customizable system and/or consult with a professional surveyor.

The online approach offers multiple advantages. If done on-site, it captures information while it is still fresh in the respondent's mind. It allows researchers to collect responses from nearly every patient instead of a sample. Whether completed on-site or off-site, it saves resources by eliminating the time and staff involved in mail or telephone interviews and the cost of paper, printing, and postage of a traditional survey form. It can be tabulated in hours, if not minutes. It is generally inexpensive and convenient (especially when a link to the survey is included in an e-mail). It is inherently attractive to those who are technologically savvy.

There are also disadvantages to online surveying. It requires access to a computer and an Internet connection, something that some people do not have. It could be intimidating to people who are unfamiliar with computers —and that fear could translate to a refusal to participate, an on-the-spot crash course or hand-holding from staff, or an incomplete survey. It could be a source of resentment for already overburdened staff, for technologically averse leaders and clinicians, or for patients who are not feeling well. It is so painless to create and implement that some marketers may be lured into developing unnecessarily lengthy questionnaires.

Online survey
A data collection technique that uses a self-administered questionnaire that can be completed and submitted via the Internet

Summary

Marketing research encompasses market, product, pricing, promotional, and distribution research. Its scope has expanded as the demand for market data has soared; data requests now come from an ever-growing variety of users. The opportunity costs of a wrong strategic decision in an increasingly competitive market are prompting some of this demand.

Marketing research should be an ongoing function in healthcare, not just an episodic action undertaken when an urgent need arises. It can take a variety of forms and does not always have to be a formal, expensive process. Marketing research is a multistep process, and the exact number and order of steps varies from one analyst to the next and from one campaign to another. Generally, the process begins with defining the issues at hand, involves developing a research plan, and ends with presenting the results to decision makers.

A number of primary research methods, each with advantages and disadvantages, can be used. The qualitative approach includes observation, interviews, and focus groups. The quantitative approach constitutes surveys, which may be conducted face to face, by mail, over the telephone, or online.

Key Points

- Any type of information gathering about the marketplace constitutes marketing research.
- Many marketing research methods applied in healthcare are borrowed from other industries.
- Strategic decisions in healthcare are more data driven today than ever before.
- Marketing research involves both primary and secondary types. The data collection technique chosen depends on the research topic, available resources, and the available data.
- Quantitative research uses objective means, such as experiments and sample surveys.
- Qualitative research uses subjective means, such as observations, interviews, and focus groups.
- Marketing research, like other aspects of marketing, benefits from contemporary technology (as evidenced by GIS and online surveys).

Discussion Questions

1. What developments have made marketing research increasingly important in healthcare?

2. In what ways has the scope of marketing research in healthcare broadened, and what accounts for the expanded scope?

3. What is the explanation for the growing influence of market research on the decision-making process in healthcare?

4. What are the relative advantages and disadvantages of primary research and secondary research?

5. Why has most research in healthcare been descriptive rather than causal or predictive?

6. What are the relative merits of quantitative and qualitative research, and why are both important to marketing researchers in healthcare?

7. How has contemporary technology improved the effectiveness of marketing research in healthcare?

8. What are the advantages of using more than one method to research a topic?

Additional Resources

Academy Health: www.academyhealth.org

Aday, L. A., and L. J. Cornelius. 2006. *Designing and Conducting Health Surveys: A Comprehensive Guide*, 3rd ed. San Francisco: Jossey-Bass.

American Marketing Association Special Interest Groups: www.ama.org/academics /Pages/ama_sigs.aspx

Dewey, A., A. Drahota, C. Fogg, S. Halson-Brown, S. Kilburn, H. Mackenzie, C. Markham, R. Stores, and A. Tremlett. 2011. "Conducting Health Services Research." *South Sudan Medical Journal*. www.southsudanmedicaljournal .com/archive/august-2011/conducting-health-services-research.html.

Quirk's Marketing Research Media. 2014. *How to Conduct Healthcare Market Research*. www.quirks.com/market_research_topics/health_care.aspx.

MARKETING PLANNING

Although most healthcare organizations have some level of marketing expertise, they are not necessarily skilled in marketing planning. Even today, healthcare marketers are often brought in at the eleventh hour to implement a marketing campaign in which they had no previous involvement. This chapter examines the marketing planning process and its importance in the development of any marketing initiative.

Marketing planning is the development of a systematic process for promoting an organization, a good, a service, or a program. This straightforward definition masks the wide variety of activities and the complexity that characterizes this activity. Marketing planning may be limited to a short-term promotional project or may be a component of a long-term strategic plan. Because the systematic implementation of a marketing initiative is not possible without a marketing plan, a plan should be in place before any marketing activities begin, regardless of whether they are intended to be broad or narrow in scope or long or short in duration. This chapter explores the importance of marketing planning and its role in the marketing endeavor. (For additional information on marketing plans, see Thomas [2003a].)

The Nature of Marketing Planning

Of the types of planning healthcare organizations undertake, marketing planning is most directly related to the consumer. Whether the targeted consumer is a patient, a referring physician, an employer, a health plan, or another category of consumer, the marketing plan is built around the needs of someone or something. Although internal factors are often considered (internal marketing is a component of many marketing plans), the marketing plan focuses on the characteristics of the external market with the objective of influencing change in one or more of these characteristics.

Marketing plans geared toward changing the image of an organization are often broad in scope, while plans that focus on a particular good or service are typically narrow in scope. All planning activities should be time delimited, and marketing plans are often rigid in this regard. Clear-cut target dates are almost always included, as the content of a marketing campaign is usually time sensitive. A marketing plan that seeks to establish consumer awareness before the opening of a new clinic, for example, does not allow much margin for error in terms of timing.

The approach to marketing planning varies according to the focus of the project and whether the plan is being developed for a new or an existing organization or product. In the former case, the intent of the marketing plan is to create awareness, generate initial business, and establish a customer base. The primary emphasis is on attracting new customers. In the latter case, the intent may be to enhance or improve the organization's image. Objectives may include changing behaviors by, for example, convincing existing customers to switch their business to the organization or product or by encouraging them to use more services. Generally, information on existing customers is readily accessible, so the planner can capitalize on this resource not only to generate as much additional business as possible but also to expand the customer base.

Although marketing planning is often considered a stand-alone activity, it should fit within the context of the organization's overall strategic initiatives. Thus, the objectives of the marketing plan should correspond to those outlined in the strategic plan. A marketing plan should be an inherent component of any formal business plan as well, even if the organization has an established customer base. Potential funders of a healthcare project are not likely to consider a business proposition that does not include a marketing plan.

Levels of Planning

Marketing planning can take place at different levels, the highest of which is the facility or the health system. A hospital branding itself might develop a master marketing plan that encompasses most aspects of its marketing effort. Such a plan is comprehensive in approach and broad in scope, and its time horizon may be relatively long—say, a multiyear implementation period. Plans formulated at the highest level are likely to be strategic (rather than tactical) in that they aim to effect large-scale change.

Most marketing plans are geared toward the operational level, focusing on a good, a service, a program, or an event. Such plans are developed to introduce a new product, an office site, a piece of equipment, or a series of patient education seminars; these plans aim at increasing patient volume or market share and are narrow in scope and short in duration. Low- or middle-level plans are considered tactical (rather than strategic) because they support relatively specific marketing goals. Their objectives are more restrictive than those of a facility-level plan and are measured, for example, by consumer awareness of the new product, attendance at patient education sessions, and/or increased patient volume.

The Marketing Planning Process

Although the marketing planning process is similar for both facility and operational levels—and those in between—it varies slightly for each level. These differences are noted in this section, along with the steps involved in the process. The sequence of steps is depicted in Exhibit 15.1. (Note that these steps are similar to those of the strategic planning process described in Chapter 8—as marketing and organizational strategies should be aligned—as well as those of the marketing campaign outlined in Chapter 13.)

Plan for Planning

The first step in any planning process is to identify the mandate under which the planners are to operate. A marketing campaign may be initiated for any number of reasons. It may be driven by competitors' actions, a political motive, or an immediate financial consideration.

Much of early marketing planning activity is organizational in nature. In addition to specifying the "why" of the initiative is the important task of identifying the key stakeholders, decision makers, and resources involved. If the organization has an established marketing department, much of the initial work (e.g., background research) may already be completed and the key players may already be in place. However, in the case of a newly installed marketing function or the marketing of an unfamiliar service, additional organizational effort is likely to be required.

Although there is no foolproof combination of team members that will ensure success, certain categories of participants should be involved. The first category includes those familiar with the service, the market, and the distribution channels. Representatives of the target audience should be involved—whether they be patients, physicians, or employers.

Internal participants in the planning process should be drawn from different functional areas, starting with management. Certainly, the marketing department should play a key role and its efforts should be combined with those of the research department (if such a unit exists). Other key departments may participate, including the finance, human resources, and clinical departments (depending on the issues at hand). The planning process is also unlikely to run smoothly without the cooperation of the information systems department.

At this point, the mechanics of the planning process must be specified. Mechanics include the process format, objectives, and the frequency and purpose of team meetings (e.g., progress reporting, decision making). Note that the objectives here are the items expected to be achieved during the planning process, not during the implementation process.

EXHIBIT 15.1
Steps in the
Marketing
Planning
Process

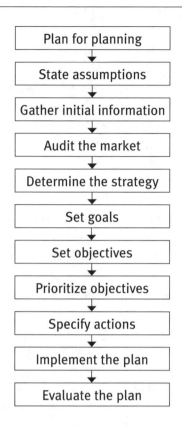

State Assumptions

Marketers must consider and state assumptions that could have potential consequences for the marketing initiative. This must be done not only at the outset but also throughout the planning process. For example, marketers might make an assumption about the image the organization wants to convey. That image could be vastly different—from an aggressive, profit-seeking enterprise driven by hard-bitten business principles to a humble, community-based organization intent on serving the needs of the population.

The assumptions made at the outset reflect the degree to which a service has already penetrated the market. The extent to which marketing activities have previously been initiated for the service affects the assumptions under which the planner operates. The approach or appeal to be used in the campaign is another element about which assumptions might be made. The intent—whether to educate, motivate, entice, or frighten the target audience—determines the nature of the appeal.

Gather Initial Information

If a healthcare organization has a marketing function in place, the tasks associated with initial information gathering may have already been completed. Typically, the marketing staff examines most aspects of the environment as part of ongoing market research; at most, the staff just needs to update some of the data collected. A newly formed marketing department or an external marketing consultant, however, may have to undertake a significant data collection effort.

This step requires planners to assemble and review general background information on the organization or the product to be marketed for a number of reasons. First, planners need to identify and then differentiate the salient attributes of the organization or product from others in the market. Distinctive features should be highlighted in the plan. Little or no differentiation creates a challenge for the marketer.

Second, planners need to be familiar with all of an organization's existing services—especially those that have not been marketed in the past. Hospitals and other large organizations frequently add new services and tend not to promote all of their offerings. Thus, marketers need to do additional background research.

Third, planners must understand the history of the organization or product being marketed. Planning is futuristic by nature, and the future is often inextricably intertwined with the past. Current relationships, for one, evolved from old experiences, occurrences, decisions, and so on; these relationships will further develop in the future on the basis of events and choices that take place today (which quickly turns into the past). The same can be said of an organization's past, present, and future trajectory. History is both instructive and influential for the future.

To minimize duplicate effort, planners typically inventory marketing resources and determine the extent to which current marketing activities relate to the proposed project. Ongoing marketing activities are easy to overlook, especially if they are informal or not labeled as marketing. At the same time, planners should determine whether the new initiative would contradict or otherwise conflict with existing marketing activities.

Planners need to note barriers to plan development—both known and potential. First, immutable patterns of behavior in the organization should be identified, particularly if the campaign is to involve internal marketing. Second, problems may crop up if the campaign pits two organizational entities against each other. For example, the director of the emergency department may not react favorably to a marketing campaign that is focused on directing patients away from the emergency department to urgent care centers affiliated with the hospital. Third, regardless of the type of organization, any environmental constraints likely to affect the organization and the provision of its services need to be identified. Some barriers may be surmountable, but others might not be. This understanding can be used to refine the assumptions previously stated.

Planners may benefit from information on similar marketing initiatives in other markets, especially if the initiative involves a product, a market, or an approach with which the marketer has limited familiarity. Planners should be able to incorporate information about marketing approaches that have and have not worked when similar organizations or services were marketed in other contexts.

As the planning process moves forward, formal data collection is likely to be required. The extent of this data collection effort will depend on the nature of the organization and the type of marketing initiative. A national organization courting a mass market (e.g., a pharmaceutical company promoting an over-the-counter product) probably would perform a detailed, national-level market analysis. On the other hand, a home health agency licensed to practice in a single county is not likely to need detailed, national home health trends to develop a marketing plan. If appropriate to the initiative, marketers may identify relevant societal developments, lifestyle trends, changes in consumer attitudes, health industry trends, and industry or product life cycle information. They may also consider regulatory, political, legal, and technological developments.

Audit the Market

Typically, planners gain an in-depth understanding of the organization's products, customers, and marketing practices through internal and external audits. An internal audit reveals the answers to the following questions:

- *Products.* What goods or services does the organization produce and distribute? What are the characteristics of these products?
- *Customer characteristics.* How many customers does the organization have, and what are their characteristics? What demographic characteristics are most pertinent? Where do these customers live, and what is the organization's market area? What is the case mix of current customers? What are the financial circumstances of the patient base?
- *Utilization patterns.* What volume of services do the organization's customers consume? How does this volume break down by service line or procedure?
- *Pricing structure.* How does the organization set prices for its products? How does this price structure compare to that of competitors or the industry average? How price sensitive are the products offered?

- *Marketing arrangements.* What marketing programs are currently in place, and how is marketing structured? What type and level of resources are available for marketing? Are processes in place for internal marketing?
- *Locations.* To what extent are operations centralized or decentralized? How many satellite locations are in operation, and how were the locations chosen? Are there markets that existing outlets are not serving?
- *Referral relationships.* How are customers referred to the organization? To what extent are there formal referral relationships?

Meanwhile, an external audit provides information about the environment in which the healthcare organization operates, including the following factors:

- Social, economic, and political environment
- Demographic, psychographic, and socioeconomic characteristics of the target population
- Health status of the target population
- Health service utilization patterns
- Characteristics and offerings of competitors within the market

Determine the Strategy

The strategy developed during the planning process sets the tone for subsequent planning activities and the parameters within which the planner must operate. Ideally, the strategy used in a marketing initiative will support the organization's mission statement and align with the organization's strategic plan. For example, if the organization's strategy is to position itself as a "caring" organization, marketing initiatives should support this approach.

Likewise, strategic considerations should guide the marketing planning process. The marketing strategy could, for example, be framed as an educational initiative, a public relations rather than an advertising approach, or a soft-sell versus a hard-sell approach, ultimately reflecting the overall corporate strategy.

Set Goals

The goal(s) of the marketing plan should reflect the information generated by the initial research; should align with the organization's mission statement; and should be broad in scope and limited in detail—for example, "to establish Hospital X as the most prominent inpatient facility in this market area." Alternatively, for a product-oriented initiative, the goal might be "to dominate the niche for occupational medicine in this market area." Organizational goal setting is somewhat problematic given the diffuseness of healthcare goals. Exhibit 15.2 discusses the variety of marketing goals found in healthcare.

Set Objectives

Goals are general statements, whereas objectives are specific. Objectives should be clearly and concisely stated. They must be time bound; clear deadlines for accomplishing objectives must be established. Finally, they must be measurable, given that the marketing plan is typically evaluated on the extent to which its objectives have been achieved. For example, an objective of the goal stated for Hospital X (see the previous step) might be as follows: "The proportion of the general population for whom Hospital X was deemed 'best' will increase from 10 percent to 25 percent within six months." A number of objectives may be specified for each goal, as each is likely to require action on several different fronts.

Any barriers to accomplishing the organization's stated objectives should be identified and assessed at this point. A lack of resources or talent is a common barrier to any type of plan. Ethical or legal considerations may be associated with some types of marketing—for example, certain health professionals may be prohibited from using advertising. Issues of appropriateness and taste may also pose problems. For example, the educational level of the target audience might be a barrier to introducing a new high-tech procedure, or the public perception that a new procedure is experimental could make potential patients apprehensive.

Prioritize Objectives

The objectives specified to support a goal are likely to address different dimensions of the initiative. Although all of the objectives may be considered important or even essential, pursuing all of the objectives may not be feasible —at least not all at the same time. Some objectives could even operate at cross-purposes.

As an example of a potential dilemma, imagine a situation in which a project has multiple objectives that support the goal of establishing a new facility as the dominant provider in a market area. One objective involves increasing public awareness of the facility and another focuses on increasing patient volume. Although these efforts might overlap, the approach the facility would take to make its name a household brand would likely be different from the approach it would take to induce patients to try the new facility. If the facility does not have the resources it needs to pursue these two objectives simultaneously, it may need to prioritize its marketing efforts.

To prioritize the objectives of a marketing plan, planners might envision the initiative according to the four Ps: product, price, place, and

EXHIBIT 15.2
The Diffuse
Goals of
Healthcare
Marketing

The mission of a healthcare organization is likely to be different from that of an organization in another industry. A healthcare organization may emphasize its charitable mission or service orientation rather than profits. Its mission is also likely to be more diffuse. A mission of improving the health status of the community, for example, is a lot different from the profit-maximization goals of corporations in most other industries.

The goals of a healthcare organization are also likely to be much more diverse than those of an organization in another industry. Hospitals, with their myriad functions and interests, are the epitome of the multipurpose organization. A marketing plan for an organization this complex must include a wide range of perspectives given that health services are often established without consideration of the potential profit.

The constituencies of healthcare organizations are different as well. Although a growing number of healthcare organizations must satisfy stockholders, most are more directly accountable to other types of constituencies. For example, a public hospital may have to cater to politicians, consumer interest groups, the medical community, and other entities. A church-affiliated hospital may be accountable not only to its board of directors but also to the denomination's leadership.

Furthermore, healthcare organizations are different in that they often provide mandated services. In other industries, an unprofitable product line can simply be eliminated. Hospitals and certain other healthcare organizations, however, may not be able to compete on equal terms unless they are comprehensive in their service offerings. If a hospital drops an unprofitable obstetrics service, other aspects of the organization may be negatively affected. State regulations may even mandate the existence of the unit, in which case eliminating it would not be an option.

promotion. For example, they could decide to focus on the product dimension of the marketing mix at the expense of price, place, and promotion. Thus, objectives most related to promoting the characteristics of the product would receive priority. Alternatively, they might capitalize on the price advantage of the product, thereby prioritizing objectives that focus on the pricing dimension.

One last consideration is the possibility of unanticipated consequences resulting from the pursuit of stated objectives. However tedious the job may be, planners need to specify both the intended and unintended consequences of carrying out each objective. Too often, planners examine only the intended outcomes, neglecting the potential negative ramifications.

Specify Actions

Actions might range from securing postage for a direct-mail initiative to enlisting a celebrity spokesperson. For example, if the objective of a specialty practice is to increase public awareness of its new sports medicine program by 50 percent, actions might include selecting an advertising agency, allocating funds for marketing, packaging the program, and scheduling press conferences. Many actions fall naturally into a sequence, so planners may want to refine the plan by specifying the timing of each action. Case Study 15.1 presents examples of plan goals, objectives, and actions.

Implement the Plan

Planning is ultimately only an exercise, albeit a meaningful one. The payoff comes when the plan is implemented. To a certain extent, planning is talk, but implementation is action. Fortunately, the handoff from planning to implementation is typically smooth in that the same parties are likely to be involved in both functions.

Implementation matrix
The list of specific actions, tasks, or activities needed to accomplish goals and objectives

In addition to a detailed marketing project plan, an **implementation matrix** is essential. The implementation matrix lists every action specified in the previous step and, if appropriate, breaks each action down into tasks. For each action, task, or activity, a number of details need to be specified, such as the following:

- Primary party responsible, along with any secondary parties
- Resources (e.g., staff time, money)
- Start and end dates
- Prerequisites
- Benchmarks

The resource requirements from the implementation matrix should be combined to determine total project resource requirements.

Evaluate the Plan

Evaluation of the plan should be top of mind from the beginning of the planning process. It should be ongoing and should use benchmarks and/ or milestones to measure progress toward goals and objectives. As discussed in Chapter 13, both process evaluation and outcome evaluation are used to assess marketing efforts.

Also discussed in Chapter 13 is the practice of calculating return on investment (ROI) to justify a marketing initiative. To determine ROI,

CASE STUDY 15.1
Sample Goals, Objectives, and Actions

Southern Neuroscience Center (SNC) completed a strategic plan and set this goal: to be recognized as the premier neurological specialty group in the region. To this end, SNC developed a marketing plan that detailed the objectives and actions to support the achievement of this goal:

Marketing Goal

To establish SNC as the premier neurological specialty center in the minds of consumers in its market area

Marketing Objectives

1. Increase awareness of SNC from 40 percent to 60 percent of consumers within 12 months.
2. Improve patient satisfaction ratings of "excellent" from 80 percent to 90 percent within 12 months.
3. Increase the number of physicians regularly referring to SNC by 25 percent within 12 months.

Marketing Actions

For objective 1, actions include the following:
- Develop an advertising campaign for local television.
- Increase SNC event sponsorship from 2 events to 4 events within the next 12 months.
- Distribute an SNC newsletter to all relevant members of the medical community.
- Establish an interactive website featuring consumer-oriented information on neurology and neurosurgery.

Case Study Discussion Questions

1. What prompted SNC to initiate marketing planning?
2. How did SNC use the marketing planning process to address its goal?
3. What indicators did SNC use to measure the success of its marketing initiative?
4. What potential barriers might SNC encounter in pursuing its marketing objectives?

marketers must not only carefully construct a marketing plan but also keep a detailed record of expenditures and revenues associated with the initiative. Some type of cost–benefit analysis should be conducted before the project is initiated, and every effort should be made to track the benefits (such as visibility, perception, market share, volume, and revenue) that accrue to the organization as a result of the campaign. Case Study 15.2 presents a simple marketing plan that includes these elements.

CASE STUDY 15.2
Marketing Planning for a New Program

SouthCoast Institute, a rehabilitation hospital, perceived an opportunity to expand its outpatient capabilities. Among SouthCoast's options was to develop an aquatherapy program that not only would supplement its existing inpatient services but also would allow it to serve a wider range of customers on an outpatient basis. The hospital's staff recognized the need to engage in the marketing planning process to successfully design, launch, and evaluate this new service.

Step 1

In organizing the process (identifying the key stakeholders, decision makers, and resources necessary), the planners had an advantage in that the development of an aquatherapy program was a proposal derived from SouthCoast's major strategic planning initiative. Many of the organizational issues had been addressed within the context of the strategic plan. A team was already in place, and a planning framework had previously been established.

Step 2

The planning team stated the following assumptions about the aquatherapy program and its relationship to the market:
- Adequate demand for aquatherapy services was present within the service area.
- SouthCoast had a captive audience for this service—its existing rehabilitation patients.
- Aquatherapy was generally unknown to the public and medical community.
- Considerable outreach was required to educate the public and raise awareness and acceptance of aquatherapy.

- If properly informed, health insurance companies would be willing to reimburse aquatherapy services.
- There was potential for significant spillover benefits from the introduction of the aquatherapy program (e.g., provide trainers for school swim teams and thereby attract student athletes needing aquatherapy).

Step 3

The team members collected background data on existing aquatherapy services in other markets. In addition, they assessed the availability of internal resources and the degree to which the general public and the external medical community were open to the idea of a new program. They also developed a general idea of what was involved in operating an aquatherapy program.

Step 4

The team performed a preliminary internal audit. Data were compiled on the types of rehabilitation procedures and services offered by most internal programs, the types of patients typically served, the reimbursement prospects, and so forth. The analysis examined the existing staff's ability to take on more responsibility, the need to add staff and to train them in aquatherapy, the available pool and the need for other equipment, and the general attitude of the staff regarding the proposed aquatherapy program.

The team also conducted an external audit. It identified potential referral sources and interviewed them to gauge their interest in the program. The team contacted local health plans to ascertain their willingness to reimburse for the service. Finally, the team conducted a competitive analysis and learned that no medically supported aquatherapy program was being offered in the community.

Step 5

On the basis of the information gathered through the initial research and the internal and external audits, the team settled on an educational strategy that would push information out to all relevant parties. Marketing efforts would focus on increasing awareness of and support for the aquatherapy program. At the same time, the strategy would emphasize

(continued)

the fact that SouthCoast was the only organization offering this therapy within the service area.

Step 6

With background data indicating significant potential for a successful and profitable service, the team set a goal of establishing South-Coast's aquatherapy service as the premier aquatherapy program in the region.

Steps 7 and 8

In support of this goal, the team established and prioritized the following objectives:

- Create and implement a comprehensive internal marketing effort for the aquatherapy program within six months.
- Directly contact all of SouthCoast's affiliates and potential external referrers within six months.
- Recruit and train a full-time marketing liaison for the aquatherapy campaign within six months.
- Identify and contact all community groups that could benefit from the aquatherapy pool within six months.
- Integrate aquatherapy into SouthCoast's sports medicine and occupational medicine programs within one year.

Step 9

The team specified the following actions needed to accomplish these objectives:

- Create promotional material to distribute to potential referral agents.
- Set up meetings with relevant internal parties (including medical staff) to explain the program.
- Identify an appropriate person to train as a marketing liaison with the community.
- Identify appropriate external targets for promotional and educational activities.

Step 10

The implementation matrix identified the required resources, the required financial commitment, the parties responsible for the tasks, and timelines for all activities. In keeping with the educational/ relationship-building approach, the marketing mix consisted of low-key promotional activities, not high-profile media advertising. For internal audiences, the marketing plan included a newsletter, articles in other internal publications, flyers in employees' pay envelopes, posters, information sessions for staff and referring physicians, and a DVD explaining to health professionals and insurance plans the purpose of the program. For external audiences, the marketing plan included a newsletter, press releases (and other media coverage as appropriate), limited print advertising, a DVD, exhibits (e.g., at schools and health fairs), and public presentations (e.g., for support groups, medical societies, voluntary health associations). A dedicated page on the SouthCoast website was created to introduce the program and its attributes. The web page featured videos illustrating the therapy process and offering testimonials from successfully rehabilitated patients.

Step 11

The team delineated an evaluation procedure to assess the progress made. Because it was a start-up operation, service utilization was easy to track. The plan also arranged for a pretest and posttest to be administered to referral agents to determine the extent to which they were made aware of the program (i.e., whether they knew enough about the program to feel confident about referring their patients to it). Satisfaction surveys were developed for patients and referrers. The extent to which the program generated secondary benefits in the community (e.g., with community groups, schools, swim clubs) was also tracked and periodically reported.

Case Study Discussion Questions

1. How did broad trends in healthcare marketing influence SouthCoast's new service development?
2. Why did SouthCoast need to assess the public's openness to the idea of an aquatherapy program during the initial information gathering?
3. What factors influenced the team's choice of strategic approach? Were there other strategies the team might have considered?
4. How did SouthCoast's promotional techniques reflect its overall strategy?
5. In what ways could the success of this marketing initiative be measured?

Summary

Most healthcare organizations have some level of marketing expertise, but that does not necessarily mean they are skilled in marketing planning. Systematic implementation of a marketing initiative is not possible without a marketing plan. A marketing plan should be in place before undertaking any marketing effort, large or small. Although marketing plans geared toward changing the image of an organization are understandably broad, most marketing initiatives focus on a particular good or service.

Marketing planning can take place at a variety of organizational levels—from the highest facility/systemwide level (strategic) to the lower operational level (tactical). The typical marketing plan focuses on a service, a program, or an event. A plan to roll out a new service, an office site, a piece of equipment, or patient education seminars is fairly narrow in scope and short in duration (i.e., tactical).

The marketing planning process involves steps that carry the planner from the initial marketing concept to plan implementation to evaluation. The organization must establish goals, objectives, and a strategy for accomplishing these ends. Objectives must be prioritized, and the intended and unintended consequences of meeting an objective must be considered. Objectives are broken down into actions, and these actions are laid out in sequence in an implementation matrix. Plan evaluation should be a consideration from the outset of the planning process, and mechanisms for evaluating the marketing effort should be built into the marketing plan.

Key Points

- Marketing planning is the development of a systematic process for promoting an organization, a good, a service, or a program.
- Marketing plans geared toward changing the image of an organization are often broad in scope, while marketing plans that focus on a particular product (either a good or a service) are typically narrow in scope. The type of marketing initiative envisioned influences the scope of the marketing plan.
- Planning can occur at different organizational levels, from the C suite to a subunit of a department.
- The marketing planning process involves a prescribed set of activities, which begins with the planning for planning and ends with evaluating the plan.
- The diffuse goals of healthcare organizations are a challenge in marketing planning.

Discussion Questions

1. In what ways does marketing planning differ from other types of planning in healthcare?
2. What determines the organizational level at which planning should occur?
3. Why do planners need to state assumptions not just on the front end but also throughout the campaign?
4. What types of data are generated through an internal audit? An external audit?
5. Within the planning context, what are the differences between goals, objectives, and actions?
6. Given that it may not be possible to pursue all possible marketing objectives, how may planners prioritize them?

Additional Resources

MailChimp. 2013. "How to Create an Email Marketing Plan." http://mailchimp .com/resources/guides/how-to-create-an-email-marketing-plan/.

Quick MBA. 2013. "Marketing Plan Outline." www.quickmba.com/marketing/plan.

Stensberg, K. 2013. "10 Steps to a Successful Health Care Marketing Plan." www .healthcarecommunication.com/Main/Articles/10_steps_to_a_successful _health_care_marketing_pla_9450.aspx#.

University of Massachusetts–Boston. 2013. "The Marketing Plan." www.sbdc.umb .edu/pdfs/marketing_plan.pdf.

MARKETING DATA

Healthcare marketers require data of various types to support marketing activities. They need data to calculate market share, profile potential markets, and initiate direct-to-consumer campaigns, all of which require extensive experience with and knowledge of data sources. This chapter examines the types of data available to healthcare marketers and describes methods of accessing, interpreting, and applying them. The importance of the Internet as a source of marketing information is also explored.

The Data Challenge

Healthcare marketers seeking data are presented with a paradox. The healthcare industry generates a wealth of data, but large portions of this bounty are inaccessible to marketers. Unlike other industries, healthcare has not yet developed a national clearinghouse or central repository for industry data. When data are available, they often are deficient in one way or another. Because data are often internally generated by private healthcare organizations, most are unpublished, proprietary, or difficult to access. The enactment of the Health Insurance Portability and Accountability Act (HIPAA) in 1996 further obstructed marketers' access to health data (see Exhibit 16.1).

Healthcare's increasingly consumer-driven approach has led to a growing demand for market data, yet the healthcare industry still lags behind other industries in collecting and disseminating market-related data. The local orientation and autonomous nature of many healthcare organizations have impeded data sharing. Increasingly, the healthcare marketer's ability (or inability) to access, manipulate, and interpret these data determines whether marketing initiatives succeed or fail. The passage of the Affordable Care Act (ACA), the implementation of its provisions, and the reimbursements and rewards related to those provisions will change the way data are shared between and among disparate providers, although it is too early to tell how this development will play out.

The primary purpose of this chapter is to outline the categories of data required for marketing activities, describe the ways in which data are generated, and indicate sites where relevant information might be accessed. This chapter, however, is not an exhaustive discussion of this topic; given

EXHIBIT 16.1
HIPAA and
Healthcare
Marketing

HIPAA protects the privacy of personal health data and guides the behavior of any entity that has access to individuals' medical information. When the legislation was first passed in 1996 and its provisions finalized in 2001, healthcare entities expressed confusion over the types of healthcare communications HIPAA exempted (and did not exempt) from the marketing definition. Questions were raised concerning customer communication activities, such as disease management information, prescription refill reminders, general health education, and wellness promotion.

Under HIPAA, every healthcare provider that communicates with its customers must address two issues. First, the definition of marketing and the kinds of communications allowed without customer (patient) authorization have to be examined. The definition of marketing worried hospitals and other providers that they could no longer use their patient records to promote services or programs that could be beneficial to those patients' health conditions. Fortunately, most kinds of communication between providers and their patients are allowable under HIPAA's marketing exclusions.

Second, the key tenets of a relationship between caregiver and patient—maintaining and improving health—have to be considered. This relationship is based on trust, and providers should be able to send information to their patients about recommended screenings and immunizations, new procedures, treatments, and healthcare seminars without fear of violating HIPAA regulations.

The US Department of Health and Human Services (HHS) conceded that when hospitals, physicians, and other providers offer such information to their patients, they advance the goal of improving their patients' health. Patients, in turn, expect their clinicians to share with them any medical knowledge and alerts that are essential to their care or healing. This concession by HHS permitted doctors, hospitals, pharmacists, and health plans to communicate freely with patients about treatment options, disease management, case management, care coordination, and myriad other healthcare issues. Thus, most of the communications programs that healthcare entities develop and implement today are not prohibited by HIPAA and do not require prior authorization.

the growing number of types and sources of health data, a comprehensive study would be unwieldy. Rather, the intent here is to elaborate on many of the data sources introduced earlier in the book and highlight these sources' important characteristics, such as frequency of release, geographic specificity, and methodological limitations.

Initially, a number of the data sets described in this chapter may not seem to be pertinent to healthcare. However, much of what affects the healthcare industry relates to other aspects of society, such as employment, housing, and crime.

Data Dimensions

The data useful to healthcare marketers can be categorized along a number of dimensions. This section addresses some of these dimensions.

Community Versus Organizational Data

Health data can be compiled on two levels: community and organizational. The community-level approach involves analyzing communitywide data—whether the "community" is a nation, state, county, or market area. Community data typically emphasize overall patterns of health service delivery and dominant practice patterns, such as information on patient flow into and out of the service area, levels of overcapacity or undercapacity affecting the area's health facilities, and the availability of different types of biomedical equipment within the service area.

The organizational-level approach focuses on the characteristics and concerns of corporate entities, such as hospitals, physician groups, and health plans. Organizational data typically detail an entity's operations in relation to competitors' activities. The focus is on the particular organization and its internal attributes, and the overall pattern of health system operation (i.e., community-level data) is important only to the extent that it affects the organization in question. A specialty physician practice, for example, may be primarily interested in the details of competing specialty practices (e.g., patient volume, market share, procedures performed) rather than general data on the health service area.

Internal Versus External Data

Marketers require data on both the internal and external environments. Although organizations usually turn first to internal information sources, data on the external environment have become increasingly important. External data are sometimes difficult to locate and access, but they are more available to the public than are internal data. See Exhibit 8.2 in Chapter 8 for examples of internal and external data used in audits.

Internally generated data are a ready source of information for healthcare marketers. Organizations routinely produce a large volume of data as a by-product of their normal operations, including information on patient characteristics, utilization patterns, referral streams, financial trends, staffing levels, and other data that have implications for marketing. Internal data are usually compiled through an *internal audit,* which typically analyzes the organization's structure, processes, customers, and resources. The internal audit may compile data from standard reports generated by the organization's data management systems (e.g., patient activity reports), but additional reports often are run to obtain the necessary data.

Even today, few data management systems in healthcare are in place to generate data for marketing purposes, although contemporary systems have a greater ability to generate custom reports that may be used by marketers. Often, marketers have to be creative in manipulating internal databases to obtain the data they require. Financial data are an increasingly important aspect of the internal data with which marketers must be familiar. Marketers must be aware of the profitability of services provided by the organization, the pricing process, and the cost–benefit breakdown associated with different marketing approaches. Benchmarking internal data against those of competitors, the community average, or some recognized indicators (e.g., Medicare performance indicators) has generated additional information marketers may use.

Today, most data collection efforts are directed toward external data. As healthcare providers have become more consumer driven and emphasis has shifted to externally oriented marketing activities, interest in external data of all types has grown. Marketing activities must address the external environment in which they operate. Marketers need to take into consideration national, state, and local trends in healthcare delivery, financing, and regulation. They also need to be aware of developments in the local market that will affect their initiatives. In particular, marketers must have an understanding of the characteristics of other organizations—especially competitors—within the market area. In fact, organizations that ignored external data in the past will need to be sensitive to communitywide data, especially in light of ACA provisions affecting not-for-profit hospitals.

Primary Versus Secondary Data

Primary research involves the use of surveys, focus groups, observational methods, and other techniques to collect original data. Secondary research, meanwhile, involves the use of data collected for some other purpose; indeed, most of the data in marketing research come from secondary sources. However, because of the lack of health data transparency, primary data collection is a concern more for marketers in healthcare than marketers in most other industries. See Exhibit 16.2 for a comparison of primary and secondary data collection.

	Primary Data	Secondary Data
Source	Collected by marketer	Collected by someone else
Reason	Collected specifically for this project	Collected for some other unrelated purpose
Usefulness	Directly applicable to the specific project	Must be interpreted to address the project
Ownership	Marketer owns	Someone else owns
Expense involved	Expensive	Free or inexpensive
Skills required	Data collection and analytic skills	Analytic skills
Time required	Significant data collection time required	Immediately available once accessed
Quality	Controlled by marketer	Potentially unknown

EXHIBIT 16.2
Comparison of Primary and Secondary Data

The Geographic Dimension

Data are available for a number of different geographic units—political or administrative, statistical, and functional. A detailed discussion of these units can be found in Chapter 4—particularly Exhibit 4.1.

- *Political or administrative units are official entities set up for administrative purposes.* States, counties, municipalities, and school districts are examples of administrative units. Much of the data available to marketers are collected for political or administrative units.
- *Statistical units are established primarily for data collection purposes.* Primary examples are the units established by the federal government for purposes of data collection during the decennial census, including census regions, metropolitan statistical areas, census tracts, and census blocks. Most demographic data are compiled from these units.
- *Functional units are established to carry out some practical function and may be unrelated to political or administrative and statistical units.* The best-known examples are the zip code areas designated by the US Postal Service. The zip codes' primary function is to support mail delivery; however, because zip codes have become such a common unit for analyzing the spatial distribution of various phenomena, they are frequently used as the geographic basis for marketing research.

Another example of a functional unit of particular significance to marketers is area of dominant influence (ADI). ADI was established by media monitoring organizations to indicate the sphere of influence of radio, television, and other forms of media. This measure is relevant to broadcast and print media that have limited geographic reach (e.g., local radio and television, local newspapers).

Healthcare marketers are likely to operate at different levels of geography, depending on the product being marketed and the type of organization involved. The Centers for Disease Control and Prevention (CDC), for example, focuses on national-level data and examines morbidity trends for the entire US population. Pharmaceutical companies with a national market also tend to examine data at that level. A large specialty group is likely to draw patients from a wide geographic area covering several counties; in this case, the county is probably the best unit for data collection. A family practitioner in a solo practice typically serves a fairly defined service area within a county. In this case, the zip code may be the level at which data would best be collected and analyzed.

The choice of geographic unit for the analysis is important not only because of its implications for the service area under study but also because of the different types of data available for various geographic areas. For many types of information, the county may offer the most extensive range of data; less data are accessible for lower levels of geography—that is, the smaller the geographic unit, the less the available data. Although use of the zip code or census tract may allow for more precise delineation of the service area, access to certain types of data becomes more limited. Thus, a trade-off is likely between the specificity of the service area and the types of data available.

The Temporal Dimension

Health professionals typically think in terms of current data—that is, data related to the present time frame or, at least, to the immediate past (e.g., the last set of lab tests). Hence, they are interested in information management systems that can provide current patient data linked to historical patient data.

From a marketing perspective, current data are important. In some ways, however, they are less important than future data and even historical data. Current data are most valuable as a baseline against which past data can be compared and from which future figures can be projected. Marketing is future oriented, and effective marketing depends on insight into likely future conditions affecting the healthcare environment. Because actual future data do not exist, conditions relevant to the community or the healthcare organization five or ten years into the future must be projected. For planning purposes, emphasis is placed on projections of the size and characteristics of populations and on trends in health service demand and utilization.

Marketers are increasingly being asked to project the future conditions of the healthcare market and the demand for health services down the road. They must either develop this capability or identify a reliable source of such data.

Data Generation Methods

The data generation methods discussed in this section are divided into four categories: (1) censuses, (2) registration systems, (3) surveys, and (4) synthetic data. The first three are traditional sources of data that support healthcare marketing activities, and the fourth—synthetic data—has become a standard marketing analysis tool.

Censuses

A census is the complete count of the persons residing in a specific place at a specific time. The US Census Bureau conducts a census every ten years (the decennial census); the 2010 enumeration was the twenty-third decennial census. The bureau collects data using the household (e.g., house, duplex, apartment, dormitory) as the means of identifying respondents.

Although a census theoretically is a complete count of the population, the usefulness of the decennial census conducted in the United States is limited in three respects:

1. *Every decade, a segment of the population is missed in the census, resulting in some level of undercount.* The undercount is typically less than 3 percent, but the fact that different segments of the population reflect different rates of undercount is problematic. The mere existence of an undercount creates myriad problems.

2. *The census's administration is infrequent.* In a society where rapid change is common, collecting data at ten-year intervals has its shortcomings. With the elapse of time after the census year, the usefulness of the data decreases. Marketers typically need the most current data possible, and even at the time of their release, census data have exceeded their shelf life.

3. *Beginning in 2010, the census no longer includes the "long form"* (which contained hundreds of population and housing items and historically was administered to one in six households). The "short form" was distributed to each household in 2010, thereby limiting the data collected to age, sex, race/ethnicity, and household composition. The remainder of the data (which were historically captured by the decennial census) are collected on an ongoing basis through the American Community Survey (described later).

Census data may be accessed through a variety of sources. Many libraries, for example, are designated as depositories of US government publications and maintain copies of most bureau reports before 2000. Census data sets in electronic format are distributed by the bureau and other data repackagers, which offer online data for free or at low cost. Virtually no print publications are produced today. The bureau gives free and relatively user-friendly online access to its data sets—see the website's American FactFinder feature at http://factfinder2.census.gov/faces/nav/jsf/pages/index.xhtml.

A lesser-known enumeration of business units—the *economic census*—is conducted every five years (currently in years ending in 2 and 7). The economic census covers businesses engaged in retail trade, wholesale trade, service activities, mineral industries, transportation, construction, manufacturing, agriculture, and government services. The information collected through the economic census includes data on sales, employment, and payroll, along with more specialized data. These data are available for a variety of geographic units, including states, metropolitan areas, counties, and places with 2,500 or more residents.

The economic census compiles extensive data on healthcare businesses as well. All businesses are assigned a code based on the North American Industry Classification System (NAICS). Aggregated data on businesses in NAICS categories that involve healthcare activities (e.g., physician practices, pharmacies, medical laboratories) are available from the bureau. No other all-inclusive source exists that indicates, for example, the number of hospitals, pharmacists, and chiropractors located in a particular area. As with population and housing data, the bulk of the data generated through the economic census is available only in electronic format.

Registration Systems

Registration system
A mechanism for systematically compiling, recording, and reporting a range of events, institutions, or individuals

Registration systems compile, record, and report on a broad range of events, institutions, and individuals in a regular, systematic, and timely fashion. Most registration systems relevant to this discussion are sponsored by some branch of government, although other types of registration systems are covered here as well.

National Center for Health Statistics (NCHS)
The federal agency charged with collecting health data in the United States

The best-known health-related registries in the United States are the *vital events* (i.e., births and deaths) registries established by the **National Center for Health Statistics (NCHS)** within the CDC. These registries are the definitive source of data on fertility and mortality, and a number of disease registries are maintained by the CDC. Registries maintained by other federal agencies may be valuable, especially when examining changes in the level and types of health services required by a population. Examples include registration systems supported by the Social Security Administration and the Centers for Medicare & Medicaid Services (CMS). Statistics from these agencies are generally available, and many provide raw data from their files.

Various agencies of state government also maintain registration systems of health conditions, reflecting the fact that many healthcare activities are regulated at the state level. State health departments typically maintain registries of health conditions (e.g., cancer cases), noteworthy public health problems (e.g., hazardous waste sites), and program participation (e.g., family planning counseling). In addition, state health departments or other designated agencies are responsible for maintaining registries of physicians and other healthcare personnel, hospitals and other health facilities, and other types of health information.

Commercial data vendors also maintain registries of various types, including registries of health personnel (often extending beyond clinical personnel to purchasing agents, chief information officers, and so on) and registries of health facilities (from urgent care centers to ambulatory care centers to hospitals). In some cases, vendors supplement registries maintained by government agencies or professional associations. In others, vendors develop proprietary registries to fill voids in the market.

Health departments at the county (or county equivalent) level are charged with filing certificates of births and deaths and thus are the initial repositories of vital statistics data. These certificates are forwarded to the vital statistics agencies of state governments, which are responsible for compiling these data for their respective state and then transmitting the information to NCHS. Exhibit 16.3 describes the work of the NCHS.

The CDC has been involved in disease surveillance activities since it was established as the Communicable Disease Center in 1946. Its surveillance activities now include programs in human reproduction, environmental health, chronic disease, risk reduction, occupational safety and health, and infectious diseases. It compiles data generated by these programs into registries, which then serve as a basis for much of the epidemiologic information in the United States.

Data registries are the main source of data on many categories of health personnel. Most health professionals must be registered in the state in which they practice. In addition, most belong to professional associations whose rosters become *de facto* registries. Like the registration of other types of data, the registration of healthcare personnel involves regular, timely recording of people entering a given profession. Updating registries of health personnel is difficult, making them more prone to error than most other registries.

Commercial data vendors maintain databases of physicians and other personnel. Some of these databases are comparable to the traditional databases maintained by professional organizations and government agencies. Data vendors may identify emerging professions or marginal practitioners that do not have an association base or are not tracked by the government.

The federal government is a major source of nationwide data on health facilities. The National Master Facility Inventory (NMFI) is a comprehensive

EXHIBIT 16.3
The National
Center for
Health
Statistics

Many consider the NCHS, a division of the CDC, to be the Census Bureau of healthcare. For more than 50 years, this agency has been charged with the collection, analysis, and dissemination of data about and related to health and healthcare in the United States and relevant subareas.

The massive amounts of data the NCHS compiles, analyzes, and makes available are the building blocks for calculating fertility, mortality, and morbidity rates as well as for producing population estimates and projections. The agency generates much of the available epidemiologic data on chronic diseases in the nation. In addition, it is the foremost administrator of health surveys in the United States. Its sample surveys are generally large scale and take two forms: community based and facility based.

The agency's most important community-based survey is the National Health Interview Survey (NHIS), which collects data annually from approximately 50,000 households. These data provide insight into the incidence and prevalence of health conditions, health status, injuries and disabilities, health services utilization, and other health indicators in the population. Other NCHS surveys that use samples of participants from the community include the Medical Expenditure Panel Survey, the National Health and Nutrition Examination Survey, and the National Survey of Family Growth. The National Maternal and Infant Health Survey involves a sampling of birth, fetal death, and infant death certificates.

Important facility-based surveys include the National Hospital Discharge Survey, the National Nursing Home Survey, and the National Ambulatory Medical Care Survey (NAMCS). The NAMCS samples the patient records of 2,500 office-based physicians to obtain data on diagnoses, treatments, medications prescribed, and characteristics of physicians and patients.

The agency's publications include annual books such as *Health, United States* (the official government compendium of statistics on the nation's health) and periodicals such as *Vital and Health Statistics*. It sponsors conferences and workshops and offers not only the findings from its research but also training in its research methodologies.

By contacting the appropriate NCHS division, health data users (including marketers) can obtain detailed statistics (many of which are unpublished) on any of the extensive number of topics the agency monitors. Staff members also are available to help with any data issues. In short, NCHS performs an invaluable service for those who require data on health and healthcare.

file of inpatient operations, including hospitals, nursing homes and related facilities, and other custodial or remedial care centers. The federal government keeps the NMFI current by periodically adding the names and addresses of new establishments licensed by state boards and other agencies and by conducting annual surveys.

Local organizations—such as marketing firms, regulatory agencies, and business coalitions—maintain databases on healthcare facilities as well. Some private data vendors collect, disseminate, and even sell data on nonhospital businesses, such as health maintenance organizations, urgent care centers, freestanding surgery centers, and other provider groups.

Arguably, the most complete hospital registry is maintained by the American Hospital Association (AHA). AHA annually compiles data on the availability of services, utilization patterns, financial activity, management, and personnel in US hospitals. It updates this database through an ongoing survey. Certain commercial data vendors also have established hospital databases.

Administrative records are a variation of the registries used in healthcare research. They are not intended to be registries of all enrollees or members of an organization or a group; rather, they are records of transactions involving these individuals. Thus, a list of all Medicare enrollees is a registry, but the recorded healthcare encounters of Medicare enrollees constitute an administrative system.

Administrative record
A registration system for the transactions involving members or enrollees of a registry

Surveys

Sample surveys are frequently used to supplement data from other sources. A sample survey involves the administration of a survey form or questionnaire to a systematically selected segment of a target population. The sample comprises respondents who are representative of the population being examined. Conclusions about the total population are then formed on the basis of the data collected from the sample.

The federal government—primarily through NCHS—is a major sponsor of health surveys. It administers myriad surveys focusing on different topics, such as medical care expenditures and utilization of hospital, ambulatory care, nursing home, and home health facilities and services. In addition, the National Institutes of Health (NIH) and the CDC episodically conduct surveys that generate data of interest to healthcare marketers.

Each year, the Census Bureau randomly contacts a sample of 3.5 million households in the United States to complete the American Community Survey (ACS). Designed to replace the long form that was administered through the decennial census, the ACS poses questions about the household's income, expenses, health insurance coverage, disabilities, education levels, work commute, veteran status, and so on. Answers to these questions allow the bureau to generate statistics and reports "that help determine how more than $400 billion in federal and state funds are distributed each year" (Census Bureau 2013a).

Although a supplement to the decennial census, the ACS is different from the traditional census in that it is continuous, not periodic. The demand for current data led federal policymakers to collect social, economic, and housing data on an ongoing basis. The benefits of having current data—along with the anticipated decennial-census benefits of cost savings, better planning, improved census coverage, and more efficient operations—led the Census Bureau to develop and implement the ACS.

Data generated by the ACS are presented for various levels of census geography. The lowest level is the census block group. The results of the ACS are published in three temporal versions: one-year data, combined three-year data, and combined five-year data. The more years that are combined the greater the sample size and the more reliable the estimates.

While the ACS does not have the statistical power of the one-in-six household long form used in the decennial census in the past and demographic purists raise some issues with the methodology, the benefit of having continuous data collection outweighs any drawbacks. The most direct way to access ACS data is on American FactFinder at http://factfinder2.census .gov/faces/nav/jsf/pages/index.xhtml.

Some professional associations—such as the American College of Healthcare Executives, the American Medical Association (AMA), and the American Hospital Association—regularly survey their members. Some voluntary health associations—such as the American Cancer Society and the American Heart Association—commission surveys of consumers, patients, or physicians. Foundations may fund research projects that collect health-related data. Some commercial data vendors sponsor nationwide surveys every year or two that involve as many as 100,000 households and that yield information on health status, health behavior, and healthcare preferences. Certain market research firms collect health data as part of their consumer surveys, and public opinion pollsters may compile data on health and healthcare. Some of the data collected in this manner are considered proprietary and are available only to clients of these firms. Other vendors sell data to the general public.

Synthetic Data

Synthetic data
Estimates,
projections,
and forecasts
generated in the
absence of actual
data

Synthetic data are figures—estimates, projections, and forecasts—generated in the absence of actual data through the use of statistical models. These data are created by merging existing demographic or health data with assumptions about a population. When census and survey activities are limited because of budgeting and time issues (e.g., the long lag time between official censuses), synthetic data are particularly valuable, filling the gap as needed. In the case of future data, synthetically produced projections are the only source available. The production of synthetic data has become a major business. See Case Study 16.1 for an example of synthetic data production.

Both government agencies and commercial data vendors generate synthetic data. Within the federal government, population estimates for states, metropolitan statistical areas, and counties are prepared each year as a joint effort of the Census Bureau and the state agency designated under the Federal–State Cooperative for Population Estimates. The purpose of the program is to standardize data and procedures so that generated estimates are of the highest possible quality.

Data generated by commercial vendors are available for various units of geography (e.g., zip codes, census tracts), and they often provide greater detail (e.g., sex and age breakdowns) than do government-produced figures. Vendors may also generate estimates and projections for custom geographic areas (e.g., a market area). Calculations for smaller geographic areas and population components, however, are less precise than calculations for their larger counterparts, but because these vendor-generated figures are easily accessible and timely, they have become a mainstay of healthcare marketers.

A major category of synthetic data comprises estimates and projections of health services demand. There are few sources of actual data on health services utilization, and projections of future demand are often required; thus, a number of approaches have been developed to synthetically generate data to fill this void. The general approach is to apply known utilization rates to current or projected population figures. To the extent possible, these figures are adjusted for, at a minimum, the age and sex composition of the target population. Most of these calculations are based on utilization rates generated by NCHS.

Commercial data vendors have led the way in developing demand estimates and projections. Some vendors have developed calculations for the full range of inpatient and outpatient services, although often these data are available only to the vendors' established customers. Other vendors provide select data on the demand for a particular service line, for example. See Case Study 16.2 for an example of estimating demand using synthetic data.

Sources of Data for Healthcare Marketing

Various sources of data are available to healthcare marketers today, and the number continues to grow. These sources fall into four main categories: government agencies, professional associations, private organizations, and commercial data vendors. The products available from these sources fall into two categories: reports that summarize the data and the actual data sets. Although the sources presented in this section consist of the agencies and publications responsible for disseminating these data sets, numerous compendia also exist that marketers may find useful. Exhibit 16.4 describes useful data available from the federal government.

CASE STUDY 16.1
Generating Population Data for Marketing Planning

In 2014, SunCoast Hospital began exploring the possibility of a satellite hospital in a fast-growing suburb next to its service area. SunCoast's marketing department was given the task of determining the size of the market in the targeted area. The decision to proceed with planning for a new facility was dependent on whether the market was large enough to support a 50-bed hospital.

Although the question was straightforward, the answer was difficult to determine. Data from the decennial census (last taken in 2010) were considered the most accurate, but census data were now four years old. Data this old might be accurate enough to use (with appropriate disclaimers) in a relatively stable community, but in SunCoast's target market the population had grown so rapidly in a short time that the four-year-old data were likely to be far from accurate. (The 2012 population estimates for the target population were available from the ACS, but these figures were not considered current enough.)

The marketing analysts considered techniques to estimate the current (2014) population in the target area. They could extrapolate trends from known data, assuming that present trends were a continuation of past trends. In this case, the analysts acquired data for the target area from the 2000 and 2010 censuses, assuming that figures from these two periods would be most realistic. (They could have gone back farther to the 1990 census, but given the rapid growth in the community, they thought much older data would not be appropriate.)

To estimate the population at the time of the study (2014), the analysts used a straight-line method to determine the average annual population increase for the area between 2000 and 2010 and then applied that rate of change to the 2010–2014 period. Thus, the calculation was as follows:

(2010 population – 2000 population) ÷ 10 years
= (Average annual population increase × 4) + 2010 population
= 2014 population estimate.

When the equation was solved, it yielded the following results:

$$(20,000 - 10,000 = 10,000) \div 10 = 1,000 \times 4$$
$$= 4,000 + 20,000$$
$$= 24,000.$$

Thus, the technique generated a 2014 population estimate of 24,000 residents for the service area. This approach assumed a steady population increase of 1,000 each year.

For comparison purposes, the analysts examined the year-to-year percentage increase rather than the increase in absolute numbers. The formula for that calculation was as follows:

[(2010 population − 2000 population) ÷ 2000 population] ÷ 10 years =
[(Average annual percentage increase × 4) × 2010 population] +
2000 population = 2014 population estimate.

When the equation was solved, it yielded the following results:

$$(20,000 - 10,000 = 10,000) \div 10,000 = 100\% \div 10 = 10\% \text{ per year}$$
$$\times 4 = 40\% \times 20,000 = 8,000 + 20,000 = 28,000.$$

This approach yielded an estimate of 28,000 residents rather than 24,000, reflecting that the proportionate increase was relatively greater than the absolute increase.

Both approaches were equally valid, and both indicated a rapidly growing population. From SunCoast's perspective, a population of 28,000 was considered more favorable than a population of 24,000. The experience of the analysts was brought to bear to determine which estimate appeared to be the most viable.

Case Study Discussion Questions

1. Why was a current population estimate unavailable to the SunCoast administrators?
2. What data did the anaysts choose as a basis for calculating population estimates and why?
3. To use a straight-line estimation method, what assumptions have to be made?
4. Why did the two techniques yield different estimates when the same baseline data were used?
5. Given the goal of the hospital, should it have used the more conservative figure or the larger estimate?

CASE STUDY 16.2
Methodology for Estimating Health Services Demand

For strategic planning purposes, Mountain View Hospital needed to determine the morbidity level characterizing its service area population and to estimate the health services demand that these conditions would yield. Unfortunately, these types of data were not readily available, and the market analyst had to develop estimates and projections of demand on the basis of modeled data.

To develop an estimate of the demand from the target population, the analyst needed two types of information: utilization rates that could be applied to the defined population and population estimates and/or projections. The utilization rates available reflected the population's age and sex, adjusted for region of the country. The population figures broke down the population into relevant age–sex categories. For each DRG (diagnosis-related group), for example, the utilization rate was calculated for each of 18 age–sex groups. These rates were then applied to the respective age–sex groups in the population in question, and the sum of the estimates/projections was calculated.

Utilization rates based on data collected through nationwide surveys were obtained from NCHS. When the rates of each age–sex group for each medical diagnosis for hospital patients were applied to the population estimate (broken into age–sex groups), a detailed estimation of health services utilization could be generated. The following table on cardiac catheterization services illustrates this process.

Calculation of Demand for Cardiac Catheterization

Population	<5	5–9	10–14	15–19	20–24	25–29	30–34	35–39	40–44
Males	1,000	1,050	970	270	2,580	3,530	3,170	3,270	3,230
Females	1,200	1,100	1,030	20	420	1,220	1,550	2,350	3,170

	45–49	50–54	55–59	60–64	65–69	70–74	75–79	80–84	>85
Males	3,110	2,020	1,070	690	280	130	1,050	970	270
Females	2,570	2,560	2,450	1,850	1,530	1,430	1,100	1,030	20

Utilization Rate	<5	5–9	10–14	15–19	20–24	25–29	30–34	35–39	40–44
Males	0.1	0.0	0.0	0.0	0.0	0.1	0.3	1.1	2.5
Females	0.0	0.0	0.0	0.1	0.0	0.0	0.2	0.3	0.7

	45–49	50–54	55–59	60–64	65–69	70–74	75–79	80–84	>85
Males	3.6	9.8	10.4	14.8	18.0	19.8	28.0	24.6	9.4
Females	1.7	2.6	5.2	3.9	9.3	11.7	12.8	8.2	8.9

Demand	Ages								
	<5	5–9	10–14	15–19	20–24	25–29	30–34	35–39	40–44
Males	0	0	0	0	0	0	1	4	8
Females	0	0	0	0	0	0	0	1	2

	45–49	50–54	55–59	60–64	65–69	70–74	75–79	80–84	>85	Total
Males	11	20	11	10	5	3	29	24	3	129
Females	4	7	13	7	14	17	14	8	0	88

Each age–sex category had its own utilization rate for cardiac catheterization. Because this procedure is primarily performed on older adults and senior citizens, relatively few children were affected. As this table demonstrates, the number of cases was calculated separately for each age–sex category, and the results were totaled to determine the overall demand for the population. For example, women in the 40- to 45-year-old age group reported a utilization rate of 0.7 per 1,000, compared with a rate of 2.5 per 1,000 for men in the same age group. Thus, although the populations of men and women in this age group were similar, four times as many cardiac catheterizations were predicted for men than for women in that age group. Each age–sex category was compared in a similar manner.

For this particular population, it appeared that there would be demand for 216 cardiac catheterizations annually—129 for men and 87 for women. In the absence of actual data, this model returned a reasonable approximation of the level of demand for this procedure.

Case Study Discussion Questions

1. Under what circumstances is it necessary to generate synthetic data (estimates and projections) for health services demand?
2. What assumptions were made about the utilization rates and population projections used?
3. How might the figures look different for a similar table for childbirth or breast cancer?
4. What are the dangers involved in making any type of projection with regard to health services utilization?
5. For how many years out (e.g., 5, 10, 20) should one feel comfortable making a projection?

EXHIBIT 16.4

Federal
Compendia of
Health Data

Because no national clearinghouse for health data currently exists in the United States, identifying and acquiring data is a challenge for healthcare marketers. However, certain compendia of health data are available that are useful for marketing purposes. No single publication provides all of the information a marketer needs, but the ones listed here offer a starting point and direct analysts to other relevant resources. These and similar reports are now accessible on—and increasingly only on—the Internet.

NCHS issues *Health, United States,* the best-known annual compendium of health data. This report includes data on health status, health behavior, health services utilization, healthcare resources, healthcare expenditures, and insurance coverage. These data are mostly at the national level, but some state and regional data are presented as well. A companion publication to *Health, United States* is *Behavioral Health, United States.* Although this is released less frequently, it is the primary source of data on behavioral healthcare. The statistics are based on data collected by the Center for Mental Health Services, a division of the Substance Abuse and Mental Health Services Administration.

CMS publishes *Data Compendium,* a collection of Medicaid and Medicare figures drawn primarily from CMS files and supplemented with records from other agencies. These data are at the national level, but some state-level data are also included. No substate levels of data are presented.

Until 2011, the Census Bureau produced three statistical compendia. The first was called *Statistical Abstract of the United States,* which drew data from the decennial census, the Bureau of Labor Statistics, and various other public and private sources. The abstract covered subject categories (e.g., vital statistics, nutrition) as well as data for states and metropolitan areas. The second compendium was a supplement to the abstract titled *County and City Data Book.* This publication contained data on all states, counties, and cities with 25,000 or more residents as well as all other places with a population of 100,000 or more. The third compendium was also a supplement called *State and Metropolitan Area Data Book.* It contained data for each state, variables for each metropolitan statistical area (MSA), and variables for each MSA's central city. In 2011, the bureau shuttered its compendia program, ending the publication of these three data references. Most of the data, however, are still accessible but are no longer in compendium form.

County Business Patterns, another annual publication of the bureau, presents data on the economic activities of counties and other small areas. It includes a comprehensive account of the healthcare business in a county. This work will continue to be produced by the bureau.

Government Agencies

Governments at all levels generate, compile, manipulate, and/or disseminate health data. The NCHS, the CDC, the NIH, and other organizations are prominent sources of a large share of the nation's health data. The Bureau of Health Professions (which operates under HHS's Health Resources and Services Administration) maintains the Area Health Resources File (AHRF), a master record of health data compiled by the federal government. In addition, other non-healthcare federal agencies create healthcare databases, such as the Bureau of Labor Statistics (e.g., data on health occupations) and the Department of Agriculture (e.g., nutritional data). The number and diversity of databases maintained by federal agencies are impressive, and the information covered, content, format, cost, data collection frequency, and accessibility of these disparate databases vary from agency to agency.

State and local governments also are major sources of health data. State governments generate demographic data, and each state has a data center responsible for demographic projections. At the state level, vital statistics may be obtained in the most timely fashion and state-university data centers can be involved in processing health data. Local governments may generate demographic data for use in various marketing functions. City or county governments may produce population projections, and county health departments are responsible for collecting and disseminating vital statistics data.

Professional Associations

As mentioned earlier, associations in the healthcare industry (e.g., AMA, AHA) compile an assortment of data about their members and those members' activities. This information is typically for internal use only, but some associations do make their databases available to external entities.

Reliable, accurate, credible, timely, and well-managed data are invaluable not only to the business of healthcare but also to the practice of medicine. This fact is essentially the foundation of the many information-focused healthcare associations that exist today, such as the following:

- Healthcare Information and Management Systems Society (www.himss.org)
- National Association of County and City Health Officials (www.naccho.org)
- National Association of Health Data Organizations (www.nahdo.org)

Like other professional associations, these healthcare information societies are a great source of data.

Private Organizations

Many private organizations (mostly not-for-profit) generate health data of various types. Voluntary healthcare associations often compile, repackage, or disseminate such data relevant to their organizations. The American Cancer Society, for example, distributes morbidity and mortality data related to cancer. The American Heart Association performs a similar function related to heart disease. Some private organizations commission and publish special studies on fertility or related issues.

Many organizations repackage data collected elsewhere (e.g., from the Census Bureau or NCHS) and present them in a specialized context. For example, the Population Reference Bureau—a private not-for-profit organization—distributes population statistics in various forms. Other organizations, such as AARP, not only assemble and disseminate secondary data but also conduct primary research and sponsor numerous studies.

Commercial Data Vendors

As discussed earlier in the chapter, commercial data vendors have emerged to fill perceived gaps in the availability of health data. Commercial data vendors may establish and maintain their own proprietary databases or reprocess/ repackage existing data. Also included in this group are the major data vendors (e.g., ESRI, Claritas, Experian) that incorporate healthcare databases into their business database systems.

Health Data and the Internet

As discussed throughout this book, the Internet has become a repository for health-related information—much of which is geared to healthcare consumers. Patients and their caregivers can find a doctor, schedule office visits and procedures, diagnose their own condition, research treatments for their symptoms, offer medical advice to peers and strangers, order prescription drugs and nutritional supplements, retrieve and discuss test results, and file and settle a complaint with a provider without leaving the house or picking up the phone. Over the years, as various healthcare movements matured and as information technology became even more sophisticated, more types of health-related data began appearing online. Today, health-related content on the Internet caters to more than just consumers; public and private groups, businesses, policymakers, researchers, and marketers (just to name a few) can access reports and extract demographic, psychographic, economic, and other data online.

The federal government has led the charge to make raw data available on the Internet. The Census Bureau, CDC, NCHS, and CMS have all expended significant effort posting their data files online, making them more accessible to a wider audience at any time or place. Data printed and then sold as books by private agencies in the past are now free and in PDF format (which in turn can be downloaded or viewed on a website). Few print versions are circulated today, and soon the Internet will be the only means of data distribution.

Summary

Healthcare marketers need a wide variety of data to research, plan, implement, and evaluate marketing activities. Marketers use demographic, psychographic, economic, and other data—even data that are seemingly unrelated to healthcare, such as information on housing, employment, and crime in a service area. Health data can be categorized as community or organizational, internal or external, and primary or secondary as well as in terms of geographic level and time period (i.e., past, present, or future). Health data are generated through censuses, registries, and surveys. Synthetic data in the form of estimates and projections are generated in the absence of actual data.

Healthcare marketers can access health data in a number of ways. Government agencies at all levels are important sources, and the federal government is a major collector and distributor of myriad types of data. The CDC, NCHS, and CMS are some of these federal agencies.

Professional associations, such as the AMA and AHA, compile statistics and data sets and then make them available to the public, their constituents, and various interested parties. Not-for-profit associations, such as the American Cancer Society and the American Heart Association, do the same. Educational institutions and research organizations provide a significant amount of data to health professionals. Increasingly, commercial data vendors have entered the field to supplement—or, in some cases, supplant—the data provided by other organizations.

The Internet enables massive amounts of health data to be distributed. The federal government has led the way in posting health data online, and a variety of public and private entities have followed suit.

Key Points

- Data on healthcare and other related topics are essential in researching, planning, implementing, and evaluating marketing activities.
- Because health information is often internally generated by private healthcare organizations, useful health data sets may be unpublished, proprietary, or difficult to access.
- HIPAA rules place restrictions on the use of health data.
- Most market research is based on secondary data, although primary research must be conducted in some situations.
- Marketers must be familiar with the geographic levels at which data are aggregated to effectively use this information.
- Health data are generated via censuses, registration systems, and sample surveys, and marketers need to be familiar with the characteristics of each method.
- In the absence of actual data, synthetic methods are used to generate demand estimates and projections.
- NCHS is the primary source of health data in the United States, but other federal agencies are major sources of health data as well.
- Other sources of health data include governments at all levels, professional associations, private organizations, and commercial data vendors.
- The Internet makes it easy to distribute health data to a wider audience.

Discussion Questions

1. Why hasn't the healthcare industry developed data clearinghouses and nationwide sources of market data as other industries have?
2. Under what circumstances might primary rather than secondary data need to be collected?
3. What are the disadvantages of using the decennial census as a data collection method?
4. Why are registration systems and administrative records important sources of data for healthcare marketers?
5. What function does NCHS serve, and why is it an important resource for healthcare marketers?
6. Under what circumstances do marketers need to access synthetic data generated by government agencies or commercial data vendors?

7. Why do healthcare marketers frequently use health data generated by state agencies?

8. What are the advantages of accessing health data online?

Additional Resources

AHA Guide, published annually by the American Hospital Association

Bureau of Health Professions: bhpr.hrsa.gov

Census Bureau: www.census.gov

Centers for Disease Control and Prevention: www.cdc.gov

County Business Patterns, published annually by the US Census Bureau

Health Resources and Services Administration: www.hrsa.gov

Health, United States, published annually by the Centers for Disease Control and Prevention

Morbidity and Mortality Weekly Review, published by the Centers for Disease Control and Prevention

National Center for Health Statistics: www.cdc.gov/nchs

Physician Characteristics and Distribution in the US, published annually by the American Medical Association

Socioeconomic Characteristics of Medical Practice, published annually by the American Medical Association

THE FUTURE OF HEALTHCARE MARKETING

Part V is a summary of both the current and future status of healthcare marketing. Its sole chapter proposes factors likely to influence this future and identifies the areas of growth on which healthcare marketers may wish to capitalize.

A LOOK AHEAD

As healthcare marketing continues to mature, it will undoubtedly undergo substantial change. The highly fluid and unpredictable environment in which healthcare marketers operate, however, makes it difficult to predict just what those changes will be. This chapter reviews the current status of healthcare marketing and considers the factors that will influence its future.

Where Healthcare Marketing Is Today

Healthcare marketers have learned much from past successes and failures. They now have better data, tools, and techniques at their disposal, and their expertise has increased dramatically. They are highly skilled at monitoring and assessing initiatives, collecting reliable and relevant data and then incorporating those data into activities, harnessing the Internet and other contemporary technologies to reach target audiences, and seeking out and responding to consumer needs and wants.

Because more and more healthcare organizations have integrated their marketing activities into their business development function, marketing is now considered an inherent part of corporate operations. The question is no longer "to market or not to market?" but "to what extent will marketing contribute to the success of the organization?" To this end, new hires are likely to receive a marketing orientation regardless of their position, and incentive programs that reward superior customer service are turning employees into marketers. In addition, the marketing department works closely with the fund development department and initiates co-marketing activities with the community relations department. Marketers foster customer-friendly facilities and develop affinity programs for target populations. While not all healthcare entities share the same enthusiasm for marketing, every single one of them benefits from marketing activities—especially in today's cash-poor but regulatory-rich environment.

The passage and implementation of the Affordable Care Act (ACA) have opened up new opportunities but introduced new threats at the same time. This reality has required marketers to develop new strategies. Before the ACA, for example, health plans marketed mostly to employers or businesses

Search engine optimization
A set of activities performed to increase a brand's or product's position on a search engine results page

New media
A catchall term for technological channels for creating, storing, distributing, transmitting, and accessing content; also known as *digital media*

Co-marketing
An agreement between two or more organizations to combine their efforts to achieve their respective objectives

that provided insurance benefits to their workforce. Today, health plans are marketing directly to individuals and households, who are required by the ACA to have medical insurance coverage or pay a tax penalty. Some of the strategies that health plans employ include **search engine optimization** (such as attaching a popular, descriptive tag to posted content), educational content production, and data collection and analysis (Tribune Media Group 2014).

New media (also known as *digital media*) and social media play a big role in disseminating promotions and other marketing initiatives. The opposite of analog or old/traditional media (e.g., print, TV, radio), new or digital media (e.g., Internet, e-mail, smartphone, data cloud, CD, MP3) are no longer an emerging technology in healthcare. Their continued evolution keeps marketers chasing ways to apply or incorporate them to healthcare campaigns—big or small. As stated in Chapter 11, social media tools (part of new media) are invaluable to healthcare marketers striving to influence their target markets and strengthen their organization's brand and products. Healthcare executives, administrators, and clinicians have become increasingly comfortable with social media, and many hospital and system CEOs are blogging and tweeting. Many health professionals (managers, researchers, nurses, physicians, allied health practitioners, policymakers, professors, consultants, pharmacists, vendors, and so on) are active users of Twitter and LinkedIn; they log in not only to share and follow healthcare-related news and debates but also to promote their own organizations and professional achievements.

Financial pressures continue to plague many healthcare organizations—and, by extension, their marketing function. Although pharmaceutical and biotech companies, among others, have robust marketing budgets (reaching up to tens of millions of dollars), other sectors of the healthcare industry have cut back. Some hospitals and other providers have eliminated their in-house marketing departments, opting instead to outsource the function to an agency or hire external consultants on an as needed basis.

Co-marketing, co-branding, co-sponsorship, and other partnerships are not new to healthcare marketing, but the present environment is ripe for more of these endeavors. The cost of marketing is always an issue, and this trend is driven in part by the spate of mergers and acquisitions that require the standardization and coordination of marketing initiatives for disparate healthcare entities. Pharmaceutical, diagnostics, and biotechnology companies as well as hospitals and health systems have entered into co-marketing deals for a number of reasons, including

- to share resources and expertise,
- to cross specific areas or expand market reach,
- to increase visibility,

- to gain credibility in another market, and
- to boost sales and revenue.

The two keys to a successful marketing partnership are the compatibility or the business alignment between the parties and the complementarity between their products. Organizations, with guidance from marketing, must identify conflicting interests, possible complications, and other opposing factors before pursuing such deals with each other.

Being optimistic about where healthcare marketing will be in the future is not hard. Judging from its continued evolution and accepted use in the industry (especially in the care delivery sector), it seems to only be moving forward.

Current Trends That Could Affect Future Practices

The trends described in this section represent some possible future realities for healthcare marketers. However, as stated repeatedly in this book, rapid changes occur in healthcare. Thus, the priorities that demand attention today may not be as urgent tomorrow. Healthcare marketers, nonetheless, must be vigilant of these trends and similar shifts in the industry.

Expected Rise in Healthcare Demand

During the first open-enrollment period of the ACA (October 1, 2013 to March 31, 2014), tens of millions of Americans enrolled in health plans through state and federal health insurance exchanges (Henry J. Kaiser Family Foundation 2014). Many of these enrollees were deemed eligible for state Medicaid programs. These newly insured individuals, not to mention those who bought coverage on their own, are expected to increase demand—not just for primary care but also for preventive and mental/behavioral health services.

Other present realities that likely will drive up future demand include the following:

- Healthcare practitioner shortages (including primary care physicians and specialists, nurses, and allied health professionals)
- Increase in older, high–health risk populations
- Longer lifespans involving chronic illness and disability
- Prevalence of various illnesses and their complications

Experienced healthcare marketers anticipate and study demand (as explained in earlier chapters) to develop and implement initiatives that will reach the right audience at the most opportune time.

Continued Consumer Involvement

Health plans are now trying to capture individual (not just business) purchasers of health insurance, appealing to consumers with customizable options. Meanwhile, employers (including healthcare organizations) are offering incentives to workers who improve their health or adopt a healthy lifestyle. Hospitals, systems, and other providers are creating infrastructures and tools to encourage patient and family participation in treatments, disease prevention, health maintenance, and decision making. In addition, many patients and other healthcare users have become involved in self-advocacy. They conduct their own informal research, talk to peers and access other resources, bring information to discuss with their physicians, monitor their conditions, and so on.

This consumer-driven movement requires marketers to understand both existing and prospective customers better. Target marketing, mass customization, direct-to-consumer marketing, customer relationship marketing, and social media marketing are just some of the essential techniques marketers could use.

Mergers and Acquisitions Frenzy

Over the past four years, the number of hospital consolidations has skyrocketed. In 2012, the number of deals was more than twice the total in 2009, and many of those deals involved multiple hospitals. One tends to think of for-profit chains when discussions about mergers and acquisitions arise (indeed, major acquisitions in 2013 and 2014 have significantly changed the for-profit healthcare sector), but since 2007 not-for-profit hospitals also have been aggressively involved in such transactions. Many small community hospitals are attractive to large and financially stable healthcare organizations seeking to expand. The future viability of independent hospitals in the age of the ACA is uncertain, however.

The following trends will likely emerge in the near future—especially for for-profits (Adamopoulos 2013):

1. Consolidation will accelerate.
2. Continued consolidation will give providers more bargaining power with payers.
3. Upcoming reimbursement cuts will intensify the need for scale and efficiency.
4. Hospitals will aim to diversify to control costs.
5. Healthcare will remain a local business.

Every merger or acquisition represents both a challenge and an opportunity for marketers. Disparate entities must be brought under a unitary marketing umbrella, widely varying marketing approaches must be standard-ized and coordinated, and new acquisitions must be rebranded under the aegis of their new owners. A national chain acquiring a local hospital is not likely to have an in-depth understanding of the local market and thus requires effective marketing input to develop a smooth ownership-transition process.

Ever-Advancing Technology

The electronic health record, mobile or mhealth, proprietary decision sup-port software and other clinical solutions, personal health and fitness apps, telemedicine, wearable sensors, physicians-only social networks, online medi-cal consultations, language translation application for doctors, remote and wireless patient monitoring, and voice search capability (e.g., Siri—Apple's personal assistant) are just some of the healthcare technologies that have been introduced in the recent past or are being tested today (Jayanthi 2014; Lee 2013). More health-specific tools, devices, and programs emerge and are adopted daily.

These developments indicate that many healthcare organizations are investing in technology and view it not only as a partner in improvement but also as a competitive advantage. (In addition, the HITECH Act mandates healthcare organizations to establish information systems and ensure their meaningful use.) For healthcare marketers, this means knowing the names, types, functions, and pros and cons of the technology used within the organi-zation by its clinical providers, patients, staff, leaders, and other stakeholders. Marketers do not have to be experts, but they do need proficiency in these technologies to convince others of the benefits and to capitalize on them for marketing purposes.

Emphasis on Outcomes

In response to concerns over the effectiveness of the healthcare delivery system and persistent disclosures of the level of medical errors in the system, an unprecedented emphasis is being placed on clinical outcomes. Healthcare providers must not only defend adverse outcomes they report but also capi-talize on favorable outcomes. As more payers turn to a pay-for-performance system, the importance of positive outcomes will further increase. Indeed, Medicare will no longer reimburse hospitals for the costs of patients read-mitted within 28 days of discharge. Patient safety issues will continue to be paramount, and a considerable groundswell of support for more controls over patient care has emerged.

Marketers will have to be front and center on the outcomes issue. They must ensure that outcomes research addresses salient issues above and beyond clinical factors (e.g., patient demographics, lifestyles, social context). They need to develop promotional campaigns based on high surgical success rates or low mortality rates. They may have to rationalize low success rates or high mortality rates. Marketers are likely to be the go-between for providers and the public, the regulators, and the policymakers.

Lingering Health Professional Shortages

The addition of the newly insured into the system, aging of the population, retirement of aging practitioners and aging faculty, length of professional training and education, changes in medical specialty distribution, and other factors all contribute to the current shortages of physicians, nurses, and other health professionals. Simply, demand exceeds the supply, and the supply is periodically tenuous.

Staff shortages in hospitals open up opportunities in other settings that are ready and able to meet increased customer demands. Retail clinics, concierge medicine practices, urgent care facilities, private practitioners, independent labs, and even health systems in other countries, for example, may see more business if the usual doctor's office or hospital unit is experiencing a long backlog of patients. The marketer's job includes finding such opportunities and capitalizing on them.

Diversified Healthcare Environment

The globalization that is widespread in other industries has affected US healthcare delivery as well. (Pharmaceutical companies, medical suppliers, health goods manufacturers, and other health-related businesses have been ahead of the commercial aspect of globalization for years.) Immigration is thriving, with the Census Bureau (2013b) projecting that immigration—not birth—will be the number-one factor in population growth in the coming decades. Over the past several decades, the patient and employee populations of many hospitals and other healthcare facilities have become less homogeneous, no longer composed of just US–born and bred citizens. In addition, foreign-trained medical personnel have become common to see in large institutions, and more continue to be recruited into the US healthcare system.

Medical tourism (or global medicine) has also added to healthcare's ethnic and racial diversity. Some US healthcare systems actively court patients from other countries, adapting their marketing techniques to the sensibilities of the foreign target markets. Other providers, meanwhile, are opening facilities overseas, exporting the typically well-respected American brand of medicine and health management. Conversely, American healthcare consumers are lured abroad to take advantage of the lower-cost but highly sophisticated medical services offered in Brazil, India, Singapore, Thailand, Turkey, and other countries. American insurance companies that recognize the cost savings of medical tourism are slowly but surely abetting this movement.

These developments represent opportunities for marketers to differentiate the organization from its competitors. A facility's diverse patient and staff makeup as well as its culturally appropriate and sensitive programs may be leveraged to attract both local and international customers. Marketers will need to be innovative, resourceful, and technologically skilled if they are to contend with global competitors.

In Chapter 2, the enterprisewide, operational, educational, and promotional functions of healthcare marketing are described (see pages 40–44). These functions will be especially salient in the future as healthcare continues to be consumer-driven, technology-enabled, and global.

Seizing Market Opportunities

Now that healthcare marketing is considered a true contributor to the success of the healthcare enterprise, marketers have the obligation and the authority to seek and pursue opportunities to promote the organization and influence its internal and external customers.

To do the best job, marketers must

- go beyond applying successful marketing approaches and shift their perspective to that of a healthcare customer or decision maker.
- get involved early in the strategic planning process to understand and influence organizational decisions.
- know enough about financial analysis to calculate and demonstrate the return on the marketing investment.
- develop an acute understanding of both the customers and the available services to match the right type of need with the right type of supply.
- check that all organizational initiatives have a marketing component and then provide evidence that those components are achieving the stated objectives.

Lastly, marketers must identify clinical areas of growth on which the organization may want to capitalize. Under the ACA, not-for-profit hospitals and other providers must conduct community health needs assessments for the purpose of population health management. Through this process, marketers could identify not only the unmet needs of the service population but also the potential business opportunities.

Anticipated Growth Areas

The following are just some of the many areas that are likely to thrive in the foreseeable future. Given the unpredictability of healthcare, however, these areas of growth are very likely to change. Thus, marketers should monitor the marketplace for similar emerging opportunities. Involvement in these (or similar) areas may help the organization fulfill the population health management provision of the ACA.

Elder Care

People are living longer—thanks to myriad factors, including better lifestyle choices and better medicine. According to the World Health Organization (2012), "within the next five years, the number of adults aged 65 and over [worldwide] will outnumber children under the age of 5." In the United States, the Census Bureau reports that the elderly population is projected to increase yearly, doubling to about 80 million by 2050. What these numbers mean is a commensurate growth in the demand for services for seniors (those aged 65 to 84), the very elderly (those aged 85 or older), and older adults (those aged 55 to 64). (Note that these age-group terms and age ranges may vary, as no standard definitions exist yet.)

Older adults typically do not require the same intensity of services as do seniors and the very elderly, but they are at an age during which chronic conditions arise and symptoms of physical and mental deterioration appear. All three groups may demand both essential and elective services, traditional and alternative therapies, physical and mental healthcare, and so on. Their medical condition and risk, health insurance, employment status, quality of life, family situation, financial assets, physical and mental acuity, technological prowess, decision-making ability, and so on vary widely. Thus, marketers should be careful about lumping the elderly together.

Rehabilitation and Disability Management

One of the paradoxes in the US healthcare system is that more people are struggling with a physical and/or mental disability now that more people are living longer. The Census Bureau (2012) found that "nearly 1 in 5 people have a disability in the U.S." The majority of the afflicted are the very elderly, followed by seniors. Part of the reason for this high disability rate is that debilitating conditions come with aging. Much, however, can be attributed to the ability of modern medicine and therapy to keep individuals (such as trauma and burn survivors, severely injured people, and premature babies) alive and functioning at some level.

The need for rehabilitation services and disability management clearly exists, and insurance companies today are more willing to reimburse for these services. In fact, some government programs mandate these services in the aftermath of various medical events.

The rehabilitation field overlaps with a variety of medical specialties (e.g., cardiology, orthopedics, neurology) and with other settings (e.g., long-term care, end-of-life care). In the future, rehabilitation is likely to be included in most medical treatment plans.

Fitness and Wellness

Wellness coaches, high-intensity interval training, anti-wheat and sugar but pro-kale diets, senior-specific and children-specific exercises, certified and educated trainers, healthy hotels, and anti-gravity movement are just among the latest trends that demonstrate Americans' never-ending devotion to fitness and wellness (an irony given that the United States is among the fattest countries in the world). Nutritionists, dietitians, sports medicine doctors, physical therapists, behavioral health practitioners, trainers or exercise instructors, bariatric surgeons, orthopedic surgeons, rehabilitation and recreational counselors, and other health professionals in the field—as well as the facilities in which they provide services—can expect to be in demand.

The advent of mobile health gave rise to mobile fitness and wellness. Wearable devices that take and record vital statistics, count steps taken and calories burned, and monitor other body inputs and outputs are the next frontier of fitness technology. On-demand personal trainers, massage therapists, nutritionists, yogis, and other wellness service providers can be arranged and paid for through a mobile app; these practitioners come to the home or business designated by the person who ordered the service.

Some fitness and wellness activities fall under the vanity services category, such as body sculpting exercises, massage, and salon and spa treatment. Vanity services are elective, paid out of pocket, and deal with the natural deterioration of the body typically caused by aging, exposure to harsh elements, or weight loss/gain. They include face and neck lifts, dental implants, tummy tucks, weight-loss surgery, hair transplant and hair removal, breast and butt augmentations, botox and collagen injections, laser eye surgery, and arthroscopic procedures, among others. Despite the slow economic recovery, the natural beauty movement, and the high cost and high risk of these procedures, the demand for vanity services is expected to surge in the coming years.

Alternative Therapy

Complementary and alternative medicine—encompassing non-Western treatments from acupuncture to chiropractic adjustments to hydrotherapy to reiki to yoga—has been around for many years now that it is considered mainstream. In fact, it has become so popular that many alternative therapies are offered in medical spas and by people with some training but no expertise. The same can be said for homeopathic vitamins, food supplements, or drug substitutes. With 22 states and the District of Columbia (as of May 2014) approving the use of medical marijuana to relieve pain and other symptoms, more forms of nontraditional remedies for all types of ailments are posed to emerge in the near future.

Alternative therapies do not appeal to a cross-section of the population but to selected subgroups. Marketers of alternative therapies should be knowledgeable about the demographic and psychographic groups that find these treatments appealing.

Pain Management

Long left out of the medical school curriculum and clinical research, pain management is finally gaining well-deserved attention. The traditional conservative approach to managing the pain of terminally ill patients, for example, is slowly being overcome, and recent research is providing guidance to doctors who administer pain medication. In addition, a number of pain management clinics have been established to address pain (like back pain) not associated with terminal disease. The growth of end-of-life care (discussed next) and the emergence of the hospice movement have heightened the interest in pain management.

End-of-Life Care

End-of-life care
The group of support services, methods, providers, and settings for managing the pain and comfort of terminally ill patients; also known as *hospice care*

A 2010 study found that Medicare spent approximately 25 to 30 percent of its annual expenditures on **end-of-life care** (Riley and Lubitz 2010). It is an eye-opening revelation, raising the question of whether providing this much care to terminally ill people is cost-effective or if the money could be spent on life-saving interventions instead. Furthermore, reports of fraudulent practices by hospice companies have surfaced. Despite its financial, ethical, and other implications, hospice care can be a profitable business and is expected to experience significant growth in the years ahead. Given the cost of end-of-life care, this expense is likely to be an ongoing issue in a society with a growing elderly population and during a period of financial constraints.

Summary

Although healthcare marketing has encountered some fits and starts during its nearly 40 years of history, it appears to be stronger today than ever. The industry has come to recognize that marketing is not an optional activity. As more and more organizations couple their marketing function with their business development function, marketing is becoming an inherent part of corporate operations. The data, analytical techniques, and technology available today offer capabilities that past healthcare marketers could not have imagined.

Currently, the US healthcare environment is marked by the ACA, consumer-driven (instead of business-driven) commerce, new media, financial pressures, and partnerships. In addition, it is experiencing trends that will likely influence how marketers do their job in the near future—trends such as increased demand, consumer involvement, technological advances, health professional shortages, and population diversity.

Today, many healthcare marketers are highly skilled, knowledgeable, and experienced. They are well positioned to help their organization improve the outcomes—clinical or otherwise—received by customers in their service areas.

Key Points

- Marketing has moved from the fringes of healthcare to a central position in the C-suite.
- Healthcare marketing will continue to evolve in response to developments in the healthcare industry.
- One of the strategies that health plans—which now market directly to individuals because of the ACA—employ is search engine optimization.
- New media and social media play a big role in disseminating promotions and other marketing initiatives.
- Health professional shortages, the aging but growing population, longer lifespans, and chronic illness are some of the factors that will drive up healthcare demand in the near future.
- Investment in technology indicates that healthcare organizations view technology not only as a partner in improvement but also as a competitive advantage.
- Marketers have the obligation and the authority to seek and pursue opportunities to promote the organization and influence its internal and external customers.

Discussion Questions

1. In what ways is healthcare marketing now considered part of corporate operations?
2. Where is healthcare marketing today, and what are some of the changes that have occurred in the past five years?

3. What are some of the current trends in the industry, and what are their implications for the future of healthcare marketing?
4. How is marketing uniquely positioned to address some of the challenging aspects of contemporary healthcare?
5. What developments indicate that marketing is becoming more of a core function in healthcare organizations?
6. What responsibilities do marketers have in promoting the field of marketing to internal customers in their organizations?
7. How can marketers respond to areas of growth or opportunities?

Additional Resources

Feldman, M. 2013. "Healthcare Marketing Automation Can Lower Readmission Rates, Increase Adherence." Fathom's Blog. www.fathomdelivers.com/blog /healthcare/healthcare-marketing-automation-can-lower-readmission-rates -increase-adherence/.

Society for Healthcare Strategy & Market Development. 2014. *Futurescan: Healthcare Trends and Implications 2014–2019*. Chicago: Health Administration Press and American Hospital Association.

———. 2011. *By the Numbers: Benchmarking Study on Healthcare Marketing/Communications,* 4th ed. Chicago: American Hospital Association.

Thomas, R. K. 2008. "How to Be a Healthcare Marketing Hero." *Marketing Health Services* 27 (4): 44.

GLOSSARY

Accountable care organization: A structure involving a group of voluntary providers collectively held responsible for the overall cost and quality of care for a defined patient population

Account management department: The function that interacts and builds a relationship with a marketing client throughout a campaign

Administrative record: A registration system for the transactions involving members or enrollees of a registry

Advertising: Any paid form of presentation or promotion of ideas, goods, or services

Affordable Care Act (ACA): *See* **Patient Protection and Affordable Care Act (ACA)**

Agency: An independent organization that supports one or more marketing functions on behalf of a client

Alternative therapy: Therapeutic modalities used as alternatives or as complements to conventional allopathic medicine

American Marketing Association: The primary organization devoted to the marketing field

Area of dominant influence (ADI): The geographic territory covered by a particular form of media

Attitude: A position a person has adopted in response to a theory, a belief, an object, an event, or another person

Audience: People or organizations that read, view, hear, or are otherwise exposed to a promotional message

Awareness: Recognition of or familiarity with an organization or its product; the ultimate goal of a public relations effort

Banner ad: A small, rectangular promotional graphic that appears in printed material or on a website

Benefit segmentation: A method of dividing the target audience according to the benefits it seeks from a good or service

Brand: A name, term, symbol, or design (or combination thereof) that signifies the goods or services of one seller or group of sellers

Branding: The creation of a brand for a company, service, or product

Business-to-business marketing: The process of building profitable, value-oriented relationships among businesses

Call center: A centralized communication hub established to capture incoming customer inquiries and generate outgoing marketing messages

Call to action: A statement, usually at the end of a marketing piece, that encourages the audience to take initiative regarding the good or service being promoted

Campaign spokesperson: An individual—typically well-known—who represents the organization's marketing campaign

Causal research: Research that identifies the specific functional relationship between two or more variables

Census: A complete count of the people residing in a specific place at a specific time

Centers for Disease Control and Prevention (CDC): The federal agency charged with monitoring morbidity and mortality in the United States

Channel: The mechanism used to distribute a promotional message, good, or service

Channel management: A formal program for reaching and servicing customers through a particular marketing channel

Client: In healthcare, a customer that consumes services rather than goods; in advertising, the entity being served by the advertising agency

Coding system: A structure for classifying and recording medical diagnoses, procedures, and other events

Collateral material: Material used to reinforce an organization's image or support a media advertising campaign

Co-marketing: An agreement between two or more organizations to combine their efforts to achieve their respective objectives

Commercial data vendor: A private organization that collects, compiles, analyzes, and disseminates data

Communication: The process of conveying information to internal and external audiences

Community health needs assessment (CHNA): An in-depth assessment of a community's population, health status, health-related issues, and unmet needs

Community outreach: A presentation of an organization's programs and services to the community to establish a relationship

Competition: The effort of two or more organizations acting independently to secure the business of the same customers

Composition: Characteristics exhibited by a population, such as demographics, lifestyle patterns, and payer categories

Concierge services: Customized health services offered to customers who pay a premium for the personalized attention

Consumer: In healthcare, any individual or organization that is a potential purchaser of goods and services

Consumer behavior: The consumer's pattern of consumption of goods and services

Consumer engagement: The process of identifying and profiling consumers and subsequently involving them in desired behaviors

Consumer health products: Healthcare goods distributed through retail outlets and directly purchased by the customer

Consumerism: A movement in which consumers participate in defining their healthcare needs and how those needs are met

Convenience good: A product consumers purchase frequently without forethought

Corporate culture: The values, beliefs, and attitudes that characterize an organization and guide its practices

Cosmeceuticals: Health or beauty products that combine the attributes of a cosmetic and a drug

Cost–benefit analysis: An evaluation technique that compares the cost of a project with its anticipated benefits

Creative department: The function that generates ideas for a campaign and translates them into words, images, and other artistic content

Cross-selling: A sales approach that encourages the purchase of additional products and services related to the initial purchase

Culture: A society's tangible and intangible aspects reflecting its beliefs, values, and norms

Current procedural terminology (CPT): The coding system used to classify medical procedures for record-keeping purposes

Customer: In healthcare, the actual purchaser (but not necessarily the end user) of goods or services

Customer relationship management: A business strategy designed to optimize profitability, revenue, and customer satisfaction by focusing on customer relationships rather than transactions

Customer satisfaction: The degree to which customers' wants and needs are fulfilled

Database marketing: The use of a data set of past, current, and prospective customers to promote an organization's products

Decision making: In healthcare, the process of determining the need for a good or service, evaluating the available options, and making a choice

Decline stage: The fourth phase of a product's life cycle in which the product or industry decreases in importance and is supplanted by another

Defined benefits: The set of covered services identified by the insurer and received by every plan member

Defined contributions: The set of covered services whose combination and value are identified by every plan member and not the insurer

Demand: The extent to which a target population needs or wants a product or service

Demographics: The range of biosocial and sociocultural attributes of a population

Descriptive research: Research that describes (but does not explain) the characteristics of a community or population

Diagnosis-related group (DRG): The coding system used to classify inpatient diagnoses and procedures

Diagnostic and Statistical Manual (DSM): The coding system used to classify behavioral health problems

Direct marketing: The process of targeting groups or individuals with specific characteristics and transmitting promotions directly to them

Direct to consumer: A marketing approach that targets the end user rather than referral agents or intermediaries

Discretionary purchase: A purchase of a good or service that is elective rather than required

Display advertising: A promotional approach using posters, billboards, and other eye-catching signs

Durable good: A product used repeatedly over an extended period

Early adopter: An individual or a group willing to try new products and services before they are accepted by the general public

Earned media: The free exposures, publicity, or word of mouth that a brand, a product, an initiative, or content receives

Effective market: The portion of the potential business within a market area believed to be suitable for cultivation

Elasticity: The tendency of demand to rise and fall in response to factors inside and outside the industry

Elective procedure: A clinical service not considered medically necessary and obtained at the discretion of the customer

Electronic media: Media that transmit content electronically, such as radio, TV, and the Internet

Emergency care: Emergency treatment or services in response to an urgent medical need

End-of-life care: The group of support services, methods, providers, and settings for managing the pain and comfort of terminally ill patients; also known as *hospice care*

End user: The person or organization that ultimately consumes a good or service, regardless of who makes the purchase decision or pays for the product

Enrollee: An individual who is enrolled in a health plan

Epidemiologic transition: A change in a population's epidemiologic profile—from acute to chronic health problems—as a result of aging and changing demographic characteristics

Estimate: The calculation of a figure in a current or past period using a statistical method

Ethics: A code of behavior that specifies a moral stance, particularly in professional dealings

Ethnicity: A common racial, national, tribal, religious, linguistic, or cultural trait or background of members of a population

Exploratory research: Research that discerns the general nature of a problem or an opportunity to identify factors of importance

External audit: The examination of the outside environment in which an organization operates; also known as *environmental assessment*

Flanking strategy: A marketing approach that seeks to avoid confrontation with better-positioned competitors by bypassing their captive audiences and cultivating neglected target audiences

Focus group: A data collection technique that involves eliciting opinions and perspectives from a panel of individuals who interact under the direction of a leader

Forecast: A form of projection that incorporates likely future developments into the calculations

Functional unit: A bounded geographic area formally defined for the execution of some practical function, such as mail delivery

Gatekeeper: An individual or organization that makes decisions on behalf of an end user or otherwise controls the purchase of goods and services

Geographic information system (GIS): A computer application that collects, analyzes, and organizes data geographically for the purpose of spatial analysis and map generation

Geographic segmentation: A method of dividing a target audience on the basis of geographic location

Geographic unit: A physical area demarcated by defined boundaries and used as a basis for market analysis

Globalization: The worldwide expansion and interconnectedness of organizations and their associated economies and influence

Goal: The ideal state or position the organization strives to achieve

Goods: Tangible products typically purchased in an impersonal setting on a one-at-a-time basis

Government relations: Organizational liaison with government agencies that enact regulations, determine reimbursement levels, provide funding, and monitor activities

Growth stage: The second phase of a product's life cycle in which the product or industry gains dominance in the market

Health: Traditionally, a state reflecting the absence of biological pathology; today, a state of overall physical, social, and psychological well-being

Health behavior: Any action aimed at restoring, preserving, and enhancing an individual's health status

Health Insurance Portability and Accountability Act (HIPAA): 1996 legislation that limits access to and protects individuals' protected health information

Health plan: Public or private medical insurance

Health professional: A trained individual who performs a clinical, an allied health, an administrative or a managerial, or a technical duty

Health status: The degree to which an individual or a population is characterized by health problems; the level of ill health within a population

Health/healthcare system: A multifacility healthcare organization; also may refer to the overall healthcare system

Healthcare: Any informal or formal activity intended to restore, maintain, or enhance the health status of individuals or populations

Healthcare model: A holistic view of health and illness that includes biological, social, and psychological dimensions

Hierarchy of needs: The prioritization of personal needs, which range from basic survival to self-actualization

Image: The perception an organization wants to project about itself, its products, and its services

Image advertising: A promotional focus on the overall attributes (rather than specific services) of an organization

Impact evaluation: An assessment of the changes brought about by the marketing effort

Implementation matrix: The list of specific actions, tasks, or activities needed to accomplish goals and objectives

Incentive: An enticement offered to current or potential customers to achieve a desired result

Incidence: The number of new cases of a disease, disability, or other health-related phenomenon in a population during a specified period; used to generate an incidence rate

In-depth interview: A data collection technique whereby the interviewer asks probing questions to elicit detailed information from the interviewee

Industrial product: Product used to create or support the production of other goods

Infomercial: An in-depth advertisement that mimics the look and feel of a daytime talk show, news report, documentary, demonstration, or other presentation format

Inpatient care: Medical care provided by a hospital to patients who are admitted for at least one night

Institutional advertising: Promotion of an organization rather than its products

Integrated marketing: A marketing approach that emphasizes consistency in the promotional strategy to achieve synergy between its component parts

Internal audit: The examination of internal data to assess organizational efficiency and effectiveness

Internal marketing: The process of training and motivating customer service employees and support personnel to work as a team to generate customer satisfaction

International Classification of Diseases (ICD): The standard coding system medical practitioners use to classify diseases

Internet marketing: A marketing approach that uses the Internet to promote an idea, an organization, a good, or a service

Introductory stage: The first phase of a product's life cycle in which the product or industry is launched

Life cycle: The maturation of a population, a product, or an industry from birth to death

Lifestyle: The entirety of attitudes, preferences, and behaviors of an individual, a group, or a culture

Long-term care: Nonacute care provided for an extended period or, sometimes, until death

Mail survey: A data collection technique that uses a self-administered paper questionnaire mailed to and from a sample of respondents

Managed care: Health insurance plans that contract with providers and healthcare organizations to provide care for members at negotiated rates

Market: A setting in which (actual and potential) buyers and sellers come together to exchange goods and services

Market area: The actual or desired area from which organizations draw or intend to draw customers; also known as *service area*

Market penetration strategy: A marketing approach that emphasizes extracting more product sales or greater service utilization from an existing customer base

Market segmentation: A process for grouping individuals or households who share similar characteristics for the purpose of target marketing

Market share: The percentage of the total market captured by a company

Marketing: A multifaceted process that involves research, planning, strategy formulation, promotion, and other activities

Marketing brief: A short document that presents the specifics of a marketing campaign

Marketing budget: The itemized allocation of financial resources to the department or a campaign

Marketing campaign: A formal, organized effort to promote a product to a target audience

Marketing consulting firm: An external agency that provides various services to support an organization's marketing function

Marketing management: The analysis, planning, implementation, and control of marketing programs

Marketing mix: The combination of product, price, place, and promotion used to influence the target market

Marketing planning: The development of a systematic process for promoting an organization, a good, or a service

Marketing research: The collection of information for myriad marketing purposes, such as identifying opportunities and problems, evaluating actions, monitoring performance, and clarifying the process

Mass marketing: An approach that targets the total population—typically through network TV or newspapers—as if it were one undifferentiated conglomeration of consumers

Maturity stage: The third phase of a product's life cycle in which the product or industry reaches its apex and ceases to grow

Media: Print or electronic modes of delivering a promotional message

Media plan: A document that outlines the objectives of a marketing campaign, its target audience, and the media intended to be used

Media planning and buying department: The function that researches, selects, and negotiates with media channels to increase a campaign's media exposure

Media supplier: An entity that provides communication channels for marketing campaigns

Medicaid: The joint federal–state health insurance program for low-income individuals

Medical model: The traditional paradigm of Western medicine that is based on germ theory and emphasizes a biomedical approach

Medical tourism: The practice of traveling to another country to obtain medical care; also known as *global medicine*

Medicare: The federal health insurance program for Americans aged 65 or older

Message: The information the marketer is trying to convey; the content of a promotional piece

Micromarketing: An approach that breaks the market down to the household or even the individual level to target those most likely to consume a product

Mission: The overarching purpose of an organization; the reason an organization exists

Monopoly: One organization controls the total market for a good or service

Mystery shopper: An individual hired by an organization to pose as a customer to covertly collect information on its own or a competitor's operations, goods, or services

National Center for Health Statistics (NCHS): The federal agency charged with collecting health data in the United States

Need: A condition objectively determined as requiring a health service

Networking: The process of establishing and nurturing relationships that may result in a mutual benefit

New media: A catchall term for technological channels for creating, storing, distributing, transmitting, and accessing content; also known as *digital media*

New product strategy: A marketing approach that introduces differing quality levels or entirely new products into an existing market

Niche: A segment of a market that can be carved out because of the uniqueness of the target population, the geographic area, or the product being promoted

Nondurable good: A product used once or a few times and then disposed of

Nonelective procedure: A clinical service considered medically necessary

Not-for-profit: An organization granted tax-exempt status by the Internal Revenue Service

Nutraceuticals*:* Food or dietary supplements that contain nutritional value and provide health benefits

Objective: A specific, concise, time-bound, formally designated target in support of a goal

Observation: A data collection technique whereby the actions and/or attributes of those being studied are recorded either by an individual or a mechanical device

Oligopoly: A few organizations dominate a market or an industry

Online survey: A data collection technique that uses a self-administered questionnaire that can be completed and submitted via the Internet

Outcome: In healthcare, the consequences of a clinical episode; in marketing, the results of a promotional campaign

Outcome evaluation: An assessment of how effectively a marketing initiative reached its objectives

Outpatient care: Medical care provided outside a hospital or an inpatient facility; also known as *ambulatory care*

Owned media: Online channels that an organization develops, maintains, and cultivates for marketing and other purposes

Packaging: The presentation of the physical attributes or the positioning of a good or service

Paid media: Ads and/or sponsorships purchased to promote a brand, a product, an initiative, or content

Patient: An individual who has been officially diagnosed with a health condition and is receiving formal medical care

Patient Protection and Affordable Care Act (ACA): 2010 legislation that aims to expand health insurance coverage and improve healthcare delivery and quality

Payer: In healthcare, the individual or organization responsible for medical expenses

Payer mix: The combination of payment sources characterizing a population; the basis for payer segmentation

Personal interview: A data collection technique that involves face-to-face interaction and the administration of a survey by the interviewer to the respondent

Personal sales: An oral or conversational presentation of promotional material to a prospective purchaser for the purpose of sales

Place: The point of distribution for a healthcare product

Political or administrative unit: A bounded geographic area formally defined for administrative purposes, such as a state, county, municipality, or school district

Population health: An approach to affecting the health status and health behavior of groups rather than individuals

Positioning: The placement of an idea, an organization, or a product in the minds of the market population, relative to its competition

Predictive model: A statistical method for identifying and quantifying the likely future need for health services on the basis of known utilization patterns for a defined population

Predictive research: Research that forecasts future characteristics or actions on the basis of known present characteristics

Prevalence: The total number of cases of a disease, disability, or other health-related condition at a particular point in time; used to calculate a prevalence rate

Price: The amount of money charged for a product

Primary care: Basic, routine health services, including preventive care

Primary data: Data generated directly through surveys, focus groups, observational methods, and other techniques

Primary research: The direct collection of data for a specific use

Print media: Any ink-on-paper medium used for promotional purposes

Process evaluation: An assessment of how efficiently a marketing initiative is carried out

Product advertising: Promotion of an organization's goods and services rather than the organization itself

Production: A focus on generating (rather than distributing) goods that deemphasizes the role of marketing

Production good: A product or raw material used to produce other goods

Products: Ideas, goods, and services

Projection: The use of a statistical technique to calculate a future estimate

Promotion: Any means of informing the marketplace that the organization has developed a response to meet its needs

Promotional mix: The combination of marketing techniques used to execute a marketing campaign

Prospect: A consumer who might be swayed to buying or using a good or service

Protected health information: A patient's identifiable healthcare data, including physical and mental health status, treatment record, and insurance and payment information

Provider: A health professional or an organization that provides direct patient care or related support services

Psychographics: The lifestyle characteristics of a population; *see* **Lifestyle**

Psychographic (or lifestyle) segmentation: The process of subdividing a population into groups of like individuals on the basis of their psychographic designation

Public relations: The management of communication that uses publicity and other persuasive techniques to influence feelings, opinions, or beliefs

Publicity: Any promotion that generally draws attention to an organization but does not target a particular audience

Public service announcement (PSA): A no-cost advertisement that supports a community program or public initiative

Purchase decision: A consumer's commitment to buy a good or to use a service

Qualitative research: A data collection technique that uses subjective methods, such as observations, interviews, and focus groups

Quantitative research: A data collection technique that uses objective methods, such as experiments and sample surveys

Quaternary care: Specialized services provided in large medical centers for complex conditions

Receiver: In communication theory, the target audience of a message

Referral: The practice of one entity sending a customer to another entity for specialized or additional good or service

Referral relationship: An agreement between two or more entities that each will refer customers to the other

Registration system: A mechanism for systematically compiling, recording, and reporting a range of events, institutions, or individuals

Reimbursement: In healthcare, compensation paid by a third-party payer to a provider or customer for the cost of services rendered/received

Relationship management: A focus on cultivating long-term relationships rather than short-term or onetime transactions

Report card: A mechanism for comparing the performance and outcomes of providers and health plans

Retail healthcare: Healthcare products designed to attract discretionary consumption

Return on investment (ROI): The value and benefit received in exchange for the resources given

Sales: An approach to business that emphasizes transactions rather than promotions

Sales promotion: The process of highlighting the value of a product to induce a purchase

Sample survey: The administration of a questionnaire to a segment of a target population that has been systematically selected

Search engine optimization: A set of activities performed to increase a brand's or product's position on a search engine results page

Secondary care: Services for conditions that are moderately complex and need a moderate level of resources and skills

Secondary data: Data collected through primary data collection and used for some other purpose, such as market research

Secondary research: The analysis of data originally collected during primary research and for some other purpose

Second-fiddle strategy: A marketing approach that concedes a subsidiary position in the market in favor of being an effective runner-up

Segment: A component of a population or market defined on the basis of some characteristic relevant to marketers

Segmentation: The process of dividing a population into meaningful segments for purposes of market analysis and strategic planning

Sender: In communication theory, the party that generates and disseminates a message to the target audience

Service area: *See* **Market area**

Service line: A bundle of unique, related services

Services: Activities or processes (or sets thereof) that meet the needs of a consumer

Shopping good: A product consumers compare to competing brands (on price, style, and features) before purchasing

Social marketing: An approach to effecting behavioral change in the general population through public relations, advertising, and other techniques

Social media: A variety of communication modes that use Internet technology to support innovative forms of interaction between people

Social media marketing: The promotion of an idea, a good, a service, or a brand using various types of social media

Society for Healthcare Strategy & Market Development: A division of the American Hospital Association that serves marketing and planning professionals in healthcare

Specialty good: A product—often expensive—that carries a brand name

Spokesperson: An individual—usually a celebrity—paid to deliver the organization's message or to speak publicly on its behalf

Sponsorship: Organizational support—typically financial—of a community project or event

Statistical unit: A bounded geographic area formally defined for data collection purposes, such as the geographic units developed by the Census Bureau

Strategic plan: A comprehensive guide to action developed by an organization for carrying out a specific strategy

Strategy: A general approach to be taken to meet market challenges

Support good: A product used to supply or support the provision of goods and services

Support services: Nonclinical, operational activities that support the provision of medical care

Survey: A data collection technique that involves the use of a questionnaire administered in any number of ways

SWOT analysis: An assessment of an organization's strengths, weaknesses, opportunities, and threats

Synthetic data: Estimates, projections, and forecasts generated in the absence of actual data

Target marketing: An approach that focuses on a market segment to which an organization desires to offer goods or services

Telemarketing: Sales via telephone, through either outbound or inbound calls

Telephone interview: A data collection technique whereby a survey instrument is administered by an interviewer to a respondent over the telephone

Tertiary care: Services for conditions that are highly complex (or serious) and need specialized clinicians, equipment, and facilities

Test market: A group or population on which a marketing theme or concept is tested

Third-party payer: An entity—other than the provider and patient—that pays for the cost of goods or services

Trade show: A convention at which vendors present their products to attendees

Traffic department: The function that delivers promotional content to the appropriate media channels on time

Upselling: A sales approach that encourages the purchase of an upgraded (and more expensive) product over a lesser and cheaper option

Urgent care: Medical care for a condition that requires immediate attention but is not significant enough to warrant emergency care

Usage segmentation: A method of dividing a target audience on the basis of historical utilization of a product or an organization

User-generated content: A website model that relies on user submissions and/or comments; the discussion thread is part of the content

US Census Bureau: The federal agency responsible for the decennial census and other data collection activities

Utilization: A measure of the extent/level of health services use

Value: Anything—usually intangible—a society considers important, such as freedom and economic prosperity

Vanity services: Health services, usually elective, intended to improve physical appearance or functioning

Viral: The rapid, epidemic-like dissemination of content on the Internet

Visibility: A marketing campaign goal that raises the public's awareness of the organization, program, or product to increase consumers' top-of-mind recall

Want: A consumer's desire (rather than a need) for a health service

Word of mouth: Positive or negative communication among consumers about an organization, a good, or a service

REFERENCES

Adamopoulos, H. 2013. "Moody's: 5 Key For-Profit Hospital Consolidation Trends." Becker's Hospital Review. Accessed May 2014. www.beckershospital review.com/hospital-transactions-and-valuation/moody-s-5-key-for-profit -hospital-consolidation-trends.html.

American Academy of Family Physicians (AAFP). 2009. "National Survey of Family Doctors Shows Recession Takes Startling Toll on Patients." Press release. Accessed March 2014. www.aafp.org/online/en/home/media/releases /newsreleases-statements-2009/nationalsurvey-familydoctors-recession.html.

American Cancer Society. 2013. "Guidelines for the Early Detection of Cancer." Last revised May 3. www.cancer.org/healthy/findcancerearly/cancerscreening guidelines/american-cancer-society-guidelines-for-the-early-detection-of -cancer.

American College of Healthcare Executives (ACHE). 2013. "Top Issues Confronting Hospitals 2013." Summary. Accessed March 2014. www.ache.org/pubs /research/ceoissues.cfm.

Are, C. 2009. "Global Expansion of U.S. Health Care System and Organizations." Accessed September. www.medscape.com/viewarticle/587903.

Assael, H. 1992. *Consumer Behavior and Marketing Action*. Mason, OH: Southwestern.

Barber, F., R. K. Thomas, and M. Huang. 2001. "Developing a Profile of LASIK Surgery Customers." *Marketing Health Services* 21 (2): 32–35.

Bartlett, D. L., and J. B. Steele. 2011. "Deadly Medicine." *Vanity Fair*. Accessed March 2013. www.vanityfair.com/politics/features/2011/01/deadly -medicine-201101.

Becker, B. W., and D. O. Kaldenberg. 2000. "Factors Influencing the Recommendation of Nursing Homes." *Marketing Health Services* 20 (4): 22–28.

Benjamins, M. R. 2003. "Religion and Preventive Health Service Use Among Older Adults." Paper presented at the annual meeting of the American Sociological Association, Atlanta. http://citation.allacademic.com//meta/p_mla_apa _research_citation/1/0/7/8/9/pages107890/p107890-1.php.

Bennett, P. D. (ed.). 1995. *Dictionary of Marketing Terms*, 2nd edition. Chicago: American Marketing Association.

Berkowitz, E. N. 2010. *Essentials of Health Care Marketing*, 3rd edition. Gaithersburg, MD: Aspen.

Berkowitz, E. N., and S. G. Hillestad. 2012. *Healthcare Marketing Plans: From Strategy to Action*, 4th edition. Boston: Jones and Bartlett.

Bureau of Labor Statistics (BLS). 2013. *Recent Price Trends in the Pharmaceutical Industry*. Accessed May 2014. www.bls.gov/mxp/pharmaceutical.pdf.

Centers for Medicare & Medicaid Services (CMS). 2013. "Accountable Care Organizations." Modified March 22. www.cms.gov/Medicare/Medicare-Fee-for-Service-Payment/ACO/.

Cossman, R. E., J. S. Cossman, W. L. James, T. Blanchard, R. Thomas, L. G. Pol, and A. G. Cosby. 2010. "Correlating Pharmaceutical Data with a National Health Survey as a Proxy for Estimating Rural Population Health." *Population Health Metrics* 8: 25. www.pophealthmetrics.com/content/8/1/25.

Craig, R. P. 1998. "The Patient as a Partner in Prescribing: Direct-to-Consumer Advertising." *Journal of Managed Care Pharmacy* 4 (1): 15–24.

Demchak, E. 2007. "The Elusive Health Care Consumer: What Will It Take to Activate Patients?" Accessed January. www.rwjf.org/newsroom/product.jsp?id=23072.

Derose, K. P., J. I. Escarce, and N. Lurie. 2007. "Immigrants and Health Care: Sources of Vulnerability." *Health Affairs* 26 (5): 1258–68.

eMarketer. 2013. "Social Networking Reaches Nearly One in Four Around the World." Published June 18. www.emarketer.com/Article/Social-Networking-Reaches-Nearly-One-Four-Around-World/1009976.

Engel, G. L. 1977. "The Need for a New Medical Model: A Challenge for Biomedicine." *Science* 196: 129–36.

Fisher, E. S. 2008. *The Dartmouth Atlas of Health Care: 2008*. Hanover, NH: The Dartmouth Institute for Health Policy and Clinical Practice.

Friedmann, S. A. 2009. "Exhibit Marketing Mistakes: Ten Tips on How to Avoid Them!" Accessed March 2014. http://marketing.about.com/od/eventandseminarmarketing/a/exhibitmkrtg.htm.

Gardner, A. 2013. "Popularity of 'Walk-In' Retail Health Clinics Growing: Poll." Published January 8. http://health.usnews.com/health-news/news/articles/2013/01/08/popularity-ofwalk-in-retail-health-clinics-growing-poll.

Gombeski, W. R., J. Taylor, K. Krauss, and C. Medeiros. 2003. "Cost-Effective Advertising Through TV and Newspaper 'Banner' Ads." *Health Marketing Quarterly* 20 (3): 37–54.

Grier, S., and C. A. Bryant. 2005. "Social Marketing in Public Health." *Annual Review of Public Health* 26: 319–39.

Hawn, C. 2009. "Take Two Aspirins and Tweet Me in the Morning: How Twitter, Facebook, and Other Social Media Are Reshaping Health Care." *Health Affairs* 28 (2): 361–68.

HCPro. 2007. "Marketing to Women: Proven Techniques to Reach Key Healthcare Decision-Makers." Accessed May. www.hcmarketplace.com/prod-5800/

Marketing-to-Women-Proven-techniques-to-reach-key-healthcare-decision makers.html.

Henry J. Kaiser Family Foundation. 2014. "State Marketplace Statistics." Updated May 1. http://kff.org/health-reform/state-indicator/state-marketplace -statistics/.

Iacobucci, D., B. J. Calder, E. Malthouse, and A. Duhachek. 2002. "Did You Hear? Consumers Tune in to Multimedia Marketing." *Marketing Health Services* 22 (3): 16–20.

IMS Health. 2013. *The Global Use of Medicines: Outlook Through 2017*. Danbury, CT: IMS Health.

International Medical Travel Journal. 2013. "Medical Tourism Climate Survey 2013." Published March. www.imtj.com/resources/research-and-statistics /medical-tourism-climate-survey-2013/.

———. 2011. "Medical Tourism: Trends for 2012 and Beyond." Accessed March 2014. www.imtj.com/articles/2011/medical-tourism-trends/.

Ireland, R. C. 2003. "Service Line Management Primer." Accessed March 2014. www.snowinst.com/articles/sll-primer.htm.

Jayanthi, A. 2014. "10 Biggest Technological Advancements for Healthcare in the Last Decade." Posted January 28. www.beckershospitalreview.com/health care-information-technology/10-biggest-technological-advancements-for -healthcare-in-the-last-decade.html.

Kotler, P. 1999. *Marketing Management: Analysis, Planning, Implementation, and Control*. Upper Saddle River, NJ: Prentice Hall.

———. 1975. *Marketing for Non-Profit Organizations*. Upper Saddle River, NJ: Prentice Hall.

Kotler, P., and K. Keller. 2011. *Marketing Management*, 14th edition. Upper Saddle River, NJ: Prentice Hall.

Kutscher, B., and M. Evans. 2013. "The New Normal? Shift to Outpatient Care, Payer Pressure Hit Hospitals." *Modern Healthcare*. Accessed March 2014. www.modernhealthcare.com/article/20130810/MAGAZINE/308109974.

Lake, L. 2009. "Branding from the Inside Out." Accessed January 2013. http:// marketing.about.com/od/marketingyourbrand/a/internalbrand.htm.

Lee, E. 2013. "5 Ways Technology Is Transforming Healthcare." Posted January 24. www.forbes.com/sites/bmoharrisbank/2013/01/24/5-ways-technology -is-transforming-health-care/.

Litch, B. K. 2007. "The Re-Emergence of Clinical Service Line Management." *Healthcare Executive* 22 (4): 14–18.

MacStravic, R. E. S. 1977. *Marketing Health Care*. Gaithersburg, MD: Aspen.

Mangini, M. K. 2002. "Branding 101." *Marketing Health Services* 22 (3): 20–23.

Maslow, A. 1970. *Motivation and Personality*, 2nd edition. New York: Harper & Row.

McGee, M. K. 2008. "Hospital Takes Its Grand Opening to Second Life." Accessed September 2009. www.informationweek.com/news/internet/ebusiness /showArticle.jhtml?articleID=206801783.

Medical Tourism Association. 2013. "Compare Cost." Accessed May 2014. www .medicaltourism.com/en/compare-costs.html.

Moynihan, R., I. Heath, and D. Henry. 2002. "Selling Sickness: The Pharmaceutical Industry and Disease Mongering." *British Medical Journal* 324 (7342): 886–91.

National Center for Health Statistics (NCHS). 2012. *Health, United States, 2012: With Special Feature on Emergency Care.* Accessed May 2014. www.cdc.gov /nchs/data/hus/hus12.pdf.

———. 2009. *Health United States, 2008.* Accessed September. www.cdc.gov/nchs /data/hus/hus08.pdf.

Noonan, M. D., and R. Savolaine. 2001. "A Neighborhood of Nations." *Marketing Health Services* 21 (4): 40–43.

Organisation for Economic Co-operation and Development (OECD). 2011. *Health at a Glance: 2011.* Paris: OECD.

Pew Research Internet Project. 2013. "Social Networking Fact Sheet." Accessed March 2014. www.pewinternet.org/fact-sheets/social-networking-fact-sheet/.

Pol, L. G., and R. K. Thomas. 2013. *The Demography of Health and Healthcare*, 3rd edition. New York: Kluwer Academic/Plenum Publishers.

Powers, T. L., and M. R. Bowers. 1992. "Challenges and Opportunities for Personal Selling." *Journal of Healthcare Marketing* 12 (4): 26–32.

PricewaterhouseCoopers Health Research Institute. 2012. *Social Media "Likes" Healthcare: From Marketing to Social Business.* New York: Pricewaterhouse-Coopers.

Prochaska, J. O., J. C. Norcross, and C. C. DiClemente. 1995. *Changing for Good.* New York: HarperCollins.

Pyrek, K. M. 2002. "Retail Medicine: Hype or Hope for the 'Worried Well.'" Published December. www.surgistrategies.com/articles/2c1feat2.html.

referralMD. 2013. "24 Outstanding Statistics & Figures on How Social Media Has Impacted the Health Care Industry." Accessed July. http://medcitynews .com/2013/11/24-outstanding-statistics-figures-social-media-impacted -health-care-industry/#ixzz2r2dq6PZc.

Riley, G. F., and J. D. Lubitz. 2010. "Long-Term Trends in Medicare Payments in the Last Year of Life." *Health Services Research* 45 (2): 565–76.

Rogers, E. M. 2003. *Diffusion of Innovations*, 5th edition. New York: Free Press.

Rohde, D. 2012. "The Swelling Middle." Reuters infographic. Accessed March 2014. www.reuters.com/middle-class-infographic.

Sarasohn-Kahn, J. 2008. *The Wisdom of Patients: Health Care Meets Online Social Media.* Oakland, CA: California Health Care Foundation.

Sargent, J. J. 2011. "How Much Does Marketing Cost?" Blog post. Posted June 14. www.joeysargent.com/2011/06/how-much-does-marketing-cost/.

Scott, D. M. 2009. *The New Rules of Marketing and PR*. Hoboken, NJ: John Wiley & Sons.

Siebens, J. 2013. "Extended Measures of Well-Being: Living Conditions in the United States: 2011." Household Economic Studies. US Census Bureau. Accessed March 2013. www.census.gov/prod/2013pubs/p70-136.pdf.

SK&A. 2013. *2012 U.S. Pharmaceutical Promotion Spending*. Published January. www.skainfo.com/health_care_market_reports/2012_promotional _spending.pdf.

Sparshott, J. 2013. "More People Say Goodbye to Their Landlines." WSJ Online. Published September 13. http://online.wsj.com/news/articles/SB1000142 4127887323893004579057402031104502.

Substance Abuse and Mental Health Services Administration (SAMHSA). 2013. "Ten Steps for Developing a Social Marketing Campaign." Accessed March 2014. http://captus.samhsa.gov/access-resources/ten-steps-developing-social -marketing-campaign.

Take Care Health Services. 2009a. "Take Care Clinic." Accessed March 2014. www .walgreens.com/topic/pharmacy/healthcare-clinic.jsp.

———. 2009b. "Take Care Health Employer Solutions." Accessed March 2014. www.takecareemployersolutions.com.

Thomas, R. K. 2008. *Health Services Marketing: A Practitioner's Guide*. New York: Springer.

———. 2005. *Attributes Sought in a Family Practice Center*. Unpublished feasibility study. Memphis, TN: Medical Services Research Group.

———. 2003a. *Society and Health: Sociology for Health Professionals*. New York: Springer.

———. 2003b. *Health Services Planning*, 2nd edition. New York: Kluwer.

Thomas, R. K., and M. Calhoun. 2007. *Marketing Matters: A Guide for Healthcare Executives*. Chicago: Health Administration Press.

Tracy, B. 2008. "The 7 Ps of Marketing." Accessed December. www.healthcaresuc-cess.com/articles/the-7-ps-of-marketing.html.

Tribune Media Group. 2014. "Healthcare Marketing in the Wake of the Affordable Care Act." News and Insights. Posted April. www.tribunemediagroup.com /consumer-insights/healthcare-marketing-in-the-wake-of-the-affordable -care-act/.

US Census Bureau. 2013a. "What Is the American Community Survey?" Accessed March 2014. www.census.gov/acs/www/about_the_survey/american _community_survey/.

———. 2013b. "International Migration Is Projected to Become Primary Driver of U.S. Population Growth for First Time in Nearly Two Centuries." Accessed

May 2014. www.census.gov/newsroom/releases/archives/population/cb13 -89.html.

———. 2012. "Nearly 1 in 5 People Have a Disability in the U.S." Press release. Posted July 25. www.census.gov/newsroom/releases/archives /miscellaneous/cb12-134.html.

US Department of Health & Human Services (HHS). 2014. "Key Features of the Affordable Care Act by Year." Accessed April 1. www.hhs.gov/healthcare /facts/timeline/timeline-text.html#PAGE_2.

———. 2013. "HHS Awards $1.9 Billion in Grants for HIV/AIDS Care and Medication." Press release. Accessed April 2014. www.hrsa.gov/about/news /pressreleases/131029ryanwhite13awards.html.

Van Dusen, A. 2008. "U.S. Hospitals Worth the Trip." Accessed December. www .forbes.com/2008/05/25/health-hospitals-care-forbeslife-cx_avd_out sourcing08_0529healthoutsourcing.html.

WebMD. 2011. "Cholesterol Tests: Guideline Recommendations." Last revised July 13. www.webmd.com/cholesterol-management/national-cholesterol -education-program-ncep-panel-guidelines-for-a-cholesterol-test.

Wennberg, J., J. L. Freeman, and W. J. Culp. 1987. "Are Hospital Services Rationed in New Haven or Over-Utilised in Boston?" *Lancet* 1 (8543): 1185–89.

Woods, J. 2007. "What's Driving the Trend Towards Retail Medicine?" Accessed December. http://seekingalpha.com/article/38887-what-s-driving-the -trend-towards-retail-medicine.

World Health Organization. 2012. "Are You Ready? What You Need to Know About Ageing." Accessed March 2013. www.who.int/world-health-day/2012/tool kit/background/en/.

York, R., K. Kaufman, and M. Grube. 2013. "Decline in Utilization Rates Signals a Change in the Inpatient Business Model." *Health Affairs* blog. Accessed May 2014. http://healthaffairs.org/blog/2013/03/08/decline-in-utilization -rates-signals-a-change-in-theinpatient-business-model/.

INDEX

ABOUT THE AUTHOR

Richard K. Thomas, PhD, is vice president of Health and Performance Resources in Memphis, Tennessee. He has been involved in healthcare market research and consultation with hospitals, clinics, health plans, and other healthcare organizations in both the public and private sectors for more than 40 years.

Dr. Thomas holds MAs in sociology and geography from the University of Memphis and a PhD in medical sociology from Vanderbilt University. He holds faculty appointments at the University of Tennessee Health Science Center and the University of Mississippi, where he is also a research associate at the Center for Population Studies.

Dr. Thomas is active in publishing and has authored or coauthored 20 books on health-related topics, most notably health services planning, healthcare market research, and the demography of health and healthcare. He has authored dozens of articles on healthcare and given numerous presentations, seminars, and workshops on related subjects. He previously served as the editor of *Marketing Health Services*, the healthcare journal of the American Marketing Association.